Ryan—

Welcome to the team!
Hope this book helps
you in the care of
your patients and reminds
you that the physical
exam is the key to
diagnosis!
Best regards,
Dr Millett
March 2022
Vail, CO

Ryan J. Warth • Peter J. Millett

Physical Examination of the Shoulder

An Evidence-Based Approach

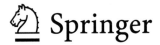 Springer

Ryan J. Warth, M.D.
Steadman Philippon Research Institute
Vail, CO, USA

Peter J. Millett, M.D., M.Sc.
The Steadman Clinic
Steadman Philippon Research Institute
Vail, CO, USA

ISBN 978-1-4939-2592-6   ISBN 978-1-4939-2593-3   (eBook)
DOI 10.1007/978-1-4939-2593-3

Library of Congress Control Number: 2015934007

Springer New York Heidelberg Dordrecht London

Printed on acid-free paper

Springer Science+Business Media LLC New York is part of Springer Science+Business Media (www.springer.com)

Preface

Proper diagnosis and treatment of the various physical ailments with which patients present to health care providers depends on accurate and efficient history and physical examination. This is arguably never more important than in the evaluation of symptoms relating to the shoulder, one of the most complicated of all the bioengineering marvels of the human body, and one of the most common sources of patient complaints.

The differential diagnosis of shoulder pain requires consideration of a very long list of potential etiologies that can range anywhere from bursitis and rotator cuff disease to cervical spine pathology in addition to any number of coexisting conditions. Appropriate performance and interpretation of the shoulder examination are essential skills that can answer many questions regarding etiologies, potential diagnoses and treatment options including surgical planning and postoperative management. This book provides an integrated approach to the diagnosis of numerous shoulder pathologies by combining discussions of pathoanatomy and the interpretation of physical examination techniques and was written for any health care professional or student who may be required to evaluate patients who present with shoulder pain. This information will allow the clinician to make informed decisions regarding further testing procedures, imaging and potential therapeutic options. The primary goal of this book is to provide readers with the knowledge and confidence required to perform an appropriate examination and to generate a succinct list of differential diagnoses using an evidence-based approach.

Vail, CO, USA

Ryan J. Warth, M.D.
Peter J. Millett, M.D., M.Sc.

Contents

About This Book

The primary purpose of this book is to provide a comprehensive guide for anyone who is required to examine the shoulder. An online version of this book is provided for easy accessibility.

While many books serve as an exhaustive list of all the available shoulder examination maneuvers, few have undertaken the task of developing a text that both simplifies and illustrates the most important pathoanatomy, procedural elements, and clinical data involved with physical examination of the shoulder. The goal of this book was to present the most relevant clinical data and examination maneuvers in a digestible, predictable manner such that the application and integration of the presented techniques can occur quickly and seamlessly.

Although there have been numerous individual studies evaluating the usefulness of the various shoulder examination techniques, it is nearly impossible to understand which maneuvers are the most relevant without a complete systematic review of each technique. This book provides a literature review that iterates the relative utility and efficacy of the various physical examination maneuvers and provides guidance as to which techniques are most important for each individual diagnosis or series of diagnoses. In addition, we provide an evaluation of current research surrounding the different examination techniques thereby identifying knowledge gaps upon which improvements can be sought.

Examination of the shoulder has historically been stigmatized as being overly difficult or intimidating, especially for the inexperienced investigator who has yet to develop the necessary fund of knowledge to adequately evaluate shoulder function. As a result, imaging studies have been relied upon to make diagnoses that should have been made during the initial physical examination. There are numerous factors that may be involved with the perceived difficulty of the shoulder exam:

1. Factors in the patient's history are often nonspecific.

   The nonspecific nature of many historical findings is particularly frustrating for the inexperienced clinician. This is especially true for physicians who are forced to care for patients with musculoskeletal problems without the necessary training. As an example, a patient with an anteroinferior labral tear (i.e., Bankart lesion) may present with a sudden onset of sharp pain with movement, a gradually intensifying dull pain or even the absence of pain in some cases. This highlights the necessity to perform a complete examination in each patient with a shoulder condition such that notable and potentially problematic conditions can be identified and properly treated.

2. Physical examination findings commonly overlap across multiple pathologies.

   There are many shoulder pathologies that present in similar ways. For example, the

R.J. Warth and P.J. Millett, *Physical Examination of the Shoulder: An Evidence-Based Approach*, DOI 10.1007/978-1-4939-2593-3_1, © Springer Science+Business Media New York 2015

active compression test, initially developed for the identification of labral pathology, is also sensitive for acromioclavicular joint pathology in certain patients. The identification of biceps tendon pathology and SLAP tears can also be difficult since there does not exist an examination maneuver with adequate sensitivity and/or specificity values. Although a positive test can be useful in many cases, it is important to recognize the ability of each test to detect various other pathologies. This book will identify these discrepancies and provide strategies for the avoidance of confusion.

3. The utility of palpation is limited due to overlying muscle and fat.

   The deltoid is a large, thick muscle that often precludes the ability to palpate normal or abnormal structures around the shoulder complex. Even though palpation is difficult, it is still a necessary portion of the physical examination process as there are certain clues that can be obtained with superficial or deep palpation. Another difficulty is that deep palpation may engender pain as a result of the pressure from the examiner's fingers rather than from the pathologic process. This is especially important when evaluating anterior shoulder pain as a result of coracoid impingement—deep palpation of the coracoid will generate pain in most patients who are not extremely thin; however, this may or may not be the result of subscapularis impingement underneath the coracoid process.

4. Specific pain patterns are variable and have not been fully defined for the shoulder.

   In most cases, the precise location, intensity, onset, timing, and quality of shoulder pain have not been firmly attached to any specific diagnosis. Although certain pain patterns are helpful and may lead the clinician to perform certain maneuvers, this information should not be considered a reliable indicator for any one condition. As an example, anterior shoulder pain can be the result of osteoarthritis, rotator cuff tears, labral lesions, acromioclavicular pathology, and/or various fractures among a long list of other potential pathologies.

5. There may be multiple coexisting conditions that present similarly.

   One of the most difficult aspects of the shoulder examination is discerning the findings of different pathologies that may be present in the same patient. These findings may overlap on many occasions, forcing the inexperienced clinician to guess at the correct diagnosis. This book will provide the reader with the tools required to make these important distinctions thus allowing for an accurate diagnosis and the development of a focused, structured treatment plan.

6. Significant pathologies may be asymptomatic.

   Sometimes the most important historical findings are those that do not exist. This is especially important for shoulder conditions that tend to progress over time—the development of symptoms often go unnoticed to the patient for a significant period of time. However, it is still important to recognize how these pathologies affect the patient's shoulder function. Thus, it is always important to complete a full, structured examination even if the patient denies symptoms. One important example is that of rotator cuff disease. While it is well recognized that the prevalence of rotator cuff disease increases with age [1–3], the development of symptoms does not always follow this pattern of progression [4]. However, studies have found that patients with asymptomatic rotator cuff tears develop changes in glenohumeral range of motion, changes in shoulder strength [5, 6], and changes in radiographic parameters [7]. As the tear biology changes and progresses, symptoms may eventually become noticeable and potentially disabling. A study by Yamaguchi et al [4]. found that patients with asymptomatic rotator cuff tears developed symptoms at an average of 2.8 years independent of whether an increase in tear size occurred. Thus, a thorough clinical evaluation beyond the patient history is necessary to identify these previously unidentified changes that may have a significant effect on the treatment approach and the final outcome.

7. Knowledge of both normal and pathologic processes around the shoulder has not been fully elucidated.

Another major difficulty is that basic knowledge of normal and pathologic processes is currently lacking; however, this is not due to a lack of research in and around the shoulder joint. Many basic science and biomechanical studies show inconsistent and inconclusive results. This is especially true for the dimensions of the rotator cuff insertion, the biomechanical function of the long head of the biceps tendon and the precise function of various ligaments around the shoulder, such as that of the coracoacromial and coracohumeral ligaments.

8. The current literature is full of studies that may or may not provide actual evidence for or against a specific maneuver.

The literature is riddled with substantially flawed studies that make comparison, analysis, and clinical integration extremely difficult. A few recent meta-analyses attempted to quantify the clinical utility and diagnostic odds ratio of the many physical examination tests; however, the major limitation of this study, as with many meta-analyses, is that the limitations of each individual study cannot be accounted for in the data analysis [8–10]. Some of these include selection bias, examiner bias, poor inter- and intra-rater reliability, publication bias, and, in some journals, the lack of an effective peer review process.

With consideration of all of these confusing factors, this book aims to provide the means to efficiently navigate the shoulder examination with confidence and accuracy. However, it is important to recognize that the examination is not always easy as there will often be challenging cases. Nevertheless, without this challenge, we would be less likely to love what we do every day.

1.1 Conclusion

Evaluation of the shoulder can be a difficult and confusing undertaking for the inexperienced examiner. The purpose of this book is to provide the reader with the pathoanatomic knowledge and examination skill to reliably and accurately evaluate the patient who presents with shoulder pain or discomfort. We do not aim to present an exhaustive list of all the physical examination tests ever to be mentioned in the literature, but rather to present and demonstrate the most relevant and useful maneuvers that can be directly integrated into clinical practice through an evaluation of current evidence.

References

1. Keener JD, Steger-May K, Stobbs G, Yamaguchi K. Asymptomatic rotator cuff tears: patient demographics and baseline shoulder function. J Shoulder Elbow Surg. 2010;19(8):1191–8.
2. Mall NA, Kim HM, Keener JD, Steger-May K, Teefey SA, Middleton WD, Stobbs G, Yamaguchi K. Symptomatic progression of asymptomatic rotator cuff tears: a prospective study of clinical and sonographic variables. J Bone Joint Surg Am. 2010;92(16):2623–33.
3. Yamaguchi K, Ditsios K, Middleton WD, Hildebolt CF, Galatz LM, Teefey SA. The demographic and morphological features of rotator cuff disease. A comparison of asymptomatic and symptomatic shoulders. J Bone Joint Surg Am. 2006;88(8):1699–704.
4. Yamaguchi K, Tetro AM, Blam O, Evanoff BA, Teefey SA, Middleton WD. Natural history of asymptomatic rotator cuff tears: a longitudinal analysis of asymptomatic tears detected sonographically. J Shoulder Elbow Surg. 2001;10(3):199–203.
5. Yamaguchi K, Sher JS, Andersen WK, Garretson R, Uribe JW, Hechtman K, Neviaser RJ. Glenohumeral motion in patients with rotator cuff tears: a comparison of asymptomatic and symptomatic shoulders. J Shoulder Elbow Surg. 2000;9(1):6–11.
6. Kim HM, Teefey SA, Zelig A, Galatz LM, Keener JD, Yamaguchi K. Shoulder strength in asymptomatic individuals with intact compared with torn rotator cuffs. J Bone Joint Surg Am. 2009;91(2):289–96.
7. Keener JD, Wei AS, Kim HM, Steger-May K, Yamaguchi K. Proximal humeral migration in shoulders with symptomatic and asymptomatic rotator cuff tears. J Bone Joint Surg Am. 2009;91(6):1405–13.
8. Hegedus EJ, Goode AP, Campbell S, Morin A, Tamaddoni M, Moorman 3rd CT, Cook C. Physical examination tests of the shoulder: a systematic review with meta-analysis of individual tests. Br J Sports Med. 2008;42(2):80–92.

9. Hegedus EJ, Goode AP, Cook CE, Michener L, Myer CA, Myer DM, Wright AA. Which physical examination tests provide clinicians with the most value when examining the shoulder? Update of a systematic review with meta-analysis of individual tests. Br J Sports Med. 2012;46(14):964–78.

10. Wright AA, Wassinger CA, Frank M, Michener LA, Hegedus EJ. Diagnostic accuracy of scapular physical examination tests for shoulder disorders: a systematic review. Br J Sports Med. 2013;47(14):886–92.

2.1 Introduction

Range of motion evaluation is a critical component of physical examination for any joint. However, the shoulder is unique in that it provides a large arc of motion in three-dimensional space which presents certain challenges for the treating physician. Determining which motions are clinically significant is perhaps the most important aspect of the range of motion examination. The clinician must then use this information to determine which static and dynamic factors are involved in the patient's pathologic processes. An understanding of the basic concepts and current evidence surrounding shoulder range of motion testing is the cornerstone for an accurate and efficient physical examination.

2.2 Glenohumeral Motion

Knowledge of a few basic concepts of glenohumeral motion is required to understand, perform, and interpret many physical examination maneuvers. As such, there exists an internationally standardized nomenclature through which basic glenohumeral motions are described to allow for reliable and reproducible communication between clinicians, physical therapists, and anyone else involved in the patient's care.

In 1923, Silver [1] made the first attempt to create a standard language for the measurement of shoulder motion. He described a "zero point" for each joint from which various motions would be measured. Cave and Roberts [2] followed in 1936 by suggesting that shoulder measurements should be made with the humerus at the side and the elbow flexed to 90°. Importantly, Cave and Roberts [2] were also the first to recommend measurement of the joints above and below the affected joint with a goniometer (discussed below).

Later in the century, further progress was made in the development of a standard nomenclature. Both the American Medical Association (AMA) [3] and the American Academy of Orthopaedic Surgeons (AAOS) [4] created committees that would eventually come to an agreement regarding this language by the early 1960s. The resulting publications defined the most important shoulder motions as flexion, abduction, adduction, extension, and internal and external rotation both with the arm at the side and at 90° of abduction.

When considering various shoulder positions, it is most useful to first note the position of the humerus alone rather than noting the position of the rest of the extremity, such as the elbow and hand. For example, pronation of the forearm does not constitute internal rotation of the shoulder in many cases. Similarly, supination of the forearm does not constitute external rotation of the shoulder. Thus, it is most important to examine the scapulohumeral relationship without regard to the rest of the extremity when evaluating shoulder motion.

R.J. Warth and P.J. Millett, *Physical Examination of the Shoulder: An Evidence-Based Approach*,
DOI 10.1007/978-1-4939-2593-3_2, © Springer Science+Business Media New York 2015

Fig. 2.1 Demonstration of forward flexion in which the humerus is elevated in front of the body (*curved arrow*).

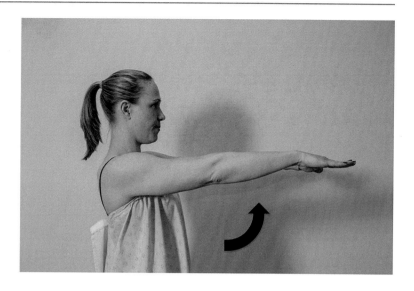

2.2.1 Forward Flexion

Forward flexion of the shoulder is defined as elevation of the humerus in front of the body in the sagittal plane (Fig. 2.1). This motion is typically governed by contraction of the anterior fibers of the deltoid muscle and weakness is often a key indicator for several different pathologies. Although the position of the elbow joint was never specified by the AMA [3] or AAOS [4] back in the 1960s, most practitioners measure flexion range of motion with the elbow extended. However, there are some other maneuvers that can be used specifically to measure deltoid strength. For example, having the patient make a fist and push anteriorly against the examiners hand would also activate the deltoid and simulate a forward elevation motion without fully elevating the shoulder overhead (see Chap. 3). This method is particularly useful when evaluating deltoid strength either before or after an arthroplasty procedure where full elevation may not be possible.

2.2.2 Abduction

Abduction of the shoulder occurs when the humerus is elevated in the coronal plane such that the extremity points directly laterally (also

known as straight lateral abduction) (Fig. 2.2). This position should be differentiated from abduction within the scapular plane which places the humerus in approximately 20–30° of forward angulation, also termed "scaption" (Fig. 2.3). This slight forward angulation facilitates examination such that surrounding soft tissues are similarly lax on both the anterior and posterior sides of the joint. For example, examination of the patient with straight lateral abduction of the shoulder would place an increased stress on anterior structures relative to posterior structures (Fig. 2.4). Thus, any evaluation of the capsular structures may produce inaccurate results when the humerus is abducted in the coronal plane. For this reason, appropriate glenohumeral and scapulothoracic resting positions should be utilized such that accurate assessment can be achieved (the scapular plane and the glenohumeral resting positions are discussed in more detail below).

2.2.3 Extension

Extension of the shoulder typically refers to any position in which the humerus rotates beyond the scapular plane (Fig. 2.5). This can be achieved with the humerus at the side or elevated. With the arm at the side, the humerus can extend posteriorly in a limited capacity. Straight

Fig. 2.2 Demonstration of humeral abduction in which the humerus is elevated in the coronal plane (*curved arrows*).

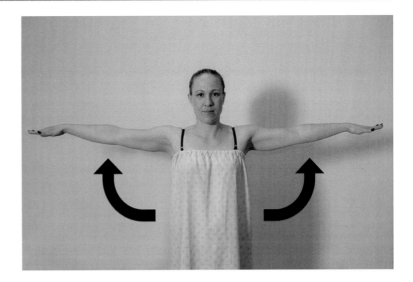

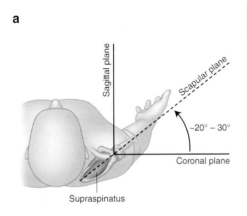

a

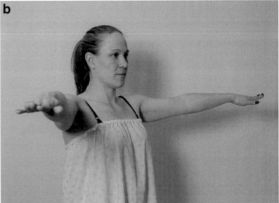

b

Fig. 2.3 (**a**) Illustration depicting the orientation of the scapular plane in which the humerus is elevated with approximately 20–30° of forward angulation relative to the coronal plane. (**b**) Demonstration of humeral abduction within the scapular plane.

lateral abduction (also known as "horizontal abduction") as discussed above is also considered a position of extension since the humerus would be angulated posterior to the plane of the scapula. Similarly, the humerus can also extend posteriorly when the arm is overhead. For example, throwing athletes require combined overhead extension and external rotation to achieve maximal torque and potential energy. Sometimes, this motion sequence can lead to pathologic problems such as symptomatic internal impingement, SLAP tears, and scapular dyskinesis.

2.2.4   Internal Rotation

Internal rotation describes motion around a center of rotation such that the angular motion vector points towards the midline. For example, when viewing a right shoulder from the superior to inferior direction, a counterclockwise rotation of the humerus would be referred to as internal rotation (Fig. 2.6). Internal rotation with the arm in a position of 90° of abduction or 90° of flexion uses the same concept. The humerus rotates in the same direction in each case, regardless of the

a 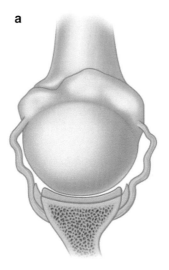   b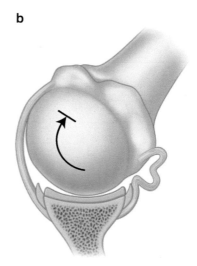

Fig. 2.4 Illustrations depicting the change in capsular tension when the humerus is elevated in the (**a**) scapular plane and (**b**) the coronal plane. Abduction in the scapular plane allows for accurate range of motion estimation because both the anterior and posterior capsular structures are similarly lax. Abduction in the coronal plane, on the other hand, can be regarded as a position of extension in which anterior capsular structures become more tight when compared to posterior capsular structures. Measuring range of motion or joint laxity in this position may produce inaccurate results.

position of the elbow, forearm, or hand. Internal rotation can also be measured with the arm in the adducted position. In this case, the patient will attempt to reach as far up the spinal column as possible while the clinician determines the most superior spinal level that the patient can reach (Fig. 2.7). This position maximizes internal rotation and has historically been a standard measure for internal rotation capacity. However, this method of measurement has recently been called to question since the vertebral level to which one reaches may be influenced by elbow, wrist, and hand motion rather than isolated internal rotation of the humerus [5].

2.2.5   External Rotation

When viewing a right shoulder from superiorly to inferiorly, external rotation would be defined as clockwise rotation of the humerus away from the midline (see Fig. 2.6). Again, similar to internal rotation, the rotational moment about the humeral anatomic axis does not change whether the humerus is abducted or flexed—it is only the scapulohumeral angle that changes.

2.2.6   Adduction

Shoulder adduction can also be described with the arm at the side or elevated. The basic resting position with the arm at the side is often referred to as "simple adduction." When the humerus is elevated to 90° followed by movement of the humerus towards the opposite shoulder, this is most often referred to as "horizontal adduction" or "cross-body adduction" (Fig. 2.8). Conversely, "horizontal extension" corresponds to the opposite motion, where the humerus is extended posteriorly beyond the scapular plane.

2.2.7   Scapular Plane

The scapular plane is generally defined as a position of neutral scapulohumeral angulation which optimizes glenohumeral joint congruity and

Fig. 2.5 (**a**) Extension
with the arms at the side
(*arrow*). (**b**) Extension
with the arms abducted
(*arrow*). (**c**) Extension with
the arms overhead (*arrow*).

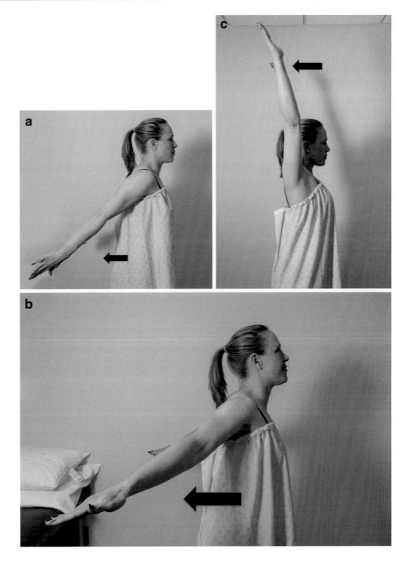

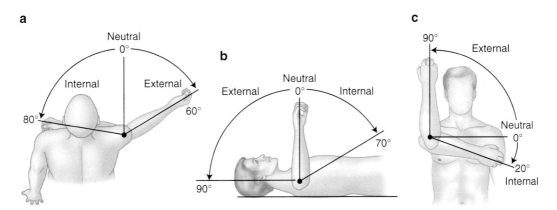

Fig. 2.6 Illustrations depicting glenohumeral internal and external rotation (**a**) with the arm at the side, (**b**) with the arm in straight lateral abduction, and (**c**) with the arm flexed.

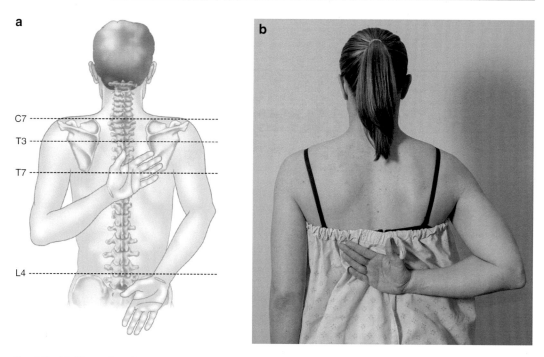

Fig. 2.7 (**a**) Illustration demonstrating the measurement of internal rotation according to vertebral levels. (**b**) Demonstration of the positioning for the measurement of internal rotation according to vertebral levels (*curved arrow*).

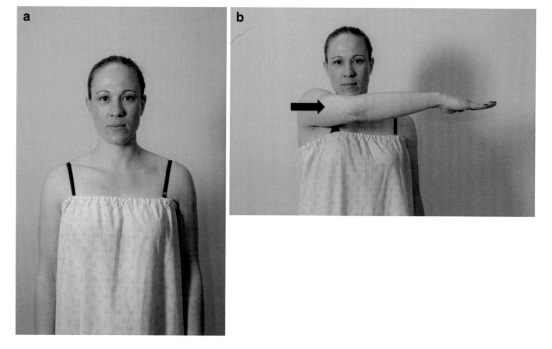

Fig. 2.8 (**a**) Demonstration of simple adduction with the humerus resting at the side. (**b**) Demonstration of horizontal adduction in which the humerus is elevated and rotated towards the contralateral shoulder (*arrow*).

facilitates accurate and consistent evaluation of the joint. This position of neutral scapulohumeral angulation is determined by the angle between a line drawn along the center axis of the scapula and second line drawn at the same level that is perpendicular to the coronal plane (see Fig. 2.3). This position, which most often occurs between 20° and 30° of forward angulation relative to the coronal plane with the humerus in various degrees of abduction, minimizes the potential for acromiohumeral contact while also allowing for the theoretical isolation of the rotator cuff musculature during various clinical examination tests. In other words, some have theorized that abduction of the humerus within the scapular plane requires zero contribution from internal or external rotators to achieve full abduction capacity [6]. Maximum capsuloligamentous laxity also occurs within the scapular plane (at the glenohumeral resting position, discussed below) which facilitates examination of these structures (instability and laxity testing are discussed in Chap. 6).

Although the scapular plane is generally defined as 20–30° of humeral forward angulation relative to the coronal plane in normal individuals, it must be recognized that patients with scapular malposition or dyskinesis, as which occurs commonly in overhead athletes, may have a scapular plane that differs from the rest of the population. For example, a throwing athlete with

scapular malposition may display increased protraction and upward rotation in the resting position (discussed below), thus altering the position of the glenoid such that the plane of the scapula occurs with greater forward angulation of the humerus. Therefore, performing physical examination tests within the "normal" scapular plane in a patient with scapular malposition may produce inaccurate results (specific examination maneuvers for evaluation of the scapulothoracic articulation are presented in Chap. 9).

2.2.8 Glenohumeral Resting Position

Also known as the "loose pack position," the resting position of a joint is the position at which surrounding soft tissues are under the least amount of tension, the joint capsule has its greatest laxity and the bony surfaces of the joint are minimally congruent [7–9]. In other words, this position is considered to allow maximal glenohumeral mobility owing to an increase in joint laxity [8]. The glenohumeral resting position in normal shoulders is thought to be between 55° and 70° of abduction with the humerus in neutral rotation within the plane of the scapula (Fig. 2.9) [10–12]. In this position, the amount of external force required to translate the humeral head is minimal

Fig. 2.9 Demonstration of the approximate glenohumeral resting position with the humerus abducted to 55–70° within scapular plane and in neutral rotation.

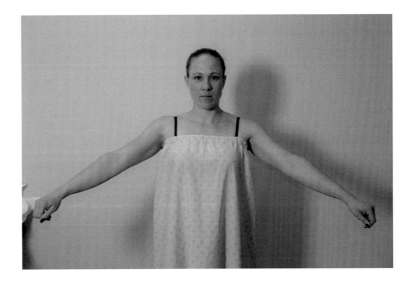

which is thought to facilitate examination accuracy. Although there is a general consensus regarding the location of the glenohumeral resting position, validation studies have seldom been conducted.

In a cadaveric study, An et al. [13] evaluated arm elevation in positions of either internal or external rotation. In this study, maximum elevation occurred with the arm externally rotated within the plane of the scapula. They could not achieve this maximal elevation with the arm internally rotated due to the acromiohumeral impingement that occurs in this position. In other words, there was bony contact between the acromion and the greater tuberosity, thus hindering the ability to further elevate the arm. When the humerus was placed in a position of 30° of forward angulation, there was little contribution from the internal and external rotators during humeral abduction.

In 2002, Hsu et al. [14] used seven cadaveric specimens to measure the translational and rotational range of motion at different angles of humeral abduction within the scapular plane. The glenohumeral resting position was calculated as the mid-point of the confidence intervals where maximal rotational and translational motion occurred. Maximal anteroposterior translation and maximal rotational range of motion occurred at approximately 39° of humeral abduction in the scapular plane and corresponded to approximately 45 % of the maximum available abduction range of motion. They also found that the glenohumeral resting position varied according to the maximal available range of motion, possibly suggesting that patients with joint hypermobility and hypomobility should be tested at greater and lesser degrees of humeral abduction, respectively. Since this was a cadaveric study, the effect of dynamic glenohumeral stabilization (which also contributes to the resting position) could not be evaluated.

More recently, Lin et al. [9] attempted to define the glenohumeral resting position in vivo in the dominant shoulders of 15 healthy patients. In that study, translational and rotational range of motion capacities were determined using an electromagnetic tracking device after an 80 N

translational load and a 4 N-m (torque) rotational load were applied. The greatest maximal rotational range of motion occurred at approximately 49.8° of abduction in the scapular plane. However, in contrast to Hsu et al. [14], the greatest maximal anterior–posterior translation occurred at approximately 23.7° of abduction in the scapular plane. These results suggested that testing for anteroposterior joint laxity should be conducted at lower degrees of abduction than when testing for rotational joint laxity.

Considered together, these studies demonstrate the complexity and potential variability that the glenohumeral resting position can have across a population, between populations or even between individuals (dominant versus non-dominant shoulders). In general, it is important to determine the maximal range of translational and rotational range of motion for each patient. In general, the rotational resting position is thought to occur at a point near 45 % of the total abduction arc [14] where half of this abduction angle is thought to represent the translational resting position [9].

2.2.9 Codman's Paradox

Codman's paradox is the observation that as the arm is flexed upward in the sagittal plane and let down in the coronal plane, the humerus appears to rotate 180° as evidenced by the orientation of the palm. In other words, when beginning the motion, the palm faces posteriorly and, at the end of the motion, the palm faces anteriorly (Fig. 2.10). Alternatively, an individual can place their hand at the top of the head through either (1) forward flexion and internal rotation or (2) abduction and external rotation. This observation has traditionally been of academic interest; however, many investigators have attempted to mathematically solve the "paradox" using complex equations and algorithms [15, 16]. Although the clinical relevance of Codman's paradox is debatable, some authors have investigated an application of Codman's paradox during manipulation of a stiff shoulder under anesthesia [17]. In addition, the quadrant test

Fig. 2.10 Illustration of Codman's paradox demonstrating that the top of the head can be reached via forward flexion and internal rotation or abduction and external rotation. (Matsen FA 3rd, Lippitt SB, Sidles JA, Harryman DT II (eds) Practical evaluation and management of the shoulder. W.B. Saunders Company, Philadelphia, 1994) Chapter 2.

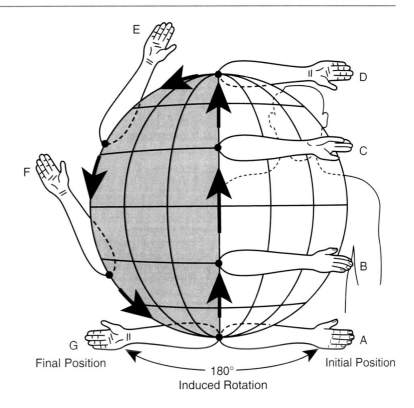

(discussed later in this chapter) is based on Codman's paradox and can be a useful measure of global shoulder motion [18].

2.3 Scapulothoracic Motion

The role of the scapula in the development and progression of various pathologies has been studied extensively over the most recent decade. Some authors have suggested that scapular malposition may be involved with both external and internal impingement mechanisms, especially in overhead athletes [19–24]. The scapula has four basic functions with regard to shoulder motion. The first function is to dynamically position the glenoid in space to facilitate the generation of a large arc of glenohumeral motion. Second, the scapula provides a stable fulcrum upon which glenohumeral motion can arise. Third, dynamic scapular positioning allows the rotator cuff tendons to glide smoothly beneath the acromion with humeral elevation. Finally, the scapula functions to transfer potential energy through the kinetic

chain, into the shoulder and, finally, to the hand thus allowing for functional overhead motion. Changes in scapular positioning as a result of alterations in the dynamic periscapular muscle force couples leads to scapular dyskinesis.

Evaluation of the scapular range of motion is one of the most difficult aspects of the shoulder examination for several reasons. One reason is that scapular motion is very complex and requires the examiner to visualize motion in three dimensions. Another reason is that the relative contributions of glenohumeral and scapulothoracic motions are difficult to distinguish, especially when abnormal motions are the result of muscle compensation for some other shoulder condition outside of the scapulothoracic articulation. The scapula is also covered with large, thick muscles making it difficult to visualize or palpate the various scapular motions. In addition, there exists a change in nomenclature when referring to scapular motion (discussed below). Specific examination maneuvers used to examine the scapulothoracic articulation are presented in Chap. 9.

To help the reader thoroughly understand scapulothoracic motion, we have organized the remainder of this section according to increasing complexity, beginning with the scapular resting position and two-dimensional motion planes followed by the interpretation of three-dimensional motion.

2.3.1 Scapular Resting Position

With the arm at rest, the scapula is predictably positioned in a specific orientation that can be used to detect scapular malposition before any motion measurements or evaluations are undertaken. There have only been a few studies that quantified the precise location of the scapula on the posterior thorax. Sobush et al. [25] quantified the normal scapular resting position in cadavers using the "Lennie test," or a series of measurements taken from the superomedial and inferomedial angles of the scapula. The distance from the superomedial angle to the midline, the distance from the inferomedial angle to the midline and also the angle of scapular inclination were determined (i.e., the angle formed between a line connecting the spinous processes and a line drawn along the margin of the medial scapular border).

This test was found to have high inter-rater reliability and accuracy when compared to post-measurement radiographs. Using similar measurements, a cadaveric study by Fung et al. [26] found that the resting position of the scapula was at approximately 3° of external rotation, 40° of internal rotation, and 2° of posterior tilt. Of note, this nomenclature does not reflect the position of the humerus. Rather, it represents the position of the scapular body relative to the coronal plane (discussed below).

2.3.2 Two-Dimensional Scapular Motion

In order to evaluate three-dimensional scapulothoracic motion, it is perhaps most advantageous to begin with an understanding of the basic two-dimensional scapular motions. In total, there are three rotational movements and two translational movements (Fig. 2.11). Although it is not possible to isolate these movements, they represent the basic components that comprise three-dimensional scapular motion.

Internal and external rotation occurs around the vertical axis of the scapula—that is, internal rotation elevates the medial scapular border away

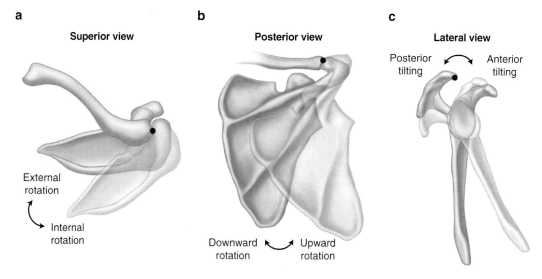

Fig. 2.11 Illustration depicting (**a**) scapular internal and external rotation, (**b**) scapular upward and downward rotation, and (**c**) scapular anterior and posterior tilting.

from the posterior thorax (i.e., the glenoid faces more anteriorly) whereas external rotation refers to the exact opposite motion (i.e., the glenoid faces less anteriorly).

Upward and downward rotation occurs along the plane of the scapula. In other words, upward rotation occurs when the inferior angle of the scapula moves laterally and the glenoid faces more superiorly. Conversely, downward rotation refers to the opposite motion in which the inferior scapular angle moves medially towards the midline and the glenoid faces more inferiorly.

Anterior and posterior rotation (i.e., tilting) occurs around the horizontal axis of the scapula. Anterior tilting of the scapula occurs when the inferior angle moves away from the thorax (and the superior border moves towards the thorax) whereas posterior tilting refers to the exact opposite motion in which the inferior angle moves towards the thorax (and the superior border moves away from the thorax).

The scapula can also translate in the medial–lateral direction (as in protraction and retraction, described below) and the superior–inferior direction (as in shrugging the shoulders). It is important to recognize that these translational motions also require intact AC and SC joints—upward and downward translation of the scapula requires upward and downward angulation of the clavicle via the SC joint whereas medial–lateral translation requires anterior–posterior motion of the clavicle through the SC joint as the scapula moves around the thorax.

2.3.3   Three-Dimensional Scapular Motion

Three-dimensional scapular motion, which is achieved by combining any of the above-mentioned two-dimensional movements, is necessary to optimize glenohumeral contact and stability throughout the entire range of shoulder motion. However, during the evaluation of an actual patient, it is most useful to consider the observed three-dimensional scapular motion as a summation of the individual rotational moments mentioned above.

The terms "protraction" and "retraction" are most often used to describe scapular movement in three-dimensional space. To understand these terms, it is perhaps easiest to first recognize that scapular motion occurs along a rounded surface (i.e., the convexity of the posterior thorax). Using this approach, one could imagine that any lateral translation of the scapular body would also require scapular internal rotation. This movement also requires some anterior tilt and downward rotation. This combination of movements is generally referred to as scapular "protraction" and can be closely simulated by having the patient thrust their shoulders anteriorly (similar to a hunchback position). Conversely, any medial translation of the scapular body would also require scapular external rotation. This movement also requires some posterior tilt and upward rotation. This combination of movements is typically referred to as scapular "retraction" which can be demonstrated by having the patient thrust their shoulders posteriorly (as in "squeezing" the scapulae together by extending the humerus posteriorly below 90° of elevation) (Fig. 2.12). Of course, neither protraction nor retraction could be achieved without some amount of upward and downward rotation along with anterior and posterior tilt; however, the purpose of the above example is to illustrate the fundamental concept of scapular translation *around* the posterior chest wall in three dimensions.

This same concept also applies when the scapula translates superiorly or inferiorly along the convex surface of the posterior thorax. In other words, inferior translation of the scapula would theoretically produce an increased posterior tilt whereas superior translation of the scapula would produce an increased anterior tilt (as in shrugging the shoulders). In reality, the shoulder shrug requires a combination of superior translation, anterior tilt, and internal rotation. Increased anterior or posterior scapular tilt is very subtle, is difficult to recognize by direct visual or tactile examination in the office setting, and generally cannot be isolated by any specific voluntary movement. Biomechanical studies suggest that scapular tilting mostly occurs during extension-type maneuvers with the arm either overhead or at the side.

Fig. 2.12 Illustration
demonstrating scapular
protraction and retraction.
Sagittal and posterior
views are shown.

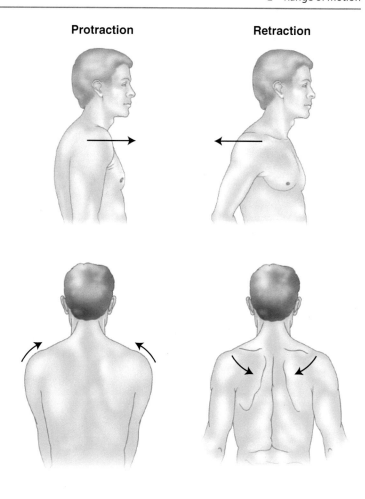

Most clinicians agree that isolated glenohu-meral motion occurs below approximately 90° of elevation whereas combined glenohumeral and scapulothoracic motion occurs above this level (discussed below). In order to maximize gleno-humeral contact and stability during this com-bined motion, the scapular stabilizers must not only contract in synchrony with each other, but also with each of the muscles that cross the glenohumeral joint along with the proprioceptive feedback obtained from surrounding soft-tissue structures (such as the glenohumeral joint cap-sule [6]). Although a thorough discussion of each possible scapular movement is beyond the scope of this book, we aim to emphasize the extreme importance of understanding the fundamental concepts related to three-dimensional scapular motion. It is with this foundational knowledge that one can begin to understand the complex dis-ease processes related to the shoulder.

2.3.4 Roles of the AC and SC Joints in Scapular Motion

The clavicle acts as a strut which allows for the strategic positioning of the shoulder girdle along the side of the thorax. In order to maximize shoulder range of motion, the clavicle must be dynamically positioned according to scapular motion via the AC and SC joints. Therefore, the health of the clavicle and the AC and SC joints is extremely important to achieve normal scapu-lar motion in three-dimensional space [26–28].

For example, arm elevation requires the clavicle to retract, elevate, translate, and rotate posteriorly along its long axis (i.e., the so-called "screw axis") where each of these movements is dependent on the function of intact, painless AC and SC joints [29, 30].

2.4 Differentiating Between Glenohumeral and Scapulothoracic Motion

The ability to elevate the arm overhead through any plane relies on dynamic scapular positioning which essentially places the glenoid in a position of maximum contact with the humeral head. Due to the three-dimensional complexity of scapular motion, it may be difficult for an inexperienced examiner to differentiate between the glenohumeral and scapulothoracic components of shoulder elevation. Many investigators have proposed methods of isolating each movement, thus allowing clinicians to more easily diagnose common shoulder problems. For example, in order to achieve normal cross-body adduction, the scapula must protract to maintain adequate glenohumeral contact and stability (i.e., the scapula must translate laterally and internally rotate to conform with the convexity of the posterior chest wall). While measuring posterior capsular tight-

ness using a cross-body adduction technique (described below), the clinician must first stabilize the scapula to minimize protraction. Otherwise, the measured amount of total combined adduction capacity will almost always be significantly greater than the true isolated glenohumeral adduction capacity as a result of the additive effect of scapular protraction.

Although complete isolation is probably not feasible in the clinical setting, clinicians can usually estimate the amount of isolated glenohumeral motion by detecting (or, in some cases, stabilizing) scapular motion. In the case of humeral elevation, the examiner can place one hand over the scapula (with the thumb over the scapular spine and the fingers wrapped anteriorly over the top of the shoulder) and ask the patient to slowly flex or abduct the humerus. During this movement, the examiner uses their hand to determine the point at which the scapula begins to translate or rotate. It is then assumed that any degree of elevation below this level would be composed of primarily glenohumeral motion whereas any motion above this level would involve a combination of glenohumeral *and* scapulothoracic motion (Fig. 2.13). The same concept can theoretically be applied to a variety of other testing procedures where isolation of glenohumeral motion is desired. In contrast to the method of detecting scapular motion, the

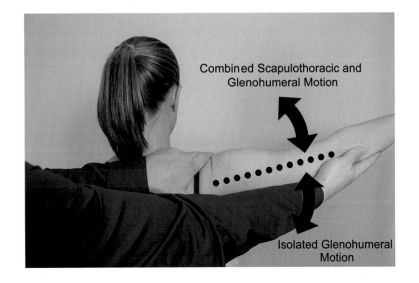

Fig. 2.13 Isolated glenohumeral motion versus combined glenohumeral and scapulothoracic motion. In this subject, the scapula began to rotate at approximately 100° of humeral abduction. Therefore, motion above this point is considered combined glenohumeral *and* scapulothoracic motion whereas motion below this point is considered isolated glenohumeral motion.

Combined Scapulothoracic and Glenohumeral Motion

Isolated Glenohumeral Motion

examiner can also stabilize the scapula by apply-ing a downward force to the top of the shoulder during shoulder elevation. In many cases, the same effect can be achieved by performing cer-tain examination maneuvers with the patient placed supine on the examination table (i.e., lay-ing on a flat surface is thought to limit scapular motion during testing).

The exact transition point between isolated and combined motion has been debated. Clarke et al. [31] found that passive isolated glenohu-meral abduction in a series of young, healthy patients occurred below 85.6° in females and below 77.4° in males. Gagey and Gagey [32] found a similar result in which 95 % of their sub-jects with normal shoulders transitioned to com-bined scapulothoracic motion between 85° and 90° of glenohumeral elevation. In contrast, Sauers et al. [33] found that the transition occurred at approximately 112° of glenohumeral elevation and Lintner et al. [34] found that the transition occurred at approximately 109° of gle-nohumeral elevation.

Due to these conflicting results, the reliability of this method in the measurement of isolated glenohumeral motion came into question. A study by Hoving et al. [35] determined that the intra-rater reliability for isolated glenohumeral motion was only 0.35; however, the study involved a series of patients with varying degrees of shoul-der pain which may have confounded their results. In addition, the clinicians were somewhat unfamiliar with the digital inclinometers that were used in the study, potentially blurring the interpretability of their results.

Several biomechanical studies have suggested that although the majority of scapular motion occurs above 90° of glenohumeral elevation, there does exist *some* scapular motion below this level. This fact calls into question the ability of an examiner to completely isolate glenohumeral elevation. Currently, it is thought that the scapula moves throughout the total arc of shoulder eleva-tion and that complete isolation of glenohumeral motion is probably not realistic. However, when the angle of glenohumeral elevation is less than 90°, the degree and quality of glenohumeral motion can be reliably estimated.

The above discussion only considers the abil-ity of an examiner to isolate glenohumeral motion during arm elevation. No published studies have examined the ability of an examiner to isolate glenohumeral rotation. However, the results of an unpublished cadaveric study by McFarland et al. [36] and Yap et al. [37] that were presented at the 1998 annual meeting of the Orthopedic Research Society in New Orleans, LA and the annual meet-ing of the American College of Sports Medicine in Orlando, FL in the same year suggested that glenohumeral rotation may be isolated and, potentially, accurately measured to within 2° prior to initiation of scapulothoracic motion. Their methods have not been validated in the lit-erature to date.

2.5   End Feel Classification

Accurate range of motion testing requires that the examiner utilizes both visual and tactile clues that ultimately aid in the entire physical examina-tion process. While the visual clues are obvious in many cases, tactile sensations that are trans-mitted to the examiner's hands or fingers as they manipulate the upper extremity are equally important in directing future examination maneu-vers and diagnostic studies. With range of motion testing, the concept of end feel is extremely important on several levels. As the glenohumeral joint nears its maximal range of motion, the qual-ity of the end feel can give the clinician an idea of what is happening anatomically.

In 1947, Cyriax and Cyriax [38] described a basic classification system in which normal end feel was characterized as bony, capsular or soft-tissue approximation and abnormal end feel was characterized as spasm, springy block, and empty (Table 2.1). These sensations occurred near the extremes of shoulder motion as a result of bony architecture, muscle contraction, and/or soft-tissue stretching.

A bony end feel occurs when an abrupt end point is reached as two hard surfaces come into contact (e.g., terminal extension of the elbow). Capsular end feel occurs as the joint approaches an extreme motion plane—further motion becomes

Table 2.1 Cyriax and Cyriax end feel classification

End-feel	Description
Capsular	Motion ends gradually, as if a leather band were being stretched.
Tissue approximation	Motion ends in a manner suggesting that motion would continue if not prevented by another structure.
Springy block	Motion ends with a noticeable rebound sensation.
Bony	Motion ends immediately when two hard surfaces come into contact.
Spasm	Motion ends in a "vibrant twang," or when motion is counteracted by muscle contraction.
Empty	Motion does not end, but patient asks examiner to stop maneuver as a result of pain.

increasingly difficult to obtain as the capsule stretches. Cyriax and Cyriax [38] suggested that capsular feel was analogous to a thick leather band being stretched. Soft-tissue approximation occurs when soft tissues prevent further motion, such as in the instance of cross-body adduction or extreme elbow flexion. Muscle spasm can often have a hard end feel and was characterized as a "vibrant twang" towards the extremes of motion. This can especially occur in the evaluation of a patient with instability who demonstrates a positive apprehension sign (the apprehension sign is discussed in Chap. 6). A springy block is felt when an intra-articular block prevents motion, followed by an episode of rebound. An empty end feel occurs when the examiner cannot discern a palpable end point; however, significant pain often prevents further motion.

In 2001, Hayes and Petersen [39] examined the inter- and intra-rater reliability of end feel in patients with painful shoulders and knees. Two physical therapists evaluated each patient twice, measuring two knee motions and five shoulder motions. The examiners noted the character and quality of the end feel at the extremes of range of motion while patients vocalized the exact moment of pain reproduction. The inter-rater κ coefficients for end feel ranged from 0.65–1.00 to 0.59–0.87 for the pain/resistance sequence. However, their study also demonstrated large variations in end feel when the shoulder was abducted. The authors suggested that this discrepancy was related to the fact that the scapulae of the subjects were variably stabilized which may have produced differences in end feel in these patients. In addition to this variation, it is thought that the presence of pain may also have a significant effect on different end feel characteristics [40].

The clinical applicability or validity of the various end feel characteristics has not been evaluated in the literature. The difficulty is that different end feel characteristics probably represent combinations of anatomic variables and pathologic lesions that likely cannot be differentiated by tactile sensation alone. Therefore, despite its widespread application in clinical practice, further study is needed to validate this method of examination before it can be formally advocated.

2.6 Methods of Measurement

Range of motion is defined as the magnitude of motion capacity that exists across a joint. Because most major joints in the body achieve angular (or rotational) movements, range of motion is typically measured in degrees relative to some normative plane. Range of motion measurement is a particularly important aspect of the physical examination that is often overlooked in clinical practice. These measurements can have significant implications regarding treatment approaches and outcomes and should not be omitted when evaluating a new patient with a shoulder complaint. Shoulder range of motion is typically quantified using one of four basic techniques; these include estimation via visual inspection, the use of an inclinometer, the use of a goniometer, the use of a gyroscope or, more recently, digital photography using a high resolution camera or smart phone.

2.6.1 Visual Inspection

Unfortunately, visual estimation is the most commonly used method for the measurement of shoulder range of motion. Although several studies have found that experienced practitioners can estimate range of motion with a similar accuracy to standardized measurement devices [41, 42], the lack of teaching regarding the fundamentals of range of motion testing is disappointing. This results in inaccurate measurement estimations by the novice examiner who was never properly taught to use goniometers or inclinometers. Although formal measurement requires more time to complete, it is suggested that inexperienced examiners use standard measurement devices to aid in accurate patient assessment until they become more knowledgeable and experienced with the examination process. In a busy clinical practice, however, the experienced clinician can usually make rapid range of motion estimations without sacrificing accuracy or precision. Visual inspection and estimation of range of motion is therefore a standard of practice in most cases, but formal measurements are required when a study involving range of motion data is being conducted.

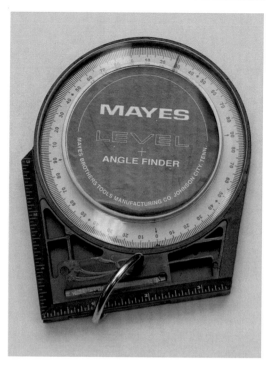

Fig. 2.14 Photograph of a mechanical inclinometer.

2.6.2 Inclinometers

An inclinometer is essentially a leveling device, similar to that which is used by a carpenter to measure the degree of inclination of a surface relative to the horizontal plane, that is occasionally used in clinical practice to quantify shoulder range of motion or, in some cases, the degree of spinal deformity such as kyphosis or scoliosis [43–45]. Both mechanical and digital inclinometers have been described as reliable and valid tools for the measurement of shoulder range of motion.

Mechanical inclinometers, or hygrometers, use gravity and a fluid-level indicator to measure the inclination of the humerus relative to the horizontal plane in degrees (Fig. 2.14). The first reported use of a mechanical inclinometer to measure range of motion was in 1975 by Clarke et al. [31]. In their study, the inter-observer reliability was approximately 0.93. Similarly, Dover et al. [46] calculated inter- and intra-rater reliability values of approximately 0.99 in the measurement of shoulder range of motion using a mechanical inclinometer. In an adjunct study [47], the same group found that the ability of the inclinometer to detect changes in joint proprioception was also pronounced. In that study, they calculated inter- and intra-observer reliabilities ranging from 0.978 to 0.984.

Currently, digital inclinometers are more commonly used to assess shoulder range of motion [48–57] and function by calculating the angle of inclination relative to the horizontal plane using an implanted gravity sensor. Kolber et al. [51] determined that the inter- and intra-observer reliabilities of digital inclinometry was greater than 0.95 and found that this method was interchangeable with goniometry (intra-class correlation [ICC] coefficients for goniometry were >0.94) [51]. Scibek and Carcia [54] studied 13 healthy collegiate subjects in an attempt to quantify scapulohumeral rhythm using a digital inclinometer. In that study, the investigators found that the scapula contributed to 2.5 % of shoulder motion in the first 30° of shoulder abduction. This proportion dramatically increased to between 20.9 and 37.5 % when measured between 30° and 90°

of humeral abduction, respectively. Johnson et al. [58] calculated the reliability and validity of a digital inclinometer to measure scapular upward rotation during humeral abduction in the scapular plane. They found that the digital inclinometer had excellent reliability and validity in the assessment of scapular motion with inter- and intra-observer ICCs ranging from 0.89 to 0.96. A similar study by Tucker and Ingram [56] calculated ICCs of >0.89 after using a digital inclinometer to quantify scapular upward rotation with static humeral elevation.

More recently, studies by Shin et al. [59] and Mitchell et al. [60] demonstrated the ability of smart phone inclinometers (and goniometers) to accurately measure range of motion with excellent inter- and intra-observer reliability (ICC >0.9). One other study [61] demonstrated the capability of smart phones to measure cervical range of motion. This method of measurement eliminates the cost of standard digital inclinometers, a factor that has limited their widespread use. Nevertheless, these studies demonstrate the utility and practicality of digital inclinometers in the accurate measurement of scapulohumeral rhythm in addition to glenohumeral range of motion capacity.

2.6.3 Goniometers

The use of a standard handheld goniometer is still the most commonly used device for the measurement of shoulder range of motion, especially since it produces results comparable to more expensive devices that measure the same variables [51, 52, 62]. Goniometers come in various shapes and sizes; however, the general setup has two movable arms where one arm is place in line within a normalized vertical or horizontal plane (or the "zero position" as defined by Clarke et al. [31]) and the other arm is used to measure the degrees of deviation from the chosen plane of reference. To use a goniometer, the fulcrum of the device is aligned over the center of rotation of the joint to be measured. The stationary arm of the goniometer is aligned with the limb being measured, generally over proximal muscle origins. The goniometer is held in place while the joint is moved through its range of motion. The degree of angulation between the two arms of the device represents the total range of motion achieved by the joint. It is important to maintain stabilization of the limb proximal to the center of rotation of the joint to avoid measurement errors. In addition, it is best practice to read the goniometer measurement before removing the device from the joint. Goniometric mastery requires extensive practice and anatomic knowledge which will eventually result in measurement consistency and reproducibility. It is therefore recommended for the novice examiner to learn the proper range of motion measurement techniques early in their orthopaedic career.

2.6.4 Gyroscopes

A gyroscope is essentially a spinning wheel that changes in three-dimensional orientation with changes in angular momentum. Gyroscopes have numerous potential applications such as inertial navigation systems (e.g., orbiting satellites) and various types of flying vehicles (e.g., helicopters). With regard to the shoulder, gyroscopes can also be used to precisely measure range of motion as shown in a few preliminary studies [63, 64].

El-Zayat et al. [63, 64] reported good reproducibility and reliability with regard to range of motion measurements in two separate studies. Penning et al. [65] evaluated 58 patients with either subacromial impingement (27) or glenohumeral osteoarthritis (31) and determined the reproducibility of a three-dimensional gyroscope to measure shoulder abduction. They also found that use of the gyroscope was a reproducible method to measure shoulder range of motion; however, they recommended repeating the measurements for improved accuracy. Further studies are needed to define how and when gyroscopes should be used for accurate range of motion assessment.

2.6.5 Digital Photography

Digital photography has been shown on multiple occasions to be an accurate method of making range of motion measurements [66–70]. Although

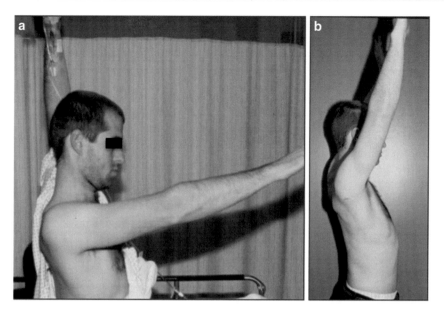

Fig. 2.15 Clinical photographs demonstrating maximal forward flexion in a patient both before (**a**) and after (**b**) an interposition arthroplasty procedure. (Courtesy of J.P. Warner, MD).

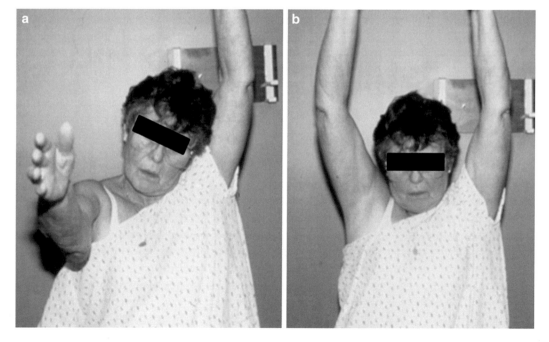

Fig. 2.16 Clinical photographs demonstrating maximal forward flexion in a patient both before (**a**) and after (**b**) subacromial injection with local anesthetic. (Courtesy of Christian Gerber, MD).

standardized photographic methods that place the patient and the camera in the correct position to allow for accurate and reproducible two-dimensional measurements have yet to be established, digital photography offers several patient advantages that should be recognized. The first advantage centers around documentation as the photograph becomes part of the patient's medical record which can be referred to at a later date (Figs. 2.15 and 2.16). Second, digital photographs can be sent through the internet to distant clinics, especially when there is a geographic constraint to proper medical care. Third, standardized range of motion photographs of any given patient can be compared and reviewed over a period of time to determine the progress of rehabilitation or physical therapy. In addition to these patient advantages, taking digital photographs or video allows for the routine documentation of uncommon pathologies which may facilitate inter-clinician communication and education.

2.7 Measuring Active and Passive Shoulder Elevation

Shoulder elevation is an umbrella term used to describe either flexion or abduction depending on the scapulohumeral angle, whether in the coronal plane (i.e., horizontal abduction), the sagittal plane (i.e., forward flexion), the scapular plane (i.e., scaption) or somewhere in between these reference points. Shoulder elevation includes the most important shoulder motions that are necessary for activities of daily living, occupations, sports, and recreational activities.

2.7.1 Measuring Shoulder Abduction

Shoulder abduction can be measured with the patient either standing or, less commonly, lying supine on the examination table. Sabari et al. [71] found changes in abduction capacity with the patient sitting due to compensatory contralateral muscle activation. It is important to note that although the patient may be able to abduct their shoulders to an overhead position, they may also utilize compensatory scapulothoracic motions to achieve this position. Thus, it is vitally important to evaluate the scapula in conjunction with any shoulder motion. Assessment of scapular motion and scapular dyskinesis is presented later in this chapter and in Chap. 9.

It is most prudent to measure abduction capacity within the plane of the scapula; that is, abduction with approximately 20–30° of forward angulation. It is nearly physiologically impossible to achieve maximal abduction with the humerus in the coronal plane. It is also best to perform this movement with the humerus externally rotated to avoid acromiohumeral impingement, thus allowing the patient to maximally elevate the humerus within the scapular plane. Attempting to abduct the humerus while internally rotated will result in an inaccurate measurement of abduction capacity.

With the humerus abducted, the goniometer is centered over the glenohumeral joint with one arm of the device perpendicular to the floor and the other arm aligned according to the angulation of the proximal humerus. Sometimes, the patient may experience pain during this maneuver. In these cases, an assistant can hold the arm in abduction while the measurement is made. After measurement, the examiner can passively assist the arm to determine whether additional motion is available. If there is a considerable remaining proportion of motion available with passive assistance, it is possible that the shoulder is weak in this position. On the contrary, if abduction capacity is limited both actively and passively, it is possible that either the shoulder is stiff or the patient is guarding from potential discomfort. It is best to measure the degree of stiffness during an examination under anesthesia, especially when stiffness comprises a large proportion of the patient's total range of motion.

2.7.2 Measuring Shoulder Flexion

Forward flexion of the humerus typically does not require a completely intact rotator cuff to achieve sufficient motion, especially when the deltoid muscle is intact. Thus, patients with rotator cuff deficiency may have full flexion capability with poor abduction capacity. Forward flexion of the humerus is typically measured with the humerus and the forearm in neutral rotation. The patient is then asked to actively and maximally forward flex the shoulder. Once full, maximal forward flexion has been achieved, the goniometer is centered over the glenohumeral joint with one arm perpendicular to the floor and the other arm in-line with the angulation of the proximal humerus. Once this measurement has been made, the arm can be passively flexed further to measure any additional motion that may be available. The inability of the patient to achieve satisfactory active or passive forward flexion may be the result of a stiff shoulder and may require an examination and manipulation under anesthesia.

2.8   Measuring Active and Passive Shoulder Rotation

Shoulder rotation has traditionally been measured in the supine position; however, there are several variations in patient positioning that can be used to answer specific clinical questions or to facilitate patient comfort. In addition to the supine position, shoulder rotation can be measured with the patient standing, sitting or in the lateral decubitus position.

2.8.1   Measuring External Rotation

2.8.1.1 Supine Position

Numerous studies have examined the reliability of isolated glenohumeral or combined glenohumeral and scapulothoracic rotational measured in the supine position. However, variability in scapular stabilization across these studies makes comparison difficult since it has been shown that scapular stabilization affects range of motion measurements along with inter- and intra-rater reliability [48, 72, 73]. When the examiner seeks information regarding glenohumeral range of motion alone, it is necessary to determine the point at which scapular motion begins. As mentioned above, the examiner places the palm of their hand over the anterior shoulder, thus stabilizing the scapula while the humerus is rotated externally at the side of the body (Fig. 2.17). The end point for glenohumeral motion occurs when the shoulder begins to lift off the table as scapular motion is initiated. The patient's position is held while the goniometric measurement is made. In the second technique, the examiner places their hand underneath the patient's scapula and simultaneously externally rotates the humerus. When the scapula begins to move, the end point has been reached and the measurement is made.

Fig. 2.17 Demonstration of the position used to measure passive external rotation in the supine position.

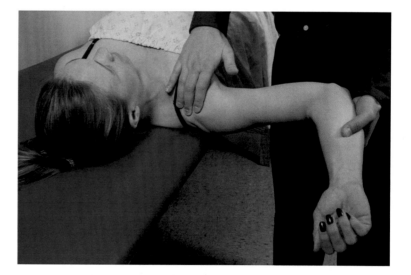

A third way to measure isolated glenohumeral external rotation in the supine position is to simply visualize the point at which the shoulder complex begins to move in response to the rotational moment. This is done while simultaneously feeling for an endpoint as the examiner externally rotates the humerus.

2.8.1.2 Sitting or Standing Position

In the sitting or standing position, measurements are made with the elbows flexed to 90° with the humerus either at the side or abducted to 90° depending on the information sought by the examiner. It is often useful to obtain multiple measurements such that a complete evaluation can be achieved. In addition, distinguishing between glenohumeral and scapulothoracic contributions to shoulder motion can also provide powerful evidence for or against a specific pathology.

Passive glenohumeral external rotation can be isolated when the arm is either at the side or abducted to 90°. When the arm is at the side, the examiner stabilizes the flexed elbow and passively externally rotates the humerus until the glenohumeral joint reaches its first end point. This generally occurs when shoulder tightness develops and the patient begins compensatory rotation of the torso. The examiner then asks the patient to hold their position at the end point so that measurements can be made with a goniometer. An assistant can also hold the arm in place while measurements are made.

When the shoulder is abducted to 90°, isolated glenohumeral external rotation capacity is measured by passively externally rotating the humerus until the first end point is detected. The end point is usually reached when the patient begins to bend backwards at the waist to compensate for the force being placed on the arm. The examiner can also simultaneously inspect the scapula to determine the point of external rotation at which the scapula begins to retract.

Passive combined glenohumeral and scapulothoracic range of motion can be assessed by simply externally rotating the humerus until its final end point is reached. It is important to prevent the patient from extending the shoulder or turning the body to increase this measurement. When the humerus is abducted to 90°, the examiner passively externally rotates the humerus as far as the patient will allow while also preventing a hyperlordotic posture. The examiner then asks the patient to hold this position while the measurement is made. In some cases, an assistant examiner may be required to assist the patient in holding this position, especially in those with joint hyperlaxity who display a large external rotation arc.

Although less commonly performed, combined scapulothoracic and glenohumeral range of motion can also be measured actively. With the arm at the side, the patient attempts to externally rotate the humerus maximally without extending the shoulder or increasing lordosis. A similar maneuver is performed with the arm abducted to 90°, taking care to prevent ancillary muscular contraction. An assistant can help hold the final position while a goniometric measurement is made.

2.8.1.3 Lateral Decubitus Position

With the patient in the lateral decubitus position and lying on the affected arm, passive external rotation capacity can be measured. The arm is first abducted to 90° and then passive external rotation is measured with a goniometer once the first end point has been reached (scapula begins to move or resistance is felt).

2.8.2 Measuring Internal Rotation

Internal rotation of the shoulder can also be quantified using methods similar to that of external rotation, differentiating between glenohumeral and scapulothoracic contributions. The various techniques for measuring active and passive internal rotation are described below.

2.8.2.1 Supine Position

Isolated glenohumeral or combined glenohumeral and scapulothoracic internal rotation in the supine position can be performed exactly as described for external rotation above (Fig. 2.18). This method is especially helpful for the

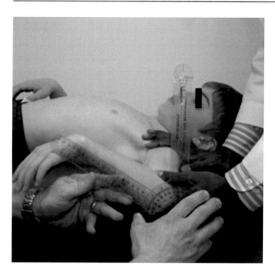

Fig. 2.18 Demonstration of the measurement of passive internal rotation in the supine position with the arm abducted to 90°. (Courtesy of Craig Morgan, MD.).

examination of overhead athletes who may have developed hyperexternal rotation with a glenohumeral internal rotation deficit (GIRD) resulting in a pathologically diminished total arc of rotation compared to the contralateral shoulder.

2.8.2.2 Sitting or Standing Position

With the patient sitting or standing, passive glenohumeral internal rotation capacity is generally measured with the arm abducted to 90° and the elbow flexed to 90°. From this position, the humerus is passively and gently internally rotated until the examiner notes compensatory scapular or bodily movements. The patient is then asked to hold this position while a measurement is recorded with a goniometer. If necessary, an assistant can hold the patient's arm in place while the measurement is being made. The zero position is defined as the plane in which the forearm is perpendicular to the floor—if the patient cannot internally rotate to the zero position, the goniometric measurement is recorded as a negative number.

Internal rotation involving combined glenohumeral and scapulothoracic components can be measured either actively or passively with the humerus abducted to 90° and the elbow flexed to 90°. In the passive form of the test, the examiner

stabilizes the elbow and rotates the humerus internally as far as possible without compensatory movements. The patient holds the arm in this position and a goniometer (or similar device) is used to make the measurement. Some patients with internal rotation deficits, rotator cuff disease, and/or osteoarthritis may develop pain with internal rotation. In these cases, the end point occurs at the degree of internal rotation in which the patient begins to experience pain.

A similar maneuver is performed to measure active internal rotation with the arm abducted to 90°. In this case, the patient uses his or her muscles to generate the internal rotation force until a maximum angle is reached. The patient (or an assistant) holds the arm in the maximally internally rotated position until the measurement is documented.

In clinical practice, measuring active internal rotation with the patient reaching the thumb along the dorsal aspect of the thoracic spine was originally advocated since this motion was thought to require maximal internal rotation (see Fig. 2.7). The measurement took into account the vertebral level to which the thumb could reach up the spinal column. For example, a patient may reach to a level of T7 or L4 with their thumb as they reach upwards—this system of reporting is still occasionally used. However, researchers have refuted its usefulness as a measure of internal rotation for several reasons [5]. First, the maneuver requires motion beyond the glenohumeral and scapulothoracic articulations. Adequate finger, wrist and elbow motion is also required to perform this maneuver. A study by Mallon et al. [5] found that this type of motion required glenohumeral, scapulothoracic, elbow, wrist, hand, and finger movements. Elbow flexion contributed significantly to the final internal rotation measurements in their study as the patient moved the hand from the sacrum upwards towards the thoracic spine. Thus, patients with elbow pathology may not reach the same spinal level as someone with a normal elbow; however, both of their shoulders may have normal active and passive internal rotation capacities. Second, Mallon et al. [5] also found that the relative contributions of the scapulothoracic and glenohumeral articulations was approximately 2:1 with this movement, suggesting that this test may be more appropriate in the evaluation of global shoulder function rather than glenohumeral or scapulothoracic motion. Third, a recent study by Hall et al. [74] found that when compared to the estimation of vertebral levels, internal rotation measurements using a goniometer with the arm abducted was more reliable and accurate.

2.8.2.3 Lateral Decubitus Position

Measuring passive isolated internal rotation in the lateral decubitus position is performed exactly as described above for external rotation.

2.9   Factors That Affect the Accuracy of Range of Motion Measurements

Measuring range of motion can sometimes be a difficult task, especially when challenged with various confounding variables. As such, there are many factors that can potentially influence range of motion measurements. Some of these include age [31, 75–77], gender [31, 75, 77–80], patient positioning [62, 71, 72, 81], arm dominance [31, 76, 82, 83], posture [84, 85], participation in overhead sports, and the experience of the examiner [42, 86].

2.9.1   Increasing Age

Several authors have reported a decrease in shoulder range of motion with advancing age [31, 75–77]. Barnes et al. [75] measured shoulder motion in 280 volunteers with 40 subjects in each of 7 groups ranging in age from 0–10, 10–20, 20–30, 40–50, 50–60, and 60–70 years. Not unexpectedly, the investigators found a gradual decline in active and passive range of motion with respect to increasing age; however, this was not true for internal rotation, which appeared to increase as age increased. This paradox may be attributed to external rotation weakness which was also found to increase over time. In addition,

the authors concluded that the loss of forward flexion in patients under 40 years of age should not be attributed to the aging process.

2.9.2   Gender

Gender appears to be another factor that may influence shoulder range of motion measurements since several studies have demonstrated the ability of women to achieve a greater range of active and passive motion when compared to men of the same age [31, 75, 77–80]. Clarke et al. [31] and Schwartz et al. [80] found similar results, however, neither study found a difference in internal rotation capacity between genders.

2.9.3   Patient Positioning

Several studies have found that the position of the torso may have a significant effect on range of motion measurements [62, 71, 72, 81]. The primary concern revolves around the potential differences in measurements when the patient is sitting versus standing versus supine. The sitting position removes the effect of gravity when testing internal and external rotation with the arm at the side. The effect of gravity on abduction can also be eliminated by having the patient lie in the supine position, thus potentially allowing the patient to obtain a larger arc of active shoulder abduction. In addition, scapulothoracic motion may be affected when a patient lies supine on a flat surface, thus inhibiting the ability of the scapula to move in conjunction with glenohumeral elevation.

Sabari et al. [71] studied the effect patient position on range of motion in a series of 30 healthy volunteers, specifically noting whether a sitting or supine position affects the ability of the patient to flex or abduct the shoulder. The investigators found significant differences in range of motion measurements depending on whether the subject was in the sitting or supine position. In the sitting position, subjects were found to use compensatory thoracopelvic movements to aid in shoulder motion. Although both methods can be used to measure range of motion, it is important to note the position of the subject during the examination to help with interpretation of the collected data.

2.9.4 Arm Dominance

Range of motion measurements of the dominant shoulder compared to those of the non-dominant shoulder can vary considerably [75, 80], especially with regard to rotational measurements in throwing athletes. Several studies have found no differences in range of motion between shoulders; [31, 76, 82, 83] however, Barnes et al. [75] found that the non-dominant shoulder had significantly increased active and passive internal rotation along with increased active and passive extension compared to the dominant shoulder in non-throwing athletes. Interestingly, the investigators also found that the dominant shoulder had significantly increased external rotation capacity compared to the non-dominant shoulder. The authors concluded that comparing rotational range of motion between dominant and non-dominant shoulders may not be as clinically useful as once thought.

2.9.5 Posture

The degree of thoracic curvature may also play a role in range of motion and strength measurements [80, 84, 85]. Kebaetse et al. [85] compared shoulder range of motion, strength, and scapulothoracic kinematics in a series of 34 healthy participants who were placed in either the erect or slouched position. When in the slouched posture, the investigators noted increased scapular elevation between 0° and 90° of humeral abduction and decreased posterior scapular tilt when the abduction angle was greater than 90°. In addition, active glenohumeral range of motion was significantly decreased in those with slouched postures. Bullock et al. [84] also noted a significantly decreased flexion range of motion after measurement of those positioned in a slouched posture. Therefore, range of motion measurements in patients who present with a slouched posture (e.g., those with kyphoscoliosis) may underestimate the true anatomic restraints to shoulder motion.

2.10 Specific Tests for General Shoulder Mobility

There are many physical examination maneuvers that can be used to measure general shoulder mobility and flexibility. Compared to other maneuvers that measure specific components of shoulder motion, these tests have the specific advantage of determining the overall functionality of the upper extremity with regard to the performance of activities of daily living. Of course, there exists a ceiling effect when performing these tests on athletes who require a greater degree of performance relative to the general population. Nevertheless, these tests can be useful to determine if range of motion loss has an effect on the patient's normal activities since they require combinations of basic shoulder movements in different planes. Some authors have called into question the clinical relevance of many of these tests while also suggesting other types of tests that more closely simulate activities of daily living [11, 12, 87, 88]. Patients who present with shoulder complaints are often questioned regarding these basic movements in outcomes questionnaires (such as the American Shoulder and Elbow Surgeons' [ASES] score [89] and Disabilities of the Arm, Shoulder and Hand [DASH] score [90]); however, these specific motions are infrequently tested directly by the treating physician.

Description and discussion of a few general shoulder mobility tests are described below. Note many more of these types of general motion tests exist; however, the tests described below were chosen because they are more likely to be taught and/or practiced.

2.10.1 Apley Scratch Test

The Apley scratch test is one of the more frequently taught maneuvers for the evaluation of general shoulder motion and overall function.

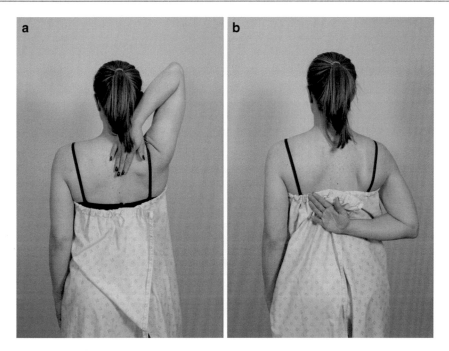

Fig. 2.19 Apley scratch test. (**a**) The subject reaches downward along the thoracic spine. (**b**) The subject reaches upwards along the lumbar spine.

The patient is first asked to place one hand on the ipsilateral shoulder and to reach as far inferiorly along the thoracic spine as possible. This motion is useful for evaluating combined abduction, flexion, and external rotation of the shoulder. Next, the patient is then asked to place the arms at the side and then to reach up the lumbar and thoracic spine as far as possible. This motion is useful for evaluating the combination of adduction, extension, and internal rotation of the shoulder (Fig. 2.19). Although the clinical utility of this test has yet to be defined, it is generally thought to be a quick and effective modality for the evaluation of global shoulder function.

2.10.2   Cross-Body Adduction Test

The cross-body adduction test is another measure of general shoulder motion that can be used more specifically to measure flexibility of the shoulder, especially with regard to the posterior capsule. In this test, the arm is forward flexed to approximately 90° of elevation followed by horizontal adduction towards the opposite shoulder. Measuring tape can be used to measure the distance from the lateral epicondyle to the AC joint at the top of the shoulder (Fig. 2.20). Once this has been completed and a measurement has been recorded, the test is repeated on the contralateral side for measurement comparison. Patients with pain related to AC joint pathology may experience pain at the top of the shoulder with this movement and, therefore, range of motion measurements may be affected (physical examination of the AC joint is discussed in Chap. 7).

2.10.3   Combined Abduction Test

The combined abduction test was first described by Pappas et al. [91] in 1985. The patient is asked to assume a supine position on the examination table. The examiner then places his or her hand behind the scapula to detect scapular motion while the arm is simultaneously elevated in using a combination of flexion and abduction until the

Fig. 2.20 Demonstration of the measurement of cross-body adduction. The arm is passively adducted across the chest until resistance is felt. The distance from the lateral epicondyle to the acromioclavicular (AC) joint is then determined using measuring tape.

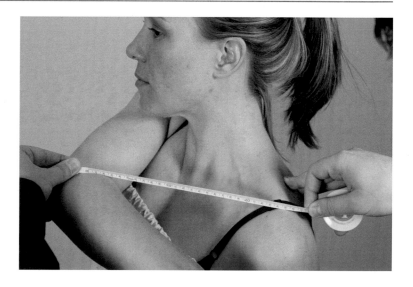

arm is fully elevated, taking care to avoid an increase in lordosis or any other compensatory movement that may increase arm elevation. If the arm cannot reach an angle that is parallel with the examination table, inflexibility is likely present and may indicate muscle or capsuloligamentous tightness. The structures involved have not been specifically evaluated, although tightness of the pectoralis major, latissimus dorsi, and teres major muscles has been implicated on one occasion [92].

2.10.4 Quadrant Test

The quadrant test, first described by Mullen et al. [18] in 1989, was designed to detect a subtle change in Codman's paradox as a result of shoulder discomfort or pathology (Codman's paradox is discussed earlier in this chapter). The test is performed with the patient in the supine position. The examiner places his or her hand over the spine of the scapula and the distal clavicle and applies a gentle inferiorly directed pressure to prevent shoulder shrugging during the test. The arm is first abducted to 90° of straight lateral abduction and 90° of external rotation. From this position, the arm is adducted until the humerus begins to internally rotate. The moment the arm begins to internally rotate is known as the quadrant position (Fig. 2.21). It should be emphasized

that this maneuver may only be clinically useful when the examiner has performed the exam on many patients with normal shoulders such that subtle changes in motion can be detected. The test has not been formally evaluated in the literature.

2.10.5 Posterior Tightness Test

Tyler et al. [93, 94] described the posterior tightness test which specifically examines the flexibility of posterior shoulder structures. In this test, the patient is placed in the lateral decubitus position with the untested arm placed beneath the head with the knees and hips flexed for comfort. The arm to be tested is then passively flexed to 90° of forward elevation and the ipsilateral scapula is stabilized with the examiner's opposite hand. The arm is then adducted across the body, taking care to prevent any rotational motion of the humerus (Fig. 2.22). When resistance is felt, a tape measure can be used to determine the distance from the lateral epicondyle to the surface of the examination table. This maneuver is typically performed with an assistant who makes the final measurement. The test is then repeated on the contralateral shoulder for comparison. The original investigators calculated an inter-rater reliability of approximately 0.80 and an intra-rater reliability of greater than

Fig. 2.21 Quadrant test.
(**a**) With the patient supine,
the scapula is stabilized
and the humerus is
abducted to 90° and
externally rotated to 90°.
The humerus is the
adducted (*curved arrow*)
until (**b**) the humerus
begins to internally rotate.
This is known as the
quadrant position.

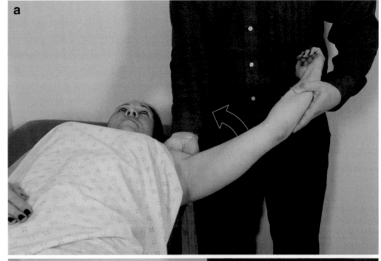

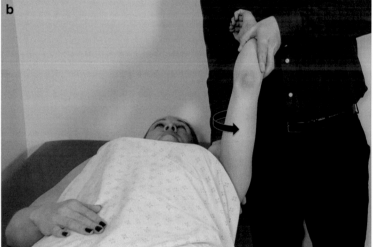

0.90 for both the dominant and non-dominant
shoulders of asymptomatic subjects.

This test was subsequently used by the same
group to evaluate a series of collegiate baseball
players and a cohort of patients with subacromial impingement syndrome. In addition, other
authors have found that the test may be useful
for comparing posterior shoulder tightness
between the dominant and non-dominant shoulders of baseball players [95] along with differences in shoulder tightness among different
baseball positions [96]. Although the test has not
been formally validated for routine practice,
several authors have confirmed the reliability

and validity of the test in overhead athletes while
also suggesting that performing the test in the
supine position may actually be more accurate
[97, 98].

2.10.6 Horizontal Flexion Test

The horizontal flexion test was also designed to
detect posterior shoulder tightness and was first
described by Pappas et al. [91] in 1985. In this
test, the patient is positioned supine and the tested
arm is flexed to 90° of elevation. Without bending
the elbow, the arm is slowly adducted until

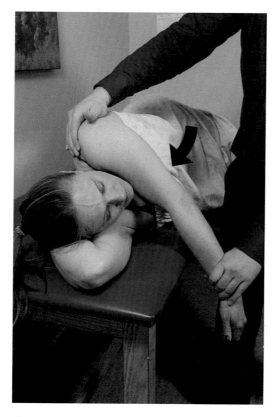

Fig. 2.22 Posterior capsular tightness. With the patient in the lateral decubitus position, the untested arm is placed under the head and the knees are bent. This positioning helps prevent the torso from rotating during the test. The humerus is placed in 90° of forward flexion. The examiner stabilizes the scapula and passively adducts the humerus until resistance is felt. A tape measure is sometimes used to measure the distance from the lateral epicondyle to the surface of the examination table.

resistance is felt. The position is held and the angle formed between the vertical axis and the arm is measured with a goniometer (Fig. 2.23). In general, when the adduction angle is less than 45°, posterior shoulder tightness should be considered. No studies have evaluated the validity of this method to diagnose posterior shoulder tightness; however, it can give the clinician a clue as to the underlying pathologic process. It is important to remember that the measured amount of adduction relative to any reference point should be corrected in patients with scapular malposition.

2.10.7 Pectoralis Minor Tightness Test

Tightness or shortening of the pectoralis minor muscle-tendon complex can have significant clinical implications and has been described a potential indirect pain generator and a cause for scapular dyskinesis with specific alterations in upward rotation, external rotation, and posterior tilt [99, 100]. As a result, the inferiorly malpositioned scapula decreases the space available for the rotator cuff tendons to travel beneath the acromion, potentially leading to subacromial impingement and subsequent rotator cuff disease [23, 101, 102].

Kendall et al. [92] described a method of determining whether pectoralis minor muscle tightness was present. In this test, the patient is

Fig. 2.23 Horizontal flexion test. With the patient supine, the humerus is flexed to 90° and slowly adducted until resistance is felt (*curved arrow*). The angle of adduction is then determined using a goniometer, using a vertical line as a reference point.

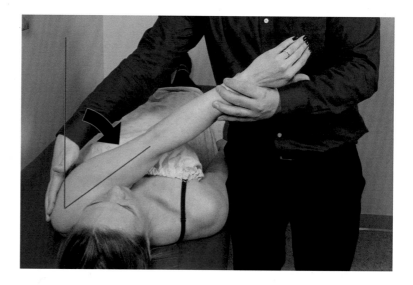

placed supine on the examination table and the examiner places one hand on the anterior shoulder. The shoulder is then pushed posteriorly towards the surface of the examination table using a gentle to moderate force. An inability to push the anterior shoulder such that the posterior shoulder lies flat on the table indicated pectoralis minor tightness. Another way of testing for pectoralis minor tightness is to simply visualize the asymmetric height of one scapula versus the contralateral scapula. In the patient with pectoralis minor tightness, the affected scapula will sit farther away from the surface of the examination table than that of the contralateral shoulder.

Borstad [103] validated a direct measurement technique in a series of cadavers that would later be used clinically to determine the actual length of the pectoralis minor muscle-tendon unit in a series of swimmers [104]. This method involves simply measuring the distance from the inferior aspect of the fourth rib to the coracoid process using a tape measure. When compared to an electromagnetic tracking system, this method resulted in inter- and intra-observer ICCs between 0.82 and 0.87 [103].

2.11   The Stiff Shoulder and the Frozen Shoulder

Skillful evaluation of the stiff shoulder is one of the most valuable skill sets that a clinician can possess. Due to the inherent complexity of the shoulder girdle, limited passive motion can have multiple potential etiologies and are typically grouped according to whether the shoulder is "stiff" or "frozen" [105–111]. These categories are independent and effort must be made to differentiate between the two categories since their treatment options vary considerably [105–107, 112–122]. In general, a "stiff shoulder" refers to any loss of joint motion from any identifiable cause including arthritis, capsule contracture, adhesion formation after surgery, or any other joint abnormality that effectively decreases the total arc of shoulder motion. A "frozen shoulder" (also known as adhesive capsulitis), on the other hand, refers to the largely idiopathic

syndrome in which shoulder pain gradually develops followed by a loss of shoulder motion. The condition is more common in women and has been associated with increased levels of cytokines and inflammatory markers within the glenohumeral synovial fluid and subacromial bursa without an identifiable cause [123–127]. Soft tissue contractures and scarring may result, leading to significant range of motion loss. While some authors have suggested an autoimmune origin and an association with thyroid disorders, systemic lupus erythematosus, and diabetes mellitus, these connections have yet to be fully substantiated [124–126, 128–131].

Clinical evaluation of the stiff shoulder thus requires a thorough history prior to initiation of the physical examination process. Patients with a history of autoimmune conditions are more likely to have a frozen shoulder whereas patients who recently had surgery on the joint are most likely to have adhesion formation and symptomatic scar tissue resulting in their loss of motion. There are a host of reasons for a stiff shoulder and most of the causes can be determined by a thorough history.

Physical examination of patients with range of motion loss should focus on the differences between active and passive shoulder motion. When the total arc of motion is the same for both active and passive motion, the patient is said to have either a stiff shoulder or a frozen shoulder, depending on the etiology. In contrast, when passive range of motion exceeds that of active range of motion, the patient is said to primarily have weakness rather than stiffness. Range of motion testing using a variety of techniques (such as those listed above) can localize the stiffness to a particular anatomic region within the shoulder. For example, a patient with identical, yet decreased, active and passive internal rotation of the shoulder with the arm at the side is likely to have stiffness of the posterior capsulolabral structures, a common finding in patients with glenohumeral osteoarthritis. Similar examinations can be performed for external rotation, abduction, forward flexion, and so on until the precise location of stiffness or scarring is surmised.

2.12 Conclusion

An understanding of glenohumeral range of motion and the various testing procedures is necessary before the clinician can implement many of the physical examination maneuvers that will be presented later in this book. A basic understanding of both traditional and modern methods of range of motion assessment is also necessary to facilitate the interpretation of clinical studies that evaluate shoulder range of motion. Therefore, this chapter provides a foundation for future learning and research that extends far beyond this text.

References

1. Silver D. Measurement of range of motion in joints. J Bone Joint Surg Am. 1923;5:569.
2. Cave EF, Roberts S. A method for measuring and recording joint function. J Bone Joint Surg Am. 1936;18(2):455–65.
3. American Medical Association. A guide to the evaluation of permanent impairment of the extremities and back. J Am Med Assn. 1958;166(15):1–109.
4. American Academy of Orthopaedic Surgeons. Joint motion: method of measuring and recording. Chicago: American Academy of Orthopaedic Surgeons; 1965.
5. Mallon WJ, Herring CL, Sallay PI, Moorman CT, Crim JR. Use of vertebral levels to measure presumed internal rotation at the shoulder: a radiographic analysis. J Shoulder Elbow Surg. 1996;5(4):299–306.
6. Jerosch J, Steinbeck J, Schröder M, Westhues M, Reer R. Intraoperative EMG response of the musculature after stimulation of the glenohumeral joint capsule. Acta Orthop Belg. 1997;63(1):8–14.
7. Debski RE, Wong EK, Woo SLY, Sakane M, Fu FH, Warner JJP. In situ force distribution in the glenohumeral joint capsule during anterior-posterior loading. J Orthop Res. 1999;17(5):769–76.
8. Inman VT, Saunders JB, Abbott LC. Observations on the function of the shoulder joint. J Bone Joint Surg. 1944;26(1):1–30.
9. Lin HT, Hsu AT, Chang GL, Chien JC, An KN, Su FC. Determining the resting position of the glenohumeral joint in subjects who are healthy. Phys Ther. 2007;87(12):1669–82.
10. Kaltenborn FM. Manual mobilization of the joints. Oslo: Olaf Nortis Bokhandel; 2002.
11. Magee D. Orthopedic physical examination, vol. 1. Philadelphia: Saunders; 2002.
12. Magee DJ. Orthopaedic physical assessment. 3rd ed. Philadelphia: WB Saunders; 1997.
13. An KN, Browne AO, Korinek S, Tanaka S, Morrey BF. Three-dimensional kinematics of glenohumeral elevation. J Orthop Res. 1991;9(1):143–9.
14. Hsu AT, Chang JG, Chang CH. Determining the resting position of the glenohumeral joint: a cadaver study. J Orthop Sports Phys Ther. 2002;32(12):605–12.
15. Mallon WJ. On the hypotheses that determine the definitions of glenohumeral joint motion: with resolution of Codman's pivotal paradox. J Shoulder Elbow Surg. 2012;21(12):e4–19.
16. Politti JC, Goroso G, Valentinuzzi ME, Bravo O. Codman's paradox of the arm rotations is not a paradox: mathematical validation. Med Eng Phys. 1998;20(4):257–60.
17. Hollis R, Lahav A, West Jr HS. Manipulation of the shoulder using Codman's paradox. Orthopedics. 2006;29(11):971–3.
18. Mullen F, Slade S, Briggs C. Bony and capsular determinants of glenohumeral 'locking' and 'quadrant' positions. Aust J Physiother. 1989;35(4):202–8.
19. Burkhart SS, Morgan CD, Kibler WB. The disabled throwing shoulder: spectrum of pathology. Part III: the SICK scapula, scapular dyskinesis, the kinetic chain, and rehabilitation. Arthroscopy. 2003;19(6):641–61.
20. Giphart JE, Brunkhorst JP, Horn NH, Shelburne KB, Torry MR, Millett PJ. Effect of plane of arm elevation on glenohumeral kinematics: a normative biplane fluoroscopy study. J Bone Joint Surg Am. 2013;95(3):238–45.
21. Giphart JE, van der Meijden OA, Millett PJ. The effects of arm elevation on the 3-dimensional acromiohumeral distance: a biplane fluoroscopy study with normative data. J Shoulder Elbow Surg. 2012;21(11):1593–600.
22. Kibler WB, McMullen J. Scapular dyskinesis and its relation to shoulder pain. J Am Acad Orthop Surg. 2003;11(2):142–51.
23. Lukasiewicz AC, McClure P, Michener L, Pratt N, Sennett B. Comparison of 3-dimensional scapular position and orientation between subjects with and without shoulder impingement. J Orthop Sports Phys Ther. 1999;29(10):574–83.
24. Warner JJ, Micheli LJ, Arslanian LE, Kennedy J, Kennedy R. Patterns of flexibility, laxity, and strength in normal shoulders and shoulders with instability and impingement. Am J Sports Med. 1990;18(4):366–75.
25. Sobush DC, Simoneau GG, Dietz KE, Levene JA, Grossman RE, Smith WB. The Lennie test for measuring scapular position in healthy young adult females: a reliability and validity study. J Orthop Sports Phys Ther. 1996;23(1):39–50.
26. Fung M, Kato S, Barrance PJ, Elias JJ, McFarland EG, Nobuhara K, Chao EY. Scapular and clavicular

kinematics during humeral elevation: a study with cadavers. J Shoulder Elbow Surg. 2001;10(3): 278–85.

27. Matsumura N, Nakamichi N, Ikegami H, Nagura T, Imanishi N, Aiso S, Toyama Y. The function of the clavicle on scapular motion: a cadaveric study. J Shoulder Elbow Surg. 2013;22(3):333–9.

28. Rubright J, Kelleher P, Beardsley C, Paller D, Shackford S, Beynnon B, Shafritz A. Long-term clinical outcomes, motion, strength, and function after total claviculectomy. J Shoulder Elbow Surg. 2014;23(2):236–44.

29. Ludewig PM, Phadke V, Braman JP, Hassett DR, Cieminski CJ, LaPrade RF. Motion of the shoulder complex during multiplanar humeral elevation. J Bone Joint Surg Am. 2009;91(2):378–89.

30. Sahara W, Sugamoto K, Murai M, Yoshikaw H. Three-dimensional clavicular and acromioclavicular rotations during arm abduction using vertically open MRI. J Orthop Res. 2007;25(9):1243–9.

31. Clarke GR, Willis LA, Fish WW, Nichols PJ. Preliminary studies in measuring range of motion in normal and painful stiff shoulders. Rheumatol Rehabil. 1975;14(1):39–46.

32. Gagey OJ, Gagey N. The hyperabduction test. J Bone Joint Surg Br. 2001;83(1):69–74.

33. Sauers EL, Borsa PA, Herling DE, Stanley RD. Instrumented measurement of glenohumeral joint laxity and its relationship to passive range of motion and generalized joint laxity. Am J Sports Med. 2001;29(2):143–50.

34. Lintner SA, Levy A, Kenter K, Speer KP. Glenohumeral translation in the asymptomatic athlete's shoulder and its relationship to other clinically measurable anthropometric variables. Am J Sports Med. 1996;25(6):716–20.

35. Hoving JL, Buchbinder R, Green S, Forbes A, Bellamy N, Brand C, Buchanan R, Hall S, Patrick M, Ryan P, Stockman A. How reliably do rheumatologists measure shoulder movement? Ann Rheum Dis. 2002;61(7):612–7.

36. McFarland EG, Fung M, Desjardins JD, Chao EYS. Glenohumeral motion can be distinguished from scapulothoracic motion in rotation. New Orleans: Orthopaedic Research Society. 1998.

37. Yap J, McFarland EG, Fung M, Kato S, Chao EYS. Glenohumeral motion can be distinguished from scapulothoracic motion in internal and external rotation. Orlando: American College of Sports Medicine Annual Meeting. 1999.

38. Cyriax JH, Cyriax PJ. Illustrated manual of orthopaedic medicine. London: Butterworth; 1993.

39. Hayes KW, Petersen CM. Reliability of assessing end-feel and pain and resistance sequence in subjects with painful shoulders and knees. J Orthop Sports Phys Ther. 2001;31(8):432–5.

40. Maitland GD. Vertebral manipulation. 5th ed. London: Butterworth; 1986.

41. Watkins MA, Riddle DL, Lamb RL, Personius WJ. Reliability of goniometric measurements and visual estimates of knee range of motion obtained in a clinical setting. Phys Ther. 1991;71(2):90–6.

42. Williams JG, Callaghan M. Comparison of visual estimation and goniometry in determination of a shoulder joint angle. Physiotherapy. 1990;76(10): 655–7.

43. Azadinia F, Kamyab M, Behtash H, Saleh Ganjavian M, Javaheri MR. The validity and reliability of non-invasive methods for measuring kyphosis. J Spinal Disord Tech. 2014;27(6):E212-8.

44. Czaprowski D, Pawłowska P, Gębicka A, Sitarski D, Kotwicki T. Intra- and interobserver repeatability of the assessment of anteroposterior curvatures of the spine using Saunders digital inclinometer. Ortop Traumatol Rehabil. 2012;14(2):145–53.

45. Siminoski K, Warshawski RS, Jen H, Lee KC. The accuracy of clinical kyphosis examination for detection of thoracic vertebral fractures: comparison of direct and indirect kyphosis measures. J Musculoskelet Neuronal Interact. 2011;11(3):249–56.

46. Dover G, Kaminski TW, Meister K, Powers ME, Horodyski M. Assessment of shoulder proprioception in the female softball athlete. Am J Sports Med. 2003;31(3):431–7.

47. Dover G, Powers ME. Reliability of joint position sense and force-reproduction measures during internal and external rotation of the shoulder. J Athl Train. 2003;38(4):304–10.

48. Awan R, Smith J, Boon AJ. Measuring shoulder internal rotation range of motion: a comparison of 3 techniques. Arch Phys Med Rehabil. 2002;83(9): 1229–34.

49. Borsa PA, Timmons MK, Sauers EL. Scapular-positioning patterns during humeral elevation in unimpaired shoulders. J Athl Train. 2003;38(1): 12–7.

50. de Winter AF, Heemskerk MA, Terwee CB, Jans MP, Deville W, van Schaardenburg DJ, Scholten RJ, Bouter LM. Inter-observer reproducibility of measurements of range of motion in patients with shoulder pain using a digital inclinometer. BMC Musculoskelet Disord. 2004;5(1):18.

51. Kolber MJ, Fuller C, Marshall J, Wright A, Hanney WJ. The reliability and concurrent validity of scapular plane shoulder elevation measurements using a digital inclinometer and goniometer. Physiother Theory Pract. 2012;28(2):161–8.

52. Kolber MJ, Hanney WJ. The reliability and concurrent validity of shoulder mobility measurements using a digital inclinometer and goniometer: a technical report. Int J Sports Phys Ther 2012;7(3):306–13.

53. Maenhout A, Van Eessel V, Van Dyck L, Vanraes A, Cools A. Quantifying acromiohumeral distance in overhead athletes with glenohumeral internal rotation loss and the influence of a stretching program. Am J Sports Med. 2012;40(9):2105–12.

54. Scibek JS, Carcia CR. Assessment of scapulohumeral rhythm for scapular plane shoulder elevation using a modified digital inclinometer. World J Orthop. 2012;3(6):87–94.

55. Scibek JS, Carcia CR. Validation and repeatability of a shoulder biomechanics data collection methodology and instrumentation. J Appl Biomech. 2012; 29(5):609–15.

56. Tucker WS, Ingram RL. Reliability and validity of measuring scapular upward rotation using an electrical inclinometer. J Electromyogr Kinesiol. 2012; 22(3):419–23.

57. Wassinger CA, Sole G, Osborne H. Clinical measurement of scapular upward rotation in response to acute subacromial pain. J Orthop Sports Phys Ther. 2013;43(4):199–203.

58. Johnson MP, McClure PW, Karduna AR. New method to assess scapular upward rotation in subjects with shoulder pathology. J Ortho Sports Phys Ther. 2001;31(2):81–9.

59. Shin SH, du Ro H, Lee OS, Oh JK, Kim SH. Within-day reliability of shoulder range of motion measurement with a smart phone. Man Ther. 2012; 17(4):298–304.

60. Mitchell K, Gutierrez SB, Sutton S, Morton S, Morgenthaler A. Reliability and validity of goniometric iPhone applications for the assessment of active shoulder external rotation. Physiother Theory Pract. 2014;30(7):521–5.

61. Tousignant-Laflamme Y, Boutin N, Dion AM, Vallée CA. Reliability and criterion validity of two applications of the iPhoneTM to measure cervical range of motion in healthy participants. J Neuroeng Rehabil. 2013;10(1):69.

62. Cools AM, De Wilde L, Van Tongel A, Ceyssens C, Ryckewaert R, Cambier DC. Measuring shoulder external and internal rotation strength and range of motion: comprehensive intra-rater and inter-rater reliability study of several testing protocols. J Shoulder Elbow Surg. 2014;23(10):1454–61.

63. El-Zayat BF, Efe T, Heidrich A, Anetsmann R, Timmesfeld N, Fuchs-Winkelmann S, Schofer MD. Objective assessment, repeatability, and agreement of shoulder ROM with a 3D gyroscope. BMC Musculoskelet Disord. 2013;14:72.

64. El-Zayat BF, Efe T, Heidrich A, Wolf U, Timmesfeld N, Heyse TJ, Lakemeier S, Fuchs-Winkelmann S, Schofer MD. Objective assessment of shoulder mobility with a new 3D gyroscope–a validation study. BMC Musculoskelet Disord. 2011;12:168.

65. Penning LI, Guldemond NA, de Bie RA, Walenkamp GH. Reproducibility of a 3-dimensional gyroscope in measuring shoulder anteflexion and abduction. BMC Musculoskelet Disord. 2012;13:135.

66. Blonna D, Zarkadas PC, Fitzsimmons JS, Odriscoll SW. Validation of a photography-based goniometry method for measuring joint range of motion. J Shoulder Elbow Surg. 2012;21(1):29–35.

67. Moncrieff MJ, Livingston LA. Reliability of a digital-photographic-goniometric method for coronal-plane lower limb measurements. J Sport Rehabil. 2009;18(2):296–315.

68. Naylor JM, Ko V, Adie S, Gaskin C, Walker R, Harris IA, Mittal R. Validity and reliability of using

69. O'Neill BJ, O'Briain D, Hirpara KM, Shaughnesy M, Yeatman EA, Kaar TK. Digital photography for assessment of shoulder range of motion: a novel clinical and research tool. Int J Shoulder Surg. 2013;7(1):23–7.

70. Verhaegen F, Ganseman Y, Arnout N, Vandenneucker H, Bellemans J. Are clinical photographs appropriate to determine the maximal range of motion of the knee? Acta Orthop Belg. 2010;76(6):794–8.

71. Sabari JS, Maltzev I, Lubarsky D, Liszkay E, Homel P. Goniometric assessment of shoulder range of motion: comparison of testing in supine and sitting positions. Arch Phys Med Rehabil. 1998;79(6): 647–51.

72. Boon AJ, Smith J. Manual scapular stabilization: its effect on shoulder rotational range of motion. Arch Phys Med Rehabil. 2000;81(7):978–83.

73. Wilk KE, Reinold MM, Macrina LC, Porterfield R, Devine KM, Suarez K, Andrews JR. Glenohumeral internal rotation measurements differ depending on stabilization techniques. Sports Health. 2009;1(2): 131–6.

74. Hall JM, Azar FM, Miller 3rd RJ, Smith R, Throckmorton TW. Accuracy and reliability testing of two methods to measure internal rotation of the glenohumeral joint. J Shoulder Elbow Surg. 2014; 23(9):1296–300.

75. Barnes CJ, Van Steyn SJ, Fischer RA. The effects of age, sex, and shoulder dominance on range of motion of the shoulder. J Shoulder Elbow Surg. 2001;10(3): 242–6.

76. Boone DC, Azen SP. Normal range of motion of joints in male subjects. J Bone Joint Surg Am. 1979;61(5):756–9.

77. Walker JM, Sue D, Miles-Elkousy N, Ford G, Trevelyan H. Active mobility of the extremities in older subjects. Phys Ther. 1984;64(6):919–23.

78. Allander E, Bjornsson OJ, Olafsson O, Sigfusson N, Thorsteinsson J. Normal range of joint movements in shoulder, hip, wrist and thumb with special reference to side: a comparison between two populations. Int J Epidemiol. 1974;3(3):253–61.

79. Murray MP, Gore DR, Gardner GM, Mollinger LA. Shoulder motion and muscle strength of normal men and women in two age groups. Clin Orthop. 1985;192:268–73.

80. Schwartz C, Croisier JL, Rigaux E, Denoël V, Brüls O, Forthomme B. Dominance effect on scapula 3-dimensional posture and kinematics in healthy male and female populations. J Shoulder Elbow Surg. 2013;23(6):873–81.

81. Kanlayanaphotporn R. Changes in sitting posture affect shoulder range of motion. J Bodyw Mov Ther. 2014;18(2):239–43.

82. Kronberg M, Brostrom LA, Soderlund V. Retroversion of the humeral head in the normal

shoulder and its relationship to the normal range of motion. Clin Orthop. 1990;253:113–7.

83. Kronberg M, Nemeth G, Brostrom LA. Muscle activity and coordination in the normal shoulder. An electromyographic study. Clin Orthop. 1990; 257:76–85.

84. Bullock MP, Foster NE, Wright CC. Shoulder impingement: the effect of sitting posture on shoulder pain and range of motion. Man Ther. 2005;10(1): 28–37.

85. Kebaetse M, McClure P, Pratt NA. Thoracic position effect on shoulder range of motion, strength, and three-dimensional scapular kinematics. Arch Phys Med Rehabil. 1999;80(8):945–50.

86. Gajdosik R, Simpson R, Smith R, DonTigny RL. Pelvic tilt. Intratester reliability of measuring the standing position and range of motion. Phys Ther. 1985;65(2):169–74.

87. Donatelli R. Physical therapy of the shoulder, vol. 1. St. Louis: Elsevier; 2004.

88. Pearl L, Jackin S, Lippit S, Sidle J, Matsen F. Humeroscapular positions in a shoulder range-of-motion-examination. J Shoulder Elbow Surg. 1992;1(6):296–305.

89. Kirkley A, Griffin S, Dainty K. Scoring systems for the functional assessment of the shoulder. Arthroscopy. 2003;19(10):1109–20.

90. Hudak PL, Amadio PC, Bombardier C. Development of an upper extremity outcome measure. The DASH (disabilities of the arm, shoulder and hand)[corrected]. The Upper Extremity Collaborative Group (UECG). Am J Ind Med. 1996;29(6):602–8.

91. Pappas AM, Zawacki RM, McCarthy CF. Rehabilitation of the pitching shoulder. Am J Sports Med. 1985;13(4):223–35.

92. Kendall SA, Kendall FP, Wadsworth GE. Muscles: testing and function, vol. 1. Baltimore: Williams and Wilkins; 1971.

93. Tyler TF, Nicholas SJ, Roy T, GLeim GW. Quantification of posterior capsule tightness and motion loss in patients with shoulder impingement. Am J Sports Med. 2000;28(5):668–73.

94. Tyler TF, Roy T, Nicholas SJ, Gleim GW. Reliability and validity of a new method of measuring posterior shoulder tightness. J Orthop Sports Phys Ther. 1999;29(4):262–9.

95. Mourtacos S, Downar J, Sauers EL. Clinical measures of shoulder mobility in the adolescent baseball player. J Athl Train. 2003;38(2):S-72.

96. Sauers EL, Koh JL, Keuter G. Scapular and glenohumeral motion in professional baseball players: effects of position and arm dominance. Orlando: Arthroscopy Association of North America Annual Meeting; 2004.

97. Borstad JD, Mathiowetz KM, Minday LE, Prabhu B, Christopherson DE, Ludewig PM. Clinical measurement of posterior shoulder flexibility. Man Ther. 2007;12(4):386–9.

98. Myers JB, Oyama S, Wassinger CA, Ricci RD, Abt JP, Conley KM, Lephart SM. Reliability, precision, accuracy, and validity of posterior shoulder tightness assessment in overhead athletes. Am J Sports Med. 2007;35(11):1922–30.

99. Borstad JD, Ludewig PM. The effect of long versus short pectoralis minor resting length on scapular kinematics in healthy individuals. J Orthop Sports Phys Ther. 2005;35(4):227–38.

100. Borstad JD, Ludewig PM. Comparison of scapular kinematics between elevation and lowering of the arm in the scapular plane. Clin Biomech. 2002; 17(9–10):650–9.

101. Hébert LJ, Moffet H, McFadyen BJ, Dionne CE. Scapular behavior in shoulder impingement syndrome. Arch Phys Med Rehabil. 2002;83(1):60–9.

102. Ludewig PM, Cook TM. Alterations in shoulder kinematics and associated muscle activity in people with symptoms of shoulder impingement. Phys Ther. 2000;80(3):276–91.

103. Borstad JD. Measurement of pectoralis minor muscle length: validation and clinical application. J Orthop Sports Phys Ther. 2008;38(4):169–74.

104. Williams JG, Laudner KG, McLoda T. The acute effects of two passive stretch maneuvers on pectoralis minor length and scapular kinematics among collegiate swimmers. Int J Sports Phys Ther. 2013; 8(1):25–33.

105. Bhargav D, Murrell GA. Shoulder stiffness: diagnosis. Aust Fam Physician. 2004;33(3):143–7.

106. Bhargav D, Murrell GA. Shoulder stiffness: management. Aust Fam Physician. 2004;33(3):149–52.

107. Chambler AF, Carr AJ. The role of surgery in frozen shoulder. J Bone Joint Surg Br. 2003;85(6):789–95.

108. Gerber C, Espinosa N, Perren TG. Arthroscopic treatment of shoulder stiffness. Clin Orthop. 2001; 390:119–28.

109. Goldberg BA, Scarlat MM, Harryman 2nd DT. Management of the stiff shoulder. J Orthop Sci. 1999;4(6):462–71.

110. Hertel R. [The frozen shoulder]. Orthopade 2000;29(10):845–51.

111. Rundquist PJ, Anderson DD, Guanche CA. Shoulder kinematics in subjects with frozen shoulder. Arch Phys Med Rehabil. 2003;84(10):1473–9.

112. Akhtar A, Gajjar S, Redfern T. MUA with steroid injection vs. arthroscopic capsular release for adhesive capsulitis: a prospective randomised study. Surgeon 2013;pii:S1479-666X(13)00060-7.

113. Bhatia S, Mather 3rd RC, Hsu AR, Ferry AT, Romeo AA, Nicholson GP, Cole BJ, Verma NN. Arthroscopic management of recalcitrant stiffness following rotator cuff repair: a retrospective analysis. Indian J Orthop. 2013;47(2):143–9.

114. Chen SK, Chien SH, Fu YC, Huang PJ, Chou PH. Idiopathic frozen shoulder treated by arthroscopic brisement. Kaohsiung J Med Sci. 2002; 18(6):289–94.

115. Chung SW, Huong CB, Kim SH, Oh JH. Shoulder stiffness after rotator cuff repair: risk factors and influence on outcome. Arthroscopy. 2013;29(2): 290–300.

116. Dehghan A, Pishgooei N, Salami MA, Zarch SM, Nafisi-Moghadam R, Rahimpour S, Soleimani H, Owlia MB. Comparison between NSAID and intra-articular corticosteroid injection in frozen shoulder of diabetic patients; a randomized clinical trial. Exp Clin Endocrinol Diabetes. 2013;121(2):75–9.

117. Doner G, Guven Z, Atalay A, Celiker R. Evaluation of Mulligan's technique for adhesive capsulitis of the shoulder. J Rehabil Med. 2013;45(1):87–91.

118. Fernandes MR. Arthroscopic capsular release for refractory shoulder stiffness. Rev Assoc Med Bras. 2013;59(4):347–53.

119. Gam AN, Schydlowsky P, Rossel I, Remvig L, Jensen EM. Treatment of "frozen shoulder" with distension and glucocorticoid compared with glucocorticoid alone. A randomized controlled trial. Scand J Rheumatol. 1998;27(6):425–30.

120. Koh ES, Chung SG, Kim TU, Kim HC. Changes in biomechanical properties of glenohumeral joint capsules with adhesive capsulitis by repeated capsule-preserving hydraulic distensions with saline solution and corticosteroid. PM R. 2012;4(12):976–84.

121. Kordella T. Frozen shoulder & diabetes. Frozen shoulder affects 20 percent of people with diabetes. Proper treatment can help you work through it. Diabetes Forecast. 2002;55(8):60–4.

122. Xu HZ, Yu B, Zhang QH, Chen XR. [Treatment of 48 cases of frozen shoulder with manual therapy under brachial plexus anesthesia through a retained tube]. Di Yi Jun Yi a Xue Xue Bao 2003;23(1):87–8.

123. Austin DC, Gans I, Park MJ, Carey JL, Kelly 4th JD. The association of metabolic syndrome markers with adhesive capsulitis. J Shoulder Elbow Surg. 2014;23(7):1043–51.

124. Kabbabe B, Ramkumar S, Richardson M. Cytogenetic analysis of the pathology of frozen shoulder. Int J Shoulder Surg. 2010;4(3):75–8.

125. Kim YS, Kim JM, Lee YG, Hong OK, Kwon HS, Ji JH. Intercellular adhesion molecule-1 (ICAM-1, CD54) is increased in adhesive capsulitis. J Bone Joint Surg Am. 2013;95(4):e181–8.

126. Lho YM, Ha E, Cho CH, Song KS, Min BW, Bae KC, Lee KJ, Hwang I, Park HB. Inflammatory cytokines are overexpressed in the subacromial bursa of frozen shoulder. J Shoulder Elbow Surg. 2013; 22(5):666–72.

127. Nago M, Mitsui Y, Gotoh M, Nakama K, Shirachi I, Higuchi F, Nagata K. Hyaluronan modulates cell proliferation and mRNA expression of adhesion-related procollagens and cytokines in glenohumeral synovial/capsular fibroblasts in adhesive capsulitis. J Orthop Res. 2010;28(6):726–31.

128. Bunker TD, Anthony PP. The pathology of frozen shoulder. A Dupuytren-like disease. J Bone Joint Surg Br. 1995;77(5):677–83.

129. Bunker TD, Reilly J, Baird KS, Hamblen DL. Expression of growth factors, cytokines and matrix metalloproteinases in frozen shoulder. J Bone Joint Surg Br. 2000;82(5):768–73.

130. Ha'eri GB, Maitland A. Arthroscopic findings in the frozen shoulder. J Rheumatol. 1981;8(1): 149–52.

131. Kilian O, Kriegsmann OJ, Berghauser K, Stahl JP, Horas U, Heerdegen R. The frozen shoulder. Arthroscopy, histological findings and transmission electron microscopy imaging. Chirurg. 2001;72(11): 1303–8.

Strength Testing

3

3.1 Introduction

The evaluation of strength is an important aspect of the shoulder examination that, when conducted properly, can provide substantial evidence for or against a suspected pathology within the differential diagnosis. To perform an adequate strength assessment, the clinician must have a basic working knowledge of anatomy and function of the skeletal muscles around the shoulder. In addition, it is important to understand the current state of research regarding shoulder strength testing to aid in the interpretation and treatment of various shoulder conditions.

3.2 General Concepts

3.2.1 Length–Force Relationship

The length–force relationship of the sarcomere was originally described by Blix in the late 1800s—a concept that was expanded upon by numerous other investigators [1–5]. In his original experiments, muscle tension during contraction was found to vary as a function of its overall length. After plotting his results, he found that this relationship took the form of a bell curve, the peak of which represented the active tension (i.e., contraction force) produced by a muscle at its resting length. As the length of the muscle was varied, the strength of contraction decreased,

even if the muscle was passively stretched prior to initiating contraction (Fig. 3.1). Therefore, suboptimal limb positioning can have a profound effect on muscular contraction strength and, as a result, may lead to inaccurate measurements during the strength evaluation. In other words, maximum contraction strength cannot be achieved when a muscle is placed in a position outside of its native resting length.

Therefore, the reliability of muscular strength testing depends on the clinician's knowledge of correct testing positions that are designed to optimize the length–force relationship of the particular muscle being tested. A few important clinical examples include strength testing of the infraspinatus, subscapularis, and deltoid muscles as described by Hertel et al. [6, 7]. In these maneuvers, the extremity is passively placed such that the muscle to be tested is in a relatively shortened position and the opposing muscle is in a relatively lengthened position (i.e. increased tension). The patient is then asked to hold the position. If the muscle being tested is weak, its contraction strength cannot overcome the passive tensile force that is applied to the opposing muscle when the arm is released by the examiner. For example, when testing for infraspinatus weakness, the humerus is passively positioned in approximately 20–30° of external rotation (also with the elbow flexed to 90°). This position decreases the passive tension across the infraspinatus muscle since its overall length has been shortened relative to its resting length. On the other hand, this position

R.J. Warth and P.J. Millett, *Physical Examination of the Shoulder: An Evidence-Based Approach*,
DOI 10.1007/978-1-4939-2593-3_3, © Springer Science+Business Media New York 2015

39

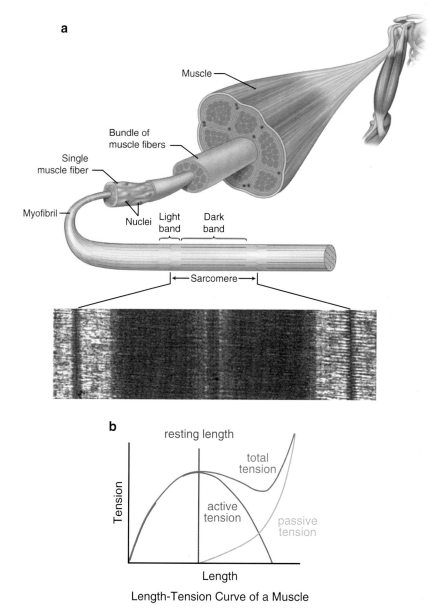

Fig. 3.1 (**a**) Skeletal muscle structure hierarchy including a scanning electron micrograph (SEM) of a typical sarcomere. (**b**) Length-tension curve of skeletal muscle (*Blix curve*). Note that active and passive tension are additive as the muscle length increases.

also *increases* the passive tension across the opposing subscapularis muscle. When the clinician releases the arm, the patient will attempt to hold the position by contracting the infraspinatus muscle. When this force of contraction cannot overcome the passive tensile force that is applied to the opposing subscapularis, the arm will internally rotate despite the patient's best efforts

(Fig. 3.2). This finding is referred to as a positive external rotation lag sign and the degrees of *internal rotation* lag (or the amount of internal rotation that occurs after the arm is released) is typically documented as a measure of infraspinatus weakness. The internal rotation lag sign [6], the deltoid lag sign [7], and the teres minor lag sign (also referred to as "Hornblower's sign" [8]

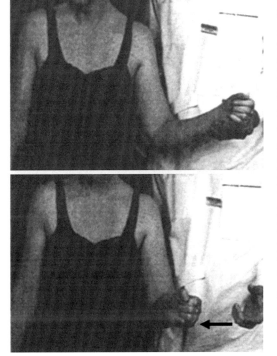

Fig. 3.2 Clinical photograph demonstrating the external rotation lag sign. When the humerus is released from a position of approximately 20–30° of external rotation, patients with infraspinatus cuff pathology may be incapable of holding the position. As a result, the humerus undergoes compensatory internal rotation by the resting tension and tone generated by the stretched subscapularis muscle. (From Hertel et al. [6]; with permission).

or "drop sign" [6]) use the same length–force relationship concepts and are discussed both later in this chapter and in Chap. 4.

3.2.2   Muscle Isolation

There are numerous muscles that cross or act upon the glenohumeral joint; however, several of these muscles produce similar force vectors which can complicate the assessment of muscular strength. As a result, shoulder motion within any plane likely involves contributions from several different muscles to produce the observed movement. While it would be ideal to isolate and test each individual muscle around the shoulder girdle, complete isolation of a single muscle for

the purpose of strength testing is a nearly impossible task. In addition, weakness of one muscle can be substituted by another similarly positioned muscle, masking the underlying weakness during physical examination. This is especially true in cases where subtle weakness is present, such as in small rotator cuff tears where, in many cases, the overlying deltoid may substitute for the deficient cuff. In fact, the ability of the deltoid to substitute for a deficient rotator cuff is the underlying principle of reverse total shoulder arthroplasty in patients with massive, irreparable rotator cuff tears with associated superior migration of the humeral head. Another example includes the levator scapulae and the superior fibers of the trapezius which have similar functions; however, the neural supply to each muscle is different. Thus, a patient with an isolated injury to the dorsal scapular nerve may still demonstrate relatively normal scapulothoracic kinematics despite levator scapulae weakness.

It is typically more advantageous to isolate the overall function of specific groups of muscles rather than attempting to isolate each muscle individually. Alternatively, the clinician can also perform tests that conceptually and theoretically isolate specific muscles with the understanding that complete isolation is probably not attainable. Regardless of the method used, it is necessary to develop a consistent, repeatable examination protocol which can improve individual diagnostic efficiency and accuracy.

3.3   Quantifying Muscle Strength

3.3.1   Manual Muscle Testing

Manual muscle testing (MMT) is the most common method by which clinicians evaluate muscle strength. MMT utilizes a standardized grading system that is determined by the ability of the tested muscle act against gravity or against resistance applied by the examiner. In 1916, Lovett and Martin [9] first described the method of manual muscle testing in newborns with infantile paralysis. Since then, abundant research has been conducted regarding its various applications, including

Table 3.1 Manual muscle testing grading system (levels 0–5)

0	No visible or palpable contraction
1	Visible or palpable contraction without motion
2	Full range of motion, gravity eliminated
3	Full range of motion against gravity
4	Full range of motion against gravity, moderate resistance
5	Full range of motion against gravity, maximal resistance

modifications of the original grading scale used to describe muscular strength. Despite these modifications, the scale that is most widely accepted is very similar to the original proposal by Lovett and Martin [9] and was devised by the Medical Research Council (MRC) [10] in 1943. The scale has six levels (0–5) and is presented in Table 3.1.

The inter- and intra-observer reliabilities of MMT in the evaluation of various pathologies resulting in muscle weakness range from 0.82 to 0.97 and 0.96 to 0.98, respectively, according to reports dating back to 1954 [11–22]. However, only a few studies have specifically examined the reliability of manual muscle testing for the evaluation of patients with various shoulder pathologies [23–25].

Although the MMT scale is still widely used in clinical practice due to its low cost and rapidity, there are several limitations that must be noted. The first limitation is that the MMT scale is subjective in nature and the score depends on the clinician's judgment [26–28]. The second limitation of MMT is the inability of the scale to detect small, between-level differences in strength. This is largely due to the stepwise design of the scale and has spurred the development of other scales that have more diagnostic levels [10]. Third, the MMT scale has been criticized for not being capable of detecting clinically relevant differences in muscle strength. MMT was originally developed to measure strength improvements in patients treated with paralytic disorders and muscular dystrophies [29, 30]. Thus, the application of MMT to a variety of clinical settings is probably due to tradition rather than sound scientific rationale. As a result of the subjectivity and reported inaccuracy of MMT, many clinicians (and insurers) prefer to measure strength with more objective means that are more sensitive, such as with hand-held dynamometers [31].

3.3.2 Dynamometry

A dynamometer is a device used to determine the mechanical force generated by a contracting muscle. While these measurements of force are generally given in Newtons or kilograms, torque can be calculated by simply multiplying Newtons or kilograms by the distance (in meters) between the dynamometer and the center of rotation of the involved joint.

Dynamometers first appeared in 1763 [32] and, since then, numerous modifications have been made. Currently, dynamometers come in a large variety of shapes, sizes, and functional mechanisms that produce the desired force measurements. Isokinetic dynamometers are large machines capable of generating numerous values including peak muscular force, power, and endurance among numerous other measurements (Fig. 3.3) [33]. Isokinetic testing has been used as a standard method of muscle strength measurement over the past 40 years since it has been

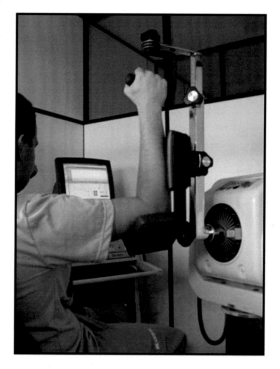

Fig. 3.3 Example of an isokinetic dynamometer which has been set up to measure shoulder internal and external rotation strength at 90° of abduction. (From Ribeiro and Oliveira [161]).

found to be reliable, reproducible, and valid on numerous occasions [34–38]. As a result, iso-kinetic devices have also been used as reference standards for the evaluation of newer devices that test muscle strength [39–42].

A large number of studies have evaluated the inter- and intra-rater reliability using handheld dynamometers to assess muscular strength. A systematic review by Stark et al. [43] identified 19 studies in which the authors compared hand-held dynamometry to isokinetic muscle strength testing. In that review, all but two studies demon-strated either good to excellent correlation with isokinetic testing or good to excellent intra-class correlation coefficient (ICCs). The study by Burnham et al. [39] found a low correlation of handheld dynamometry with isokinetic testing when measuring shoulder abduction strength in a series of football players ($r=0.28$–0.43); how-ever, the scapulae of the tested athletes in that study were not stabilized by the examiner, introducing potential confounding factors in their measurements. Reinking et al. [44] also found a poor correlation between handheld dynamometry and isokinetic testing when measuring knee extension ($r=0.43$–0.45); however, testing this group of muscles requires a sufficiently strong examiner to prevent movement of the dynamom-eter while the subject is tested.

In general, clinical dynamometry is performed with handheld devices due to their portability, simplicity, low cost, and reported excellent reli-ability and validity when compared to isokinetic dynamometry [27, 43]. Although there are numerous such devices that have been reported as both accurate and reliable for the measurement of muscular force, most handheld dynamometers fall into one of two categories depending on the mechanism of measurement. These include spring scale and strain gauge dynamometers. Spring scale dynamometers work simply by mea-suring the deformation (lengthening) of a spring as a force is applied—this deformation distance is converted to kilograms and is based on the stiffness (spring constant) of the inserted spring. Strain gauge dynamometers are more complex and work by detecting changes in electrical sig-nals caused by the deformation of an electrical

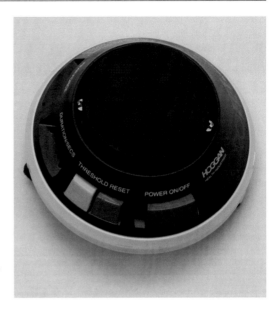

Fig. 3.4   Example of a typical strain gauge dynamometer.

insulator by an outside force (e.g., the force of muscle contraction) (Fig. 3.4).

In 1989, Bohannon and Andrews [45] studied the accuracy of two handheld spring scale and two strain gauge dynamometers using a series of certified weights ranging from 5 to 55 pounds. The dynamometers were tested by gradually increasing the applied weight by 5-pound incre-ments and comparing the readout measurement generated by each device to the actual weight applied. In their study, the spring scale dyna-mometers measured forces significantly different from the force that was actually applied. The authors also noted that the accuracy of the spring scale dynamometers diminished after extensive use, suggesting that spring fatigue or permanent deformation have been responsible for inaccurate measurements. In contrast, the strain gauge dyna-mometers measured forces that were much closer to the actual applied force.

Hayes and Zehr [46] evaluated the reliability of MMT, a manual spring scale dynamometer and a digital strain gauge dynamometer to measure rotator cuff strength using a random effects statistical model. In this group of patients with symptomatic rotator cuff disease, they found that the digital strain gauge dynamometer was the most reliable method of measuring rotator

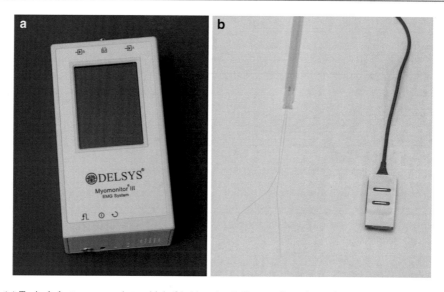

Fig. 3.5 (**a**) Typical electromyograph to which (**b**) thin wire (*left*) or surface electrodes (*right*) can be attached.

cuff strength. Hosking et al. [47] examined the test-retest reliability of handheld dynamometers in children with and without muscular disease and found that repeated testing did not cause measurement variability of more than 15 %. However, another study by Bohannon [28] found the test-retest reliability to be much higher in healthy patients compared to those who had muscle weakness, potentially suggesting that muscle fatigue may play a role in the ability to obtain an accurate measurement of peak muscle force after multiple testing sessions.

There are several other potential limitations of digital handheld dynamometry. The first is that these handheld devices are of minimal use when testing large muscle groups that can produce a much larger force than the examiner can resist. This is particularly true for large, high-output lower extremity muscles that may overcome the strength of the examiner's upper extremity [28, 48–51]. A second limitation is that an inability to adequately stabilize the device while the subject applies maximal force is quite difficult to achieve. As a result, handheld dynamometers placed in a fixed apparatus have gained popularity to eliminate the effect of examiner strength and stabilization on the reliability of strength measurements [52–55].

3.3.3 Electromyography

Electromyography (EMG) has been used extensively over the past century to evaluate the utility of various manual muscle tests. An electromyogram is obtained by placing an electrode on the skin over the muscle being tested (i.e., surface EMG) or, alternatively, a thin wire can be placed directly into the muscle of interest (i.e., intramuscular EMG) (Fig. 3.5). When the muscle is stimulated, the electrical potential that is produced by the muscle travels through the electrode and towards the connected electromyograph which interprets and displays the signal through an oscilloscope. It is important to remember that EMG readouts with higher amplitude do not necessarily indicate that the muscle is generating greater force. As an example, an eccentrically contracting muscle produces similar amplitude as a concentrically contracting muscle; however, the force produced by the eccentric contraction may be much less than that produced by the concentric contraction.

EMG is an important tool for the evaluation of skeletal muscle activity; however, its interpretation can be influenced by several factors that must be taken into account. Features of the surface electrode such as width, diameter, and electrical properties can influence the signal output.

In the case of surface EMG, increased distance or increased soft-tissue interposition between the surface electrode and the muscle being tested can also significantly influence signal interpretation [56, 57]. The primary drawback of thin-wire EMG is that the sample size is limited to the surface area of the small electrode whereas surface EMG can obtain measurements over an expanded area of muscle tissue and is also easier to implement; however, this can also introduce unwanted noise due to soft-tissue interposition and contributions from surrounding musculature. In addition, the amplitude or morphology of the EMG readout may be affected by the type of muscle being tested (fast-twitch versus slow-twitch).

Many studies have utilized a normalization technique to study muscle activity—that is, the electrical measurements are compared to a reference standard generated from a maximal voluntary contraction (MVC) of the muscle in question. The ratio of the two measurements is recorded and compared between different subjects [58]. Other methods of obtaining EMGs involve submaximal voluntary contractions and isometric measurements; however, these methods have been less reliable to date [57, 59].

3.4   Strength Screening of Specific Muscles

Anatomic characteristics of the scapular musculature are presented in Table 3.2 [60] to help guide the reader through this section.

Table 3.2 Anatomic characteristics of the periscapular musculature [8]

Muscle	Origin	Insertion	Nerve supply	Vascular supply	Action
Supraspinatus	Supraspinous fossa	Superior facet of greater tuberosity	Suprascapular nerve	Suprascapular artery	Abduction of the humerus
Infraspinatus	Infraspinous fossa	Posterior facet of greater tuberosity	Suprascapular nerve	Suprascapular artery	External rotation of the humerus
Teres minor	Inferolateral aspect of posterior scapular body	Inferior facet of greater tuberosity	Axillary nerve	Posterior circumflex humeral artery, circumflex scapular artery	External rotation of humerus in abduction
Subscapularis	Subscapular fossa	Lesser tuberosity	Upper and lower subscapular nerves	Transverse cervical artery, subscapular artery	Internal rotation of humerus
Trapezius	Spinous processes of C7-T12	Superior aspect of scapular spine	Spinal accessory nerve	Superficial branch of transverse cervical artery	Scapular rotation and elevation
Serratus Anterior	Upper nine ribs	Anterior aspect of medial scapular border	Long thoracic nerve	Thoracodorsal artery, lateral thoracic artery	Scapular protraction and upward rotation
Levator Scapulae	Transverse processes of C1-C4	Medial border of scapula superior to medial base of the scapular spine	Dorsal scapular nerve	Dorsal scapular artery	Scapular elevation
Rhomboid Minor	Spinous processes of C7-T1	Medial border of scapula at the level of the medial base of the scapular spine	Dorsal scapular nerve	Dorsal scapular artery	Scapular retraction and rotation
Rhomboid Major	Spinous processes of T2-T5	Medial border of scapula inferior to medial base of scapular spine	Dorsal scapular nerve	Dorsal scapular artery	Scapular retraction and rotation

3.4.1 Periscapular Muscles

3.4.1.1 Trapezius

Innervated by the spinal accessory nerve, the trapezius muscle is a large, flat, triangular muscle that makes up the majority of the superficial posterior cervical and thoracic musculature. The muscle is thought to have three anatomic regions—namely, the superior, middle, and inferior regions—that are thought to have specific functional attributes (Fig. 3.6). The superior fibers originate medially between the occiput and the C7 spinous processes and extend laterally to insert upon the posterior aspect of the distal clavicle, the superomedial acromion and the most distal portion of the scapular spine. The middle fibers arise medially between the C7 and T3 spinous processes and extend laterally to insert primarily along the scapular spine. The inferior fibers originate between the T4 and T12 spinous processes and extend superolaterally to insert as an aponeurosis on the medial confluence of the scapular spine.

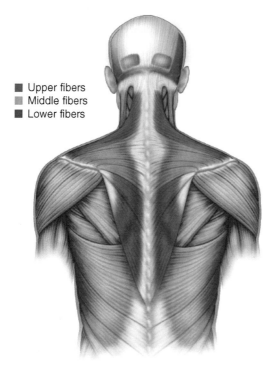

■ Upper fibers
■ Middle fibers
■ Lower fibers

Fig. 3.6 Illustration depicting the superior, middle, and lower fibers of the trapezius muscle.

In the early 1990s, Lindman et al. [61, 62] performed immunohistochemical analysis on human trapezius muscles and found significant differences in mitochondrial ATPase activity in various portions of the muscle. Specifically, the lower third of the superior region, the middle region, and the inferior region all had low concentrations of mitochondrial ATPase activity. On the other hand, the uppermost aspect of the superior region had the highest mitochondrial ATPase activity. With this information, the authors suggested that the upper aspect of the superior region was best suited for high-demand, short duration functionality (e.g., heavy lifting) whereas the rest of the muscle was best suited for low-demand, long duration functionality (e.g., posture and dynamic scapular stability). The authors concluded that the differences in ATPase activity and fiber type are likely due to both genetic factors and functional demands.

The functions of the superior, middle, and inferior fibers of the trapezius were first described by Inman et al. [63] in 1944. However, the exact function of each muscle division has been debated for many years. Based on fiber orientation, Johnson et al. [64] suggested that the trapezius largely functions as a scapular stabilizer. More specifically, it was proposed that the upper fibers draw the scapula superomedially while the middle and lower fibers antagonize the function of the serratus anterior, preventing lateral excursion of the scapula. Although others have confirmed the functions of the middle and lower trapezius with various motions (including scapular internal and external rotation [87]) [66–69], the precise role of the upper trapezius remains controversial. A study by Ruwe et al. [70] found a decrease in upper trapezius muscle activity in a series of swimmers with shoulder pain. Another study [69] found increased muscle activity of the middle and lower fibers in a series of patients with signs and symptoms of impingement. Although we understand that contraction of the upper trapezius causes upward rotation of the scapula, its precise role in the development of shoulder discomfort has not been clearly defined. However, it is widely reported that unbalanced periscapular strength and altered muscle firing patterns lead to scapular malposition and dyskinesis, both of which can

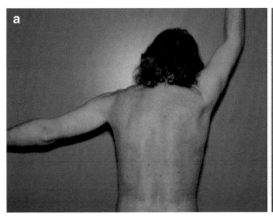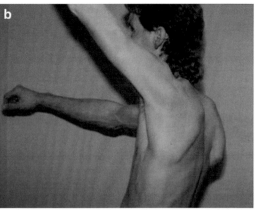

Fig. 3.7 (**a**) Subtle left-sided scapular winging due to trapezius muscle weakness. (**b**) Right-sided scapular winging due to serratus anterior muscle weakness. (Courtesy of J.P. Warner, MD).

cause and exacerbate subacromial impingement (scapular dyskinesis is discussed in further detail in Chap. 9).

Clinically, atrophy of the trapezius muscle with alteration in scapular resting position can be quite subtle and thus requires close examination (the scapular resting position is discussed in Chap. 2). Patients with trapezius muscle atrophy, most commonly due to spinal accessory nerve palsy, generally present with "scalloping" of the ipsilateral neck (due to loss of trapezius muscle mass) and superomedial displacement of the inferomedial border of the scapula (so-called "lateral" scapular winging; Fig. 3.7). Patients with trapezius weakness may also have difficulty elevating the humerus above the horizontal plane due to the inability to initiate upward rotation of the scapula [71]. This pattern of winging must be discerned from that which is produced by serratus anterior weakness as a result of long thoracic nerve palsy, which most commonly results in elevation of the medial scapular border away from the chest wall with superolateral displacement of the inferomedial angle.

The upper fibers of the trapezius muscle are tested by simply asking the patient to shrug their shoulders against resistance (Fig. 3.8). At least one study has confirmed this test as being effective for activating the uppermost fibers of the trapezius muscle using surface EMGs [72, 73]. A study by Moseley et al. [74] found that rowing exercises maximally activate the upper trapezius

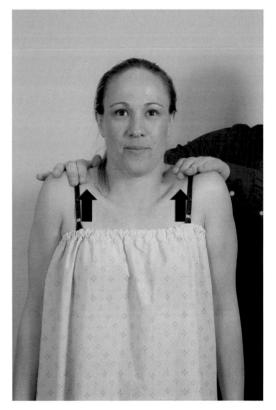

Fig. 3.8 Strength of superior trapezius. The examiner asks the patient to shrug their shoulders against resistance.

muscle; however, this type of movement also recruits ancillary muscles and is difficult to perform in the clinic setting.

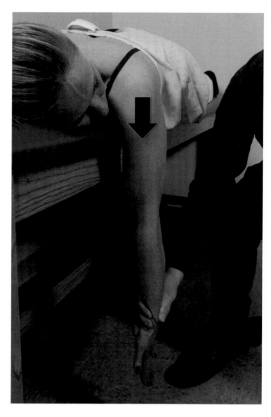

Fig. 3.9 Strength of middle trapezius. With the patient prone and the arm hanging over the edge of the table, the examiner grasps the distal arm and applies a downward force while the patient resists.

The middle trapezius is most easily tested with the patient in the prone position with the arm hanging over the side of the table in 90° of forward flexion. The examiner then places their hand distally and applies a moderate downward force while the patient resists (Fig. 3.9). While this test is effective at testing the middle fibers of the trapezius, care must be taken to rule out anterior instability before performing this test in order to avoid glenohumeral dislocation.

To test the lower fibers of the trapezius, the patient is placed in the prone position with the arm abducted to approximately 120° within the scapular plane. This position aligns the upper extremity with the superolaterally directed fibers of the lower trapezius. From this position, the subject then attempts to extend the arm upward while the examiner both applies resistance and simultaneously examines the scapula for any evidence of winging (Fig. 3.10).

Rhomboids

The rhomboid musculature consists of both the rhomboid major and minor which, on some occasions, exist as a single muscle-tendon unit [75]. The rhomboid major originates from the spinous processes between T2 and T5 and inserts along the posterior aspect of the medial border of the scapula just inferior to the medial confluence of the scapular spine and spans inferiorly towards the inferomedial angle. The rhomboid minor originates between the C7 and T1 spinous processes and inserts just superiorly to the rhomboid major at the level of the scapular spine on the posterior aspect of the medial scapular border. The dorsal scapular nerve is derived from the C5 nerve root and provides the motor innervation for both of these muscles (Fig. 3.11).

The primary functions of the rhomboid musculature are to induce superomedial migration and downward rotation of the scapula such that the glenoid surface is angled inferiorly and posteriorly (i.e., scapular retraction). To test the rhomboids, the patient is asked to place the hands on the iliac crests with the thumbs pointed posteriorly and with the elbows in neutral position. The patient is then asked to resist an anteriorly directed force applied to the medial epicondyles such that the elbows are pushed anteriorly into a flared position. It is advised to observe and/or palpate the medial scapular border while the test is being performed (Fig. 3.12).

Smith et al. [76] suggested that the above maneuver (sometimes referred to as the modified Kendall test) does not separately activate the rhomboid muscles from synergistic muscles such as the levator scapulae, middle trapezius, and latissimus dorsi muscles. The authors found that manual testing of the posterior deltoid elicited greater electromyographic activity of the rhomboids compared to that of any of the other MMT maneuvers that were tested (e.g., the Hislop–Montgomery test for rhomboid strength). According to Smith et al. [76], the posterior deltoid test (which is used to test rhomboid strength) is performed with the patient in a sitting position, facing away from the examiner. The humerus is slightly internally rotated and abducted within the plane of the body to approximately 90°. The examiner then places one hand on the posterolateral aspect of the upper

Fig. 3.10 Strength of lower trapezius. With the patient prone, the humerus is abducted to approximately 120° within the scapular plane. The patient then attempts to extend the humerus upward while resistance is applied by the examiner.

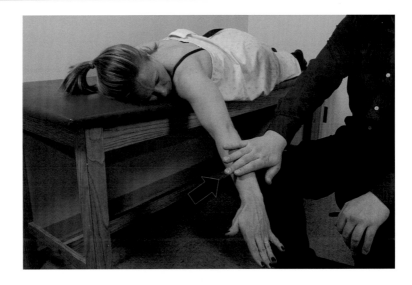

Fig. 3.11 Illustration highlighting the anatomy of the rhomboid musculature.

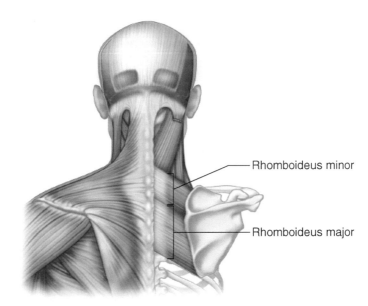

Rhomboideus minor

Rhomboideus major

arm and applies an anteromedially directed force while the patient resists (Fig. 3.13).

There are no clinical studies that have specifically evaluated the effects of isolated rhomboid or levator scapulae weakness on shoulder function. However, a case report by Hayes and Zehr [46] in 1981 described a patient with interscapular pain and scapular winging who was ultimately found to have a rhomboid muscle avulsion fracture after a traumatic injury. The patient was successfully treated by surgically reattaching the avulsed segment. More recently, Kibler et al. [66]

evaluated 64 patients with traumatic medial scapular muscle detachments. All patients that were included in that study demonstrated abnormal resting scapular positions (i.e., winging) and scapular dyskinesis with arm motion.

Serratus Anterior

The serratus anterior muscle is anatomically divided into three divisions. The first division, arising from ribs 1 and 2, inserts along the anterior aspect of the superomedial scapular angle. The second division arises from ribs 2 through 4

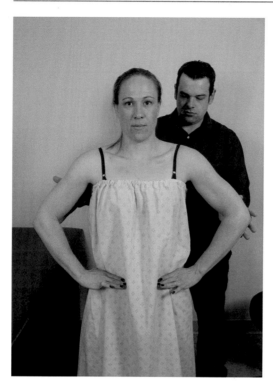

Fig. 3.12 Strength of rhomboids (modified Kendall). The patient is asked to place their hands on the "hips" or iliac crests with the elbows in a neutral position. An anteriorly directed force is applied to the medial epicondyle while the patient attempts to resist. The medial scapular border is simultaneously palpated, if possible.

and inserts along the anterior surface of the medial border of the scapula. The third division originates from ribs 5 through 9 and inserts on the anterior aspect of the inferomedial scapular angle. Although these distinct divisions are anatomically convenient, the muscle generally functions as a single unit. The muscle is innervated by the long thoracic nerve which is derived from the C5, C6, and C7 nerve roots (Fig. 3.14).

Contraction of the serratus anterior muscle results in upward rotation and protraction of the scapula. Weakness of this muscle is most commonly due to long thoracic nerve palsy and results in scapular winging with an increased distance between the medial scapular border and the posterior chest wall. This form of scapular winging must be differentiated from the scapular winging produced by spinal accessory nerve palsy with subsequent weakness of the trapezius muscle (see Fig. 3.7).

Scapular winging due to global weakness of the serratus anterior can be elicited by simply having the patient actively forward flex both arms to 90° of elevation while simultaneously observing the dynamic motion of both scapulae. The examiner can also provide resistance to forward flexion; however, using this method places the

Fig. 3.13 Strength of rhomboids (posterior deltoid test). With the patient sitting facing away from the examiner, the humerus is slightly internally rotated and abducted to approximately 90° of elevation. The examiner places one hand on the posterolateral aspect of the upper arm and applies an anteromedially directed force while the patient provides resistance.

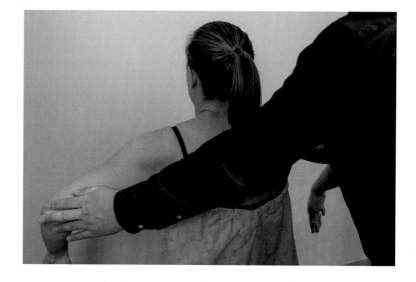

a

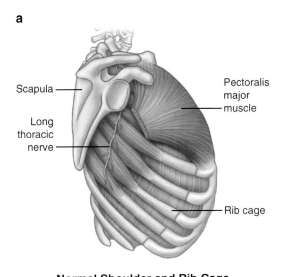

Scapula

Long
thoracic
nerve

Pectoralis
major
muscle

Rib cage

**Normal Shoulder and Rib Cage
Viewed from the Right Side**

b

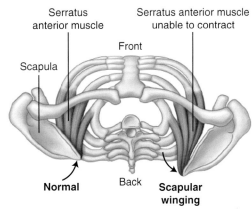

Serratus
anterior muscle

Serratus anterior muscle
unable to contract

Front

Scapula

Normal

Back

Scapular
winging

**Shoulders and Rib Cage
Viewed from Above**

Fig. 3.14 (**a**) Illustration highlighting the three divisions of the serratus anterior muscle and the associated long thoracic nerve (*lateral view*). (**b**) Orientation of the serratus anterior relative to the scapulae in both a normal shoulder and a shoulder with scapular winging (*axial view*).

examiner in an awkward position to visualize the scapula during arm motion. We prefer to have the patient perform a wall push-up as this maneuver is more sensitive for the detection of both mild and severe serratus anterior weakness in a busy clinic setting. To perform the wall push-up, the patient's hands are placed flat on a nearby wall at approximately shoulder height and shoulder width apart. The patient then performs a normal push-up as if they were in the prone position while the clinician simultaneously observes both scapulae (Fig. 3.15). Of note, this method of strength testing activates the entire serratus anterior muscle and does not differentiate between the three divisions [77].

A study by Celik et al. [78] found that several periscapular muscles, including the serratus anterior, were markedly weaker in shoulders with signs of subacromial impingement compared to healthy shoulders. This finding suggests that evaluation of periscapular musculature is necessary even in patients without perceived scapular dyskinesis. Periscapular muscle weakness can also result from fatigue, especially in those who participate in repetitive overhead activities [79–82]. Glousman [83] found that throwing athletes

with shoulder pain had significantly decreased serratus anterior activity via EMG when compared to throwing athletes without shoulder pain. As many others have suggested, the authors concluded that scapular malposition and dyskinesis was a significant contributor to the development of shoulder pain in overhead athletes. Burkhart et al. [84] later described a series of pathologic findings related to scapular motion in overhead athletes for which the term "SICK scapula syndrome" was coined.

Latissimus Dorsi

The latissimus dorsi, which receives its motor innervation from the thoracodorsal nerve, originates from the iliac crest, sacrum, and T7 through L5 spinous processes as an aponeurotic attachment. The fibers of this large, flat muscle travel superolaterally over the teres major muscle and insert just inferior to the lesser tuberosity of the humerus on the medial aspect of the bicipital groove (Fig. 3.16). This orientation has led some to infer its potential role as a humeral head stabilizer acting in synergy with the rotator cuff, especially in the rare situation of humeral avulsion of the glenohumeral ligament (HAGL) lesions [85].

Fig. 3.15 Wall push-up for the assessment of serratus anterior strength. Weakness of the serratus anterior would induce scapular winging during this maneuver.

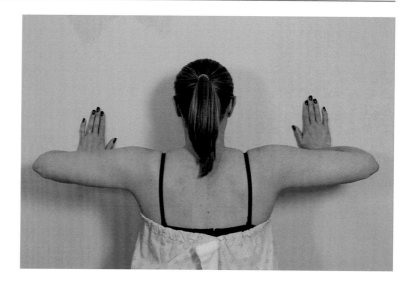

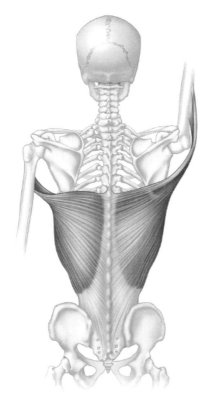

Fig. 3.16 Illustration depicting the normal anatomy and functional orientation of the latissimus dorsi muscle.

The muscle also variably attaches to the inferomedial angle of the scapula as it travels over the teres major with or without an intervening bursa [86].

The primary functions of the latissimus dorsi muscle are to adduct, extend, and internally rotate the humerus. A classic EMG study by Scheving and Pauly [87] determined that the latissimus dorsi is a more important internal rotator of the humerus than the pectoralis major in several planes.

Clinically, the latissimus dorsi is tested with the patient in the prone position and the arms at the side. The patient is then asked to simultaneously extend and internally rotate the humerus while the examiner applies resistance (Fig. 3.17). It is important to note the position of the scapulae during this movement since latissimus dorsi dysfunction has been associated with scapular dyskinesis [88]. The efficacy of this test has been confirmed in a study by Park and Yoo [89] who compared latissimus dorsi activation between six different isometric exercises using surface EMG. The authors found that extension of the humerus in the prone position activated the muscle with greater intensity than any other tested exercise, including the common "lat pull-down" exercise in the seated position.

Several authors have documented potential pathologic processes involving the latissimus dorsi muscle as it relates to the throwing shoulder [65, 90–92]. Nobuhara [91] described a "latissimus dorsi syndrome" in overhead athletes which is characterized by insertional tenderness or muscle tightness. The syndrome is thought to result from repetitive throwing as the latissimus dorsi

Fig. 3.17 Strength testing of latissimus dorsi. With the patient prone and the arm at the side, the patient is asked to extend and internally rotate the humerus against resistance applied by the examiner.

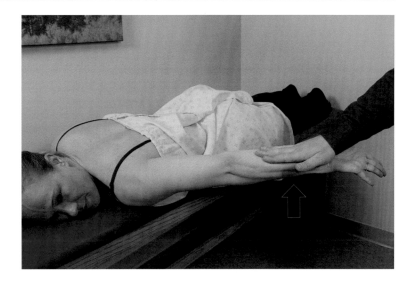

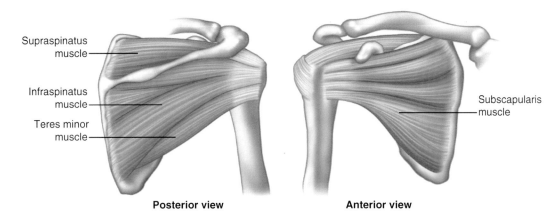

Supraspinatus muscle

Infraspinatus muscle

Teres minor muscle

Subscapularis muscle

Posterior view   **Anterior view**

Fig. 3.18 Illustration of the rotator cuff musculature viewing from both posteriorly and anteriorly.

tendon counteracts the significant external rotation torque produced by overhead athletes resulting in a type of insertional tendinitis. Although uncommon, tears of the latissimus dorsi and/or teres major have also been reported in throwing athletes [90, 93].

3.4.1.2 Rotator Cuff
Supraspinatus
Innervated by the suprascapular nerve, the supraspinatus takes origin from the supraspinous fossa of the scapula and its fibers travel laterally to insert on the greater tuberosity (Fig. 3.18).

At approximately the level of the glenohumeral joint, its tendon fibers become confluent with those of the infraspinatus to form a thick, wide tendinous insertion that envelops the humeral head (Fig. 3.19). Due to the intermingling of fibers from each tendon, data regarding the individual insertional dimensions of the supraspinatus tendon footprint have been inconsistent to date (Table 3.3) [94–100]. Further biomechanical and anatomical considerations as they relate to supraspinatus pathology are discussed in Chap. 4.

The isolated primary functions of the supraspinatus muscle are to abduct the humerus and to

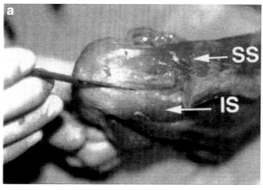 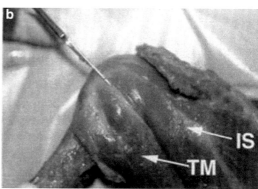

Fig. 3.19 Cadaveric photograph showing the confluence of (**a**) the supraspinatus and infraspinatus tendons and their insertion sites and (**b**) the confluence of the infraspi-

natus and teres minor tendons and their insertion sites. (From Dugas et al. [95]; with permission).

Table 3.3 Reported dimensions of the posterosuperior cuff insertion

References	Footprint dimensions Mean M-L × A-P Length in mm)	
	Supraspinatus	Infraspinatus
Minagawa et al. [96]	NR × 22.5	NR × 14.1
Roh et al. [98]	NR × 21.2	NR
Volk and Vangsness Jr [100]	27.9 × NR	NR
Dugas et al. [95]	12.7 × 16.3	13.4 × 16.4
Ruotolo et al. [99]	NR × 25	NR
Curtis et al. [94]	23 × 16	29 × 19
Mochizuki et al. [97]	6.9 × 12.6	10.2 × 32.7

M–L medial–lateral, *A–P* anterior–posterior, *NR* not reported

act as a physical barrier to prevent superior migration of the humeral head. There are numerous methods by which supraspinatus strength can be tested. Perhaps the most popular methods were proposed by Jobe [101]. According to the results of previous EMG studies [97], he recommended testing the supraspinatus with the humerus in 90° of abduction within the scapular plane and in maximal internal rotation such that the thumb pointed towards the floor (the "empty can" position). The patient then attempted to abduct the humerus further against resistance applied by the examiner (Fig. 3.20). Weakness in this position was thought to be the result of isolated supraspinatus weakness with minimal contributions from other muscles.

The assumption that the supraspinatus is isolated using the "empty can" test has been challenged on several occasions. Of note, Blackburn et al. [102] studied the electrical activation of the supraspinatus muscle in various arm positions with and without the application of resistance using surface EMG. Although the investigators did find relative isolation of the supraspinatus with the arm abducted to 90° within the scapular plane in neutral rotation, their EMG results suggested that the "empty can" position did not maximally activate the supraspinatus. Rather, maximal electrical activity occurred with the patient prone and the humerus abducted to approximately 100° in maximal external rotation; however, they also found EMG activity within the teres minor and infraspinatus muscles in this position. A later EMG study found that neither the "empty can" position nor the Blackburn position fully isolated the supraspinatus muscle and that other muscles, particularly the anterior and middle portions of the deltoid muscle, contribute significantly to strength in these positions [103].

The fact that the deltoid and the supraspinatus work synergistically to abduct the humerus has also been suggested by others [104, 105]. Colachis Jr and Strohm [105] selectively injected the suprascapular nerve with local anesthetic, thus paralyzing the supraspinatus and infraspinatus muscles. Although subjects were mildly weak with abduction, they were still able to achieve full

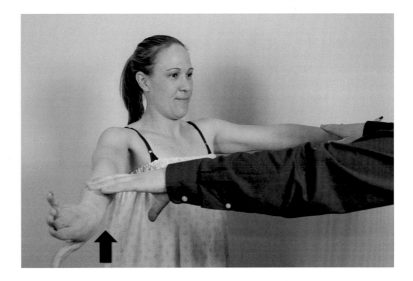

Fig. 3.20 Jobe's "empty can" position for supraspinatus strength. With both arms at approximately 90° of abduction in the scapular plane and the thumbs pointed downward, the patient attempts to further abduct the humerus against resistance applied by the examiner. The relative strength of each arm is compared.

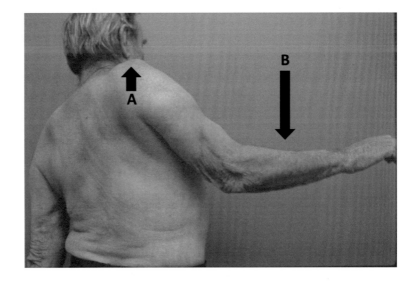

Fig. 3.21 Drop arm sign. The examiner passively places the humerus in 90° of abduction and asks the patient to hold the position. The drop arm sign occurs when (**a**) the shoulder appears to "shrug" as the humerus is displaced superiorly and (**b**) the arm falls back towards the side of the body despite the patient's best efforts. (Courtesy of Christian Gerber, MD).

humeral abduction. The investigators found a similar result after selective injection into the axillary nerve (paralyzing the deltoid muscle)— patients were still able to fully abduct the humerus despite mild weakness [104]. These studies suggested that patients with a full-thickness supraspinatus tear or deltoid dysfunction may still be able to achieve full active humeral abduction, especially when the supraspinatus tear does not extend anteriorly or posteriorly resulting in a derangement of dynamic rotator cuff force couples (see Chap. 4 for more details on rotator

cuff force couples [106]). Patients with massive rotator cuff tears involving more than one tendon often display a positive "drop arm sign" in which they are unable to hold the humerus in an abducted position against gravity. In these cases, the arm "drops" back to the patient's side (Fig. 3.21).

Patients with supraspinatus weakness are likely to have a range of other symptoms, including subacromial pain, with humeral abduction and internal rotation. Thus, the ability to achieve an "empty can" position may be difficult for some patients due to guarding or pain, making it difficult to

Fig. 3.22 Jobe's "full can" position for supraspinatus strength. With both arms at approximately 90° of abduction in the scapular plane and the thumbs pointed *upward*, the patient attempts to further abduct the humerus against resistance applied by the examiner. The relative strength of each arm is compared.

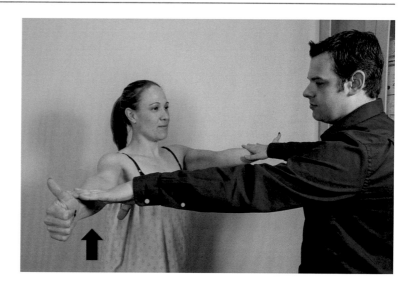

assess supraspinatus strength using this maneuver. In addition, internal rotation of the humerus places the greater tuberosity in a position that may exacerbate symptoms related to rotator cuff impingement on the undersurface of the acromion. This impingement-type of pain can be reduced by simply having the patient abduct the humerus to 90° in the plane of the scapula in either neutral rotation or external rotation (i.e., the "full can" position; Fig. 3.22). A study by Kelly et al. [24] found no difference in EMG activity between the "empty can," "full can" or neutral positions, indicating that supraspinatus testing can probably be estimated using in any of these positions. Because internal rotation in 90° of abduction also recruits the teres minor and subscapularis muscles, we prefer to test the supraspinatus in neutral rotation as a means of decreasing the potential for ancillary muscle contraction.

Infraspinatus

The infraspinatus muscle, one of the primary external rotators of the humerus, originates from the infraspinous fossa and inserts as a tendon sheet posterior and inferior to the insertion of the supraspinatus tendon (see Fig. 3.19). As mentioned above, because the tendinous fibers of the supraspinatus and infraspinatus intermingle, it is difficult to determine the exact location and/or dimensions of the infraspinatus insertional footprint (see Table 3.3).

The infraspinatus is innervated by the infraspinatus branch of the suprascapular nerve after passing through the spinoglenoid notch. Isolated atrophy of the infraspinatus muscle is most often due to a synovial or glenolabral cyst that impinges upon the nerve as it courses nearby. Other causes include traction injuries [107, 108], rotator cuff tears [109], and/or postoperative scarring. In contrast, impingement that occurs more proximally along the suprascapular nerve will cause weakness and/or atrophy of both the supraspinatus and the infraspinatus muscles (Fig. 3.23). Atrophy of the supraspinatus and/or infraspinatus can often be detected on physical examination by comparing the posterior contour of both scapulae, particularly noting the relative prominence of the scapular spine with the arms in a neutral position and in 90° of forward flexion (Fig. 3.24) [107, 110].

Isolated atrophy of the infraspinatus muscle is a common occurrence in overhead athletes, especially in volleyball players [107, 111–114] and baseball players [108, 115, 116], as a result of traction injury to the portion of the suprascapular nerve distal to the spinoglenoid notch. Lajtai et al. [107] evaluated 35 male beach volleyball players and noted that 12 players (34 %) had visible isolated infraspinatus atrophy. External rotation and elevation strength was also decreased in the dominant shoulder of all players. After correlation of these clinical findings with EMG, the

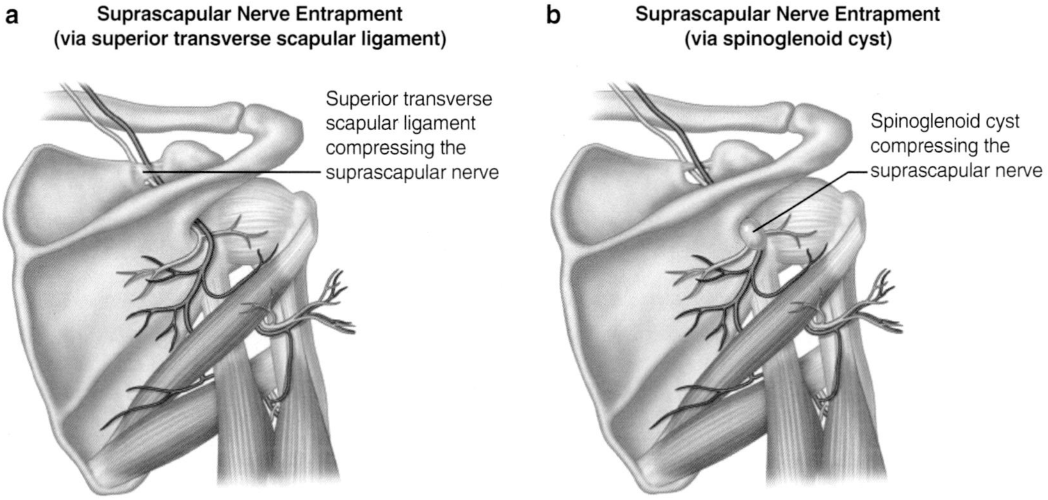

a   **Suprascapular Nerve Entrapment**
          (via superior transverse scapular ligament)

Superior transverse
scapular ligament
compressing the
suprascapular nerve

b   **Suprascapular Nerve Entrapment**
          (via spinoglenoid cyst)

Spinoglenoid cyst
compressing the
suprascapular nerve

Fig. 3.23 Posterior view of the shoulder depicting (**a**) proximal suprascapular nerve entrapment beneath the transverse scapular ligament and (**b**) distal suprascapular nerve entrapment due to a spinoglenoid cyst.

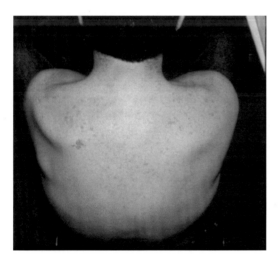

Fig. 3.24 Clinical photograph demonstrating a prominence of the left scapular spine with the arms in a neutral position which is indicative of supraspinatus and infraspinatus atrophy. (Courtesy of J.P. Warner, MD).

investigators found that nerve conduction velocities were significantly decreased and amplitudes were much lower in those shoulders with decreased volume of the infraspinatus muscle, suggesting a possible stretching mechanism during the deceleration phase of overhead motion resulting in suprascapular neuropathy in this population [107, 113].

Although challenged by several authors [24, 71], it is generally accepted that the optimal position for testing infraspinatus strength is with the humerus at the side in neutral rotation with the elbow flexed to 90°. While the patient provides resistance, the examiner then applies a medially directed force on the forearm to internally rotate the humerus (Fig. 3.25). The patient's inability to hold the humerus in neutral rotation signifies potential infraspinatus weakness. Others prefer to also test the infraspinatus in positions of internal rotation [24] and/or external rotation [71]. According to their rationale, internally rotating the humerus would force the infraspinatus to assume a stretched position thus placing the muscle at a mechanical *advantage*—weakness of the infraspinatus in this position may indicate significant pathology. On the other hand, externally rotating the humerus would force the infraspinatus to assume a less-stretched position thereby placing the muscle at a mechanical *disadvantage*—weakness in this position may therefore indicate a more subtle pathology. Testing the infraspinatus in either the internally or externally rotated positions as a method to determine the subtlety of infraspinatus weakness has not been validated or substantiated in the literature to date. This description also contradicts the length–force relationship since increasing or decreasing the passive tension within a muscle away from its resting position would each result in a decrease in muscle contraction force.

Fig. 3.25 Strength of infraspinatus. With the arms at the side and in neutral rotation, the elbows are flexed to 90°. The examiner then provides resistance as the patient attempts to externally rotate.

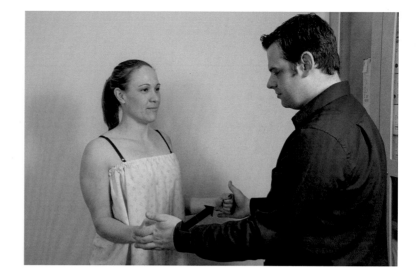

Fig. 3.26 Strength of subscapularis. With the arms at the side and in neutral rotation, the elbows are flexed to 90°. The examiner then provides resistance as the patient attempts to internally rotate.

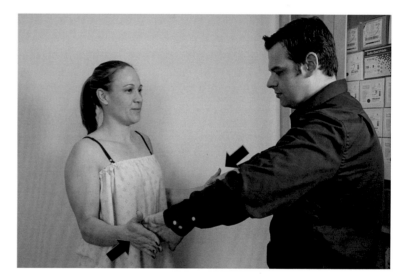

There are several other provocative maneuvers that can be utilized to test for infraspinatus strength; however, these are more sensitive for detecting specific rotator cuff pathologies and are discussed further in Chap. 4.

Subscapularis

The subscapularis is a large, thick muscle that originates from the subscapular fossa and inserts on the lesser tuberosity while also contributing to the structure and function of the bicipital sheath (see Fig. 3.18) (relevant anatomy of the bicipital sheath is discussed in Chap. 5). The muscle is innervated by the upper and lower subscapular nerves which are derived primarily from the posterior cord of the brachial plexus. Unlike the supraspinatus and infraspinatus, isolated atrophy of the subscapularis is very rare and cannot be seen by simple observation.

The subscapularis is one of several internal rotators of the humerus. Similar to infraspinatus testing, the best position for determining subscapularis strength is with the arm at the side in neutral rotation and the elbow flexed to 90°. The subject then resists a laterally directed force applied to the forearm by the examiner. In the case of subscapularis weakness, the patient will not be able to hold the neutral position and the humerus will externally rotate as a result of the force applied by the examiner (Fig. 3.26).

Although there are other muscles that provide internal rotation of the humerus (such as the pectoralis major, teres major, and latissimus dorsi) [117], the subscapularis has been identified as the primary internal rotator of the humerus in a biomechanical study by Chang et al. [118] An EMG study by Suenaga et al. [119] also found that resisted internal rotation in the neutral position (arm at the side in neutral rotation with the elbow flexed to 90°) electrically activated the subscapularis more than any other muscle at each tested position (81.7 %); however, the muscle is probably best isolated when the humerus is abducted to 90° within the scapular plane in neutral rotation [120, 121].

Gerber and Krushell [122] reported on 16 cases of isolated subscapularis tendon rupture where 15 of the patients were manually tested for internal rotation strength with the arm at the side and the elbows flexed to 90°. Fourteen of the fifteen patients (93.3 %) had at least grade 4 weakness

according to the MMT scale (see Table 6.1). In the same study, the authors proposed a new "lift-off" test and reported that it was both highly sensitive and specific for subscapularis tears. This test, along with the bear-hug test and the belly-press test, is discussed in detail in Chap. 4.

Teres Minor
The teres minor muscle, which also functions as an external rotator, originates from the posterior aspect of the scapular body, just inferior to the infraspinatus muscle, and inserts on the posterior aspect of the proximal humerus (see Fig. 3.18). The tendon fibers of the teres minor blend with those of the infraspinatus, making them indistinguishable in most cases. The teres minor is innervated by the axillary nerve as the nerve passes through the quadrilateral (or quadrangular) space towards the undersurface of the deltoid muscle (Fig. 3.27). Fatty infiltration and atrophy of the teres minor muscle from axillary nerve

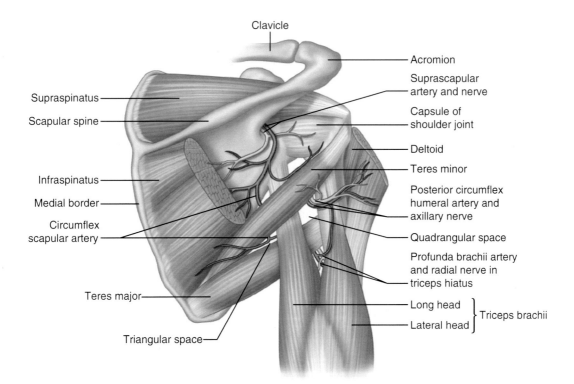

Fig. 3.27 Illustration showing the borders and contents of the quadrilateral space. The inferior margin of the teres minor defines the superior border, the humeral shaft defines the lateral border, the lateral margin of the long head of the triceps defines the medial border and the superior margin of the teres major defines the inferior border. The posterior circumflex humeral artery and the axillary nerve pass through this space.

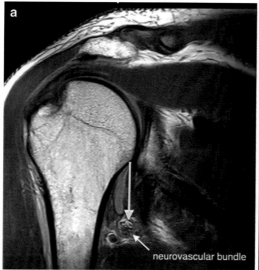
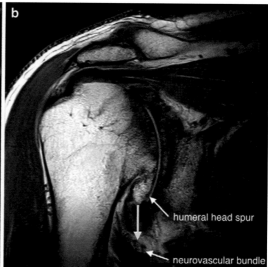

Fig. 3.28 (**a**) Coronal-oblique MRI slice showing a normal humeral head with the distance from the axillary neurovascular bundle depicted by the *yellow arrow*. (**b**) Coronal-oblique MRI slice showing a humeral head with a large inferior osteophyte in close proximity to axillary neurovascular bundle. (From Millett et al. [123]; with permission).

impingement can occur in patients with large inferior humeral head osteophytes as a result of glenohumeral osteoarthritis [123]. The inferior osteophyte can generate a mass effect or make direct contact with the axillary nerve as it passes between the superior aspect of the lateral scapular border and the humeral head before reaching the teres minor and deltoid muscles (Fig. 3.28). In contrast to atrophy involving the supraspinatus and infraspinatus muscles, atrophy of the teres minor is rarely detected by inspection or palpation of the posterior scapulae.

The teres minor is primarily an external rotator with the humerus at 90° of abduction within the scapular plane. Screening for teres minor weakness can be performed by simply having the patient abduct the humerus to 90° in neutral rotation with the elbow flexed to 90° and resisting external rotation from this position (Fig. 3.29). Blackburn et al. [102] suggested that isolation of the teres minor is best obtained when the patient is in the prone position with the arm in maximal external rotation; however, this maneuver is not quickly or easily performed in clinical practice and has not been formally validated in the literature. There are a few other maneuvers, such as the Patte test and the "Hornblower's sign," that can be used to specifically identify pathologic lesions

of the teres minor muscle and are discussed further in Chap. 4.

3.4.1.3 Other Scapulohumeral Muscles
Teres Major

Innervated by the lower subscapular nerve, the teres major originates from the posterior aspect of the inferomedial angle of the scapula and inserts on the proximal humerus just posterior to the latissimus dorsi tendon, oftentimes with an intervening bursa (Fig. 3.30). In some cases, the teres major may insert directly into the latissimus dorsi tendon [124]. Similar to the latissimus dorsi, the primary function of the teres major muscle is to adduct, extend, and internally rotate the humerus. Pearl et al. [125] found that both the latissimus dorsi and the teres major muscles fire maximally when moving the arm "obliquely downward away from the midline." Because of their identical force vectors, each muscle can be successfully transferred to the greater tuberosity as a salvage procedure in patients with massive, irreparable posterosuperior rotator cuff tears (Fig. 3.31) [126–129].

Although there have been several reports of isolated tears of the teres major muscle in high-level athletes, this injury is uncommon in the general population [93, 130, 131]. In these cases,

Fig. 3.29 Strength screening of teres minor. (**a**) The humerus is abducted to 90° in the scapular plane in neutral rotation and the elbow is flexed to 90°. The examiner then applies resistance as the patient attempts to externally rotate the humerus. (**b**) The same test, except that the patient will start at 90° of external rotation.

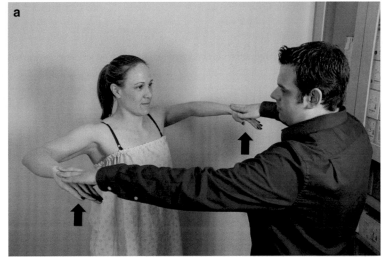

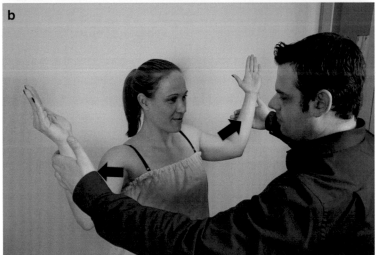

the diagnosis is most often made via imaging studies or direct visualization during surgery since physical examination maneuvers designed to specifically detect weakness of the teres major have not been developed.

Deltoid

The deltoid is the largest muscle of the shoulder girdle and consists of three separate divisions: anterior, middle, and posterior. The anterior portion of the deltoid originates from the superior aspect of the distal third of the clavicle, the middle division originates from the superior aspect of the acromion and the posterior division originates from the inferior aspect of the scapular spine. All three divisions of the deltoid muscle insert on the deltoid tubercle of the humerus and function to elevate the arm in several different planes (Fig. 3.32).

The axillary nerve branches from the posterior cord of the brachial plexus, travels through the quadrangular space, around the proximal humerus and towards the undersurface of the deltoid muscle. The nerve first gives off a branch to the teres minor muscle as it passes through the quadrilateral space and then to the posterior, middle and, finally, the anterior deltoid while also providing sensory innervation to the skin overlying the middle deltoid (i.e. the superior lateral cutaneous nerve).

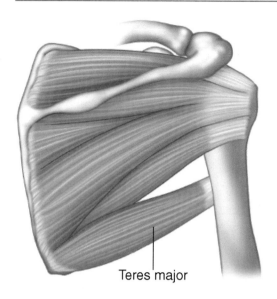

Teres major

Fig. 3.30 Illustration of a posterior right scapula highlighting the teres major muscle.

The function of the deltoid muscle is to elevate the humerus. It is usually taught that the plane of elevation depends on which of the three muscle divisions are activated. For example, forward flexion of the humerus requires activation from the anterior fibers and abduction requires activation from the middle fibers. Thus, the key to testing the strength of the individual components of the deltoid muscle is to position the humerus in line with the muscle fibers to be tested.

This model suggests that the muscle fibers not in-line with plane of elevation are relatively inactive. However, in reality, all three divisions of the muscle are active with nearly any movement of the arm in any direction [92]. In 1959, Scheving and Pauly [92] conducted an electromyographic study of several upper extremity muscles in various movement planes. With respect to the deltoid, it was found that although the entire deltoid muscle was active during humeral elevation in any plane, the anterior deltoid was most active during forward flexion, the middle deltoid was most active in abduction, and the posterior deltoid was most active during extension. It was postulated that the less active portions of the deltoid actually function to prevent humeral head translation with arm elevation. In 2002, Lee and An [132] found that the deltoid was effective at stabilizing the

glenohumeral joint during abduction within the scapular plane; however, this function was less effective and, in fact, decreased glenohumeral stability during abduction in the coronal plane. The authors also proposed that rehabilitation in patients with anterior instability should focus on strengthening the middle and posterior divisions of the deltoid muscle to enhance glenohumeral stability. More recently in 2008, Yanagawa et al. [133] used a three-dimensional model to calculate the relative contributions of the deltoid and rotator cuff to glenohumeral stability. They found that of all the muscles tested, the middle deltoid produced the greatest amount of compression between the humeral head and the glenoid; however, because of the significant shear forces produced, the middle deltoid was actually less able to maintain glenohumeral stability than the rotator cuff musculature. This study suggested that the rotator cuff is probably more effective at maintaining glenohumeral stability than the deltoid muscle which has significant implications for physical therapy and postoperative rehabilitation in patients with instability.

Testing the individual components of the deltoid muscle is probably not routinely necessary unless one suspects axillary nerve dysfunction. In these cases, the examiner can also examine the shoulder for any signs of deltoid atrophy that may localize the site of axillary involvement. The "scaphoid sign" or "scallop sign" can be observed in patients with deltoid atrophy since the loss of muscle allows the acromion, acromioclavicular joint and anterior structures to become more prominent when compared to the contralateral side (Fig. 3.33). In addition, the muscle mass over the lateral aspect of the proximal humerus diminishes, thus giving a concave appearance of the upper arm compared to the contralateral side. In some patients with deltoid atrophy, prominence of the scapular spine may also be evident—this becomes problematic in patients who have undergone shoulder arthrodesis since the resulting deltoid atrophy allows the plate over the scapular spine to irritate the overlying skin.

There are several methods that can be used to test the anterior division of the deltoid muscle. As a screening exam, we tend to place the patient

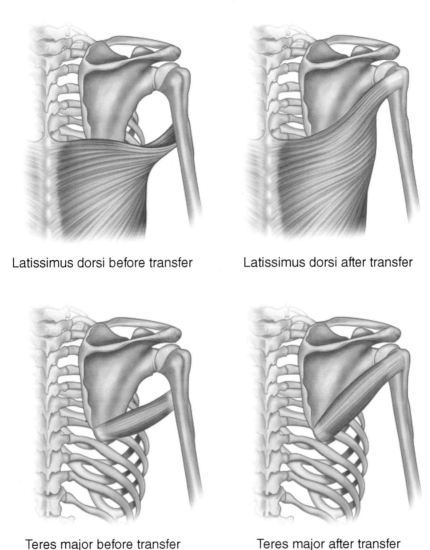

Latissimus dorsi before transfer

Latissimus dorsi after transfer

Teres major before transfer

Teres major after transfer

Fig. 3.31 Illustrations demonstrating the positions of the latissimus dorsi and teres major muscles both before and after muscle transfer procedures for the treatment of massive rotator cuff tears.

in the sitting position with the humerus at the side and the elbow flexed to 90°. We then ask the patient to make a fist and to push forward against resistance applied by the examiner (Fig. 3.34). Another way to test the anterior deltoid, as suggested by McFarland [71], is to place the humerus in approximately 70° of abduction within the scapular plane and to resist flexion and adduction (Fig. 3.35). Placing the arm in 70° of abduction is thought to more adequately isolate the deltoid muscle from the rotator cuff; however, this theory has not been proven in any clinical or biomechanical study. As discussed above, an EMG study by Colachis Jr et al. [104] found that both the rotator cuff and the deltoid function synergistically to achieve glenohumeral abduction. This test can therefore be performed with the elbow flexed or extended, depending on the subtlety of the suspected pathology. For example, applying resistance to the wrist with the elbow extended increases the contraction force necessary to flex and adduct the humerus due to lengthening of the

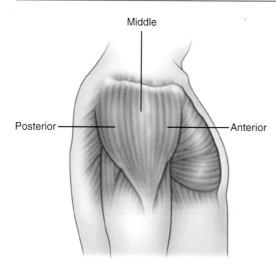

Middle

Posterior ——

—— Anterior

Fig. 3.32 Illustration of a right shoulder showing the relative positions of the anterior, middle, and posterior divisions of the deltoid muscle.

lever arm. This method is likely to detect more subtle forms of weakness as a result of axillary neuropathy or primary deltoid weakness.

The middle division of the deltoid can be tested using the same starting position—that is, 70° of straight lateral abduction. However, rather than resisting flexion and adduction, the patient is asked to further abduct the humerus against resistance. Similar to testing of the anterior deltoid, this test can be performed with the elbow flexed or extended, depending on the severity of the suspected pathology.

There are a few different ways to test the posterior division of the deltoid, both of which require the patient to be standing. One method is to position the humerus at the patient's side in neutral rotation and to resist active extension of the humerus from this position (sometimes called the "swallowtail test") (Fig. 3.36). Another method, called the "deltoid lag sign" [7], is performed by passively extending the humerus and asking the patient to hold the position once the examiner releases the arm. If the arm falls back to the side, the patient has a positive deltoid lag sign which is indicative of posterior deltoid weakness. This test is specifically designed to distinguish between axillary neuropathy and a massive rotator cuff tear since both pathologies

will result in abduction weakness. Bertelli and Ghizoni [134] described an abduction-internal rotation test to identify patients with axillary nerve lesions. In this test, the patient actively internally rotates and maximally abducts the affected shoulder. If the patient could not reach the abduction level of the contralateral shoulder, the patient was asked to hold abducted and internally rotated position. If the patient could not hold the position and the arm slowly fell back to the side, axillary nerve palsy was diagnosed. Fujihara et al. [135] devised the "akimbo test" which was designed to detect abduction weakness as a result of deltoid dysfunction; however, none of the patients with axillary neuropathy could consistently demonstrate the sign.

Biceps Brachii

The biceps muscle spans two joints and is composed of two origins (long head and short head) from the scapula with a single insertion site at the bicipital tuberosity of the proximal radius (Fig. 3.37). The distal biceps insertion may be bifurcated into their corresponding short and long head segments [136]. The distal biceps also forms an aponeurotic attachment to the muscles of the medial forearm (the "lacertus fibrosus"). The long head of the biceps travels within the bicipital groove of the proximal humerus and courses through the glenohumeral joint before variably attaching to the superior labrum and supraglenoid tubercle. Further details regarding the long head of the biceps tendon are discussed extensively in Chap. 5. The short head of the biceps converges with the coracobrachialis muscle proximally (i.e., the "conjoined tendon") and originates from the anteroinferior aspect of the coracoid process. The musculocutaneous nerve pierces the conjoined tendon approximately 8 cm distal to the coracoid tip and runs deep to the main belly of the biceps muscle and superficial to the brachialis muscle of the forearm. There have been reports of anomalous biceps musculature, such as those with three or four muscle heads; however, these cases are uncommon [137–139].

The musculocutaneous nerve (C5 and C6) provides the motor innervation to the biceps, brachialis and coracobrachialis muscles. Injury

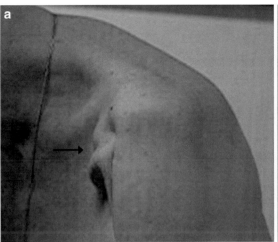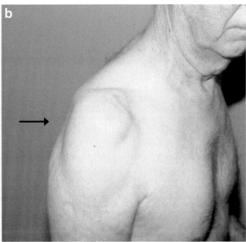

Fig. 3.33 (**a**) Clinical photograph demonstrating atrophy of the deltoid muscle. The implant from a previous hemiarthroplasty can be seen across the atrophic anterior deltoid (*arrow*). (**b**) Clinical photograph also showing atrophy of the deltoid muscle as evidenced by prominence of the acromioclavicular joint and anterior shoulder structures. This patient also had significant atrophy of the supraspinatus and infraspinatus muscles (*arrow*), possibly indicating the presence of a concurrent injury to the suprascapular nerve. (Part B courtesy of J.P. Warner, MD, and Christian Gerber, MD).

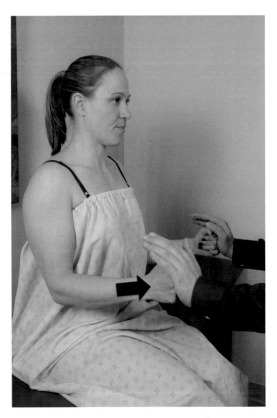

Fig. 3.34 Anterior deltoid strength. With the patient in the sitting position, the arms at the side and the elbows flexed to 90°, the patient is asked to make a fist and to push anteriorly against the examiner's hand.

to the musculocutaneous nerve often occurs as a traction injury due to overzealous surgical retraction of the coracobrachialis while approaching the glenohumeral joint using a deltopectoral approach. This injury results in weakness of the entire biceps muscle (short and long heads), the coracobrachialis and the medial half of the brachialis muscle.

The biceps muscle functions primarily to supinate the forearm and to flex the elbow. The function of the long head of the biceps tendon as it courses through the glenohumeral joint is controversial and will be discussed in detail in Chap. 5. Rupture of the long head of the biceps tendon typically results in a classic "Popeye deformity" in which the muscle belly retracts distally, forming a ball of muscle just proximal to the elbow joint. In contrast, partial or complete rupture of the distal biceps tendon causes muscle retraction that appears more proximally (Fig. 3.38). Despite the commonality of proximal and distal biceps ruptures, it is important to rule out other causes of deformity, such as tumors, that may have a similar appearance [140, 141].

Triceps Brachii

Although the triceps muscle contributes little to shoulder motion, it is considered here since it

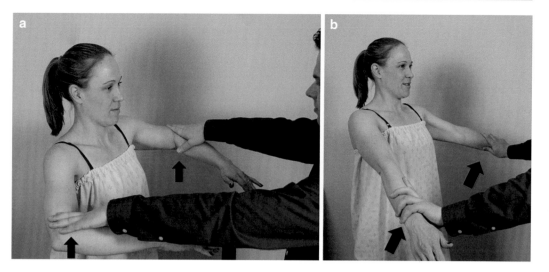

Fig. 3.35 Anterior deltoid strength. (**a**) The arms are abducted to 70° in scapular plane with the elbows flexed to approximately 90°. The patient then attempts to further elevate the arms against resistance provided by the examiner. (**b**) The test can also be performed with the elbows extended.

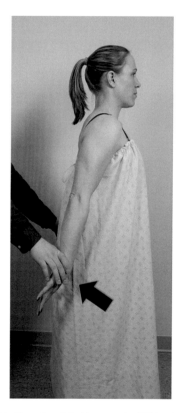

Fig. 3.36 Posterior deltoid strength. With the patient standing, the arms at the side and the elbows extended, the patient attempts to extend the humerus against resistance provided by the examiner.

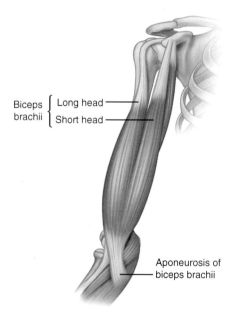

Fig. 3.37 Illustration highlighting the basic anatomy of the biceps muscle.

attaches to the scapula and may contribute to shoulder pain in overhead athletes. The triceps has three heads: a long head, a medial head, and a lateral head. The long head primarily takes ori-

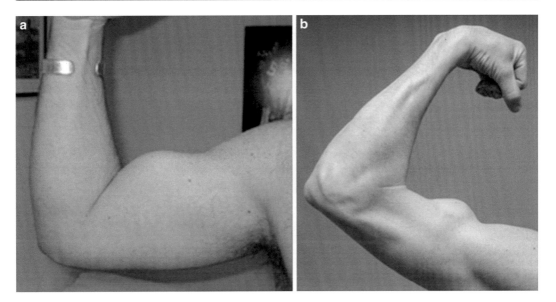

Fig. 3.38 (**a**) "Popeye" deformity due to rupture of the proximal LHB tendon (distal retraction). (**b**) "Popeye" deformity due to rupture of the distal LHB tendon (proximal retraction).

gin from the infraglenoid tubercle of the scapula; however, it can also have an attachment to the inferior capsulolabral complex of the glenohumeral joint. The lateral head originates from the posterior aspect of the proximal humerus and the medial head originates from the posterior aspect of the distal 1/3 of the humerus inferior to the radial groove. All three heads of the triceps insert posteriorly on the olecranon process of the ulna as a wide, flat tendon (Fig. 3.39). Motor innervation to the triceps is mostly provided by the radial nerve (C6 through T1) which spirals around the proximal humerus in the radial groove. The medial head of the triceps has a dual nerve supply—the medial half of the medial head is supplied by the ulnar nerve and the lateral half of the medial head is supplied by the radial nerve which forms an interneural plane that is used to facilitate deep surgical dissection.

The main function of the triceps muscle is to extend the elbow joint and to prevent hyperflexion of the elbow as a counter-regulatory mechanism. Although its role in the shoulder has not been clearly defined, several investigators have found that the triceps muscle may be involved in the development of shoulder pain in overhead athletes. Bennett [142] was perhaps the first

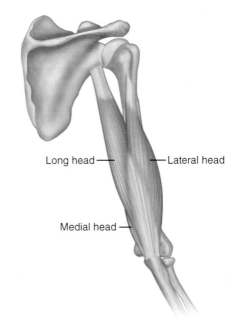

Fig. 3.39 Illustration depicting the general anatomy of the triceps muscle. The medial, lateral, and long heads of the triceps muscle are shown.

author to suggest that the deceleration phase of the throwing motion produced traction on the inferior capsule from the pull of the triceps, thus

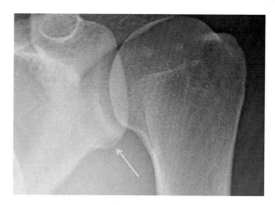

Fig. 3.40 Anteroposterior (AP) radiograph demonstrating an inferior glenoid enthesophyte (Bennett lesion) in an overhead athlete with posterior shoulder pain. (From Spiegl et al. [162]; with permission).

resulting in a traction spur at the inferior aspect of the glenoid. Although this theory has since been refuted, this so-called Bennett lesion is often an indicator of posterosuperior glenoid impingement in throwing athletes (Fig. 3.40). Nobuhara [91] later suggested that repeated traction of the triceps during the deceleration phase of the throwing motion may cause an overuse-type of tendinitis thereby resulting in posteromedial pain in the upper arm. To date, no clinical or biomechanical studies have evaluated the effects of triceps muscle function on shoulder motion and thus there are no clinical examination tests of the triceps muscle that are relevant to the shoulder.

3.4.1.4 Pectoral Muscles
Pectoralis Major
The pectoralis major has two heads that originate from the thorax—the clavicular head and the sternal head. The clavicular head arises from the inferior aspect of the medial clavicle along the pectoralis ridge and the first few ribs. The sternal head arises from the ribs and the lateral portion of the sternum. The two heads converge into a single tendon sheet that inserts over the lateral lip of the bicipital groove (Fig. 3.41). The medial and lateral pectoral nerves branch from the medial and lateral cords of the brachial plexus, respectively, to innervate the pectoralis major. The mus-

cle functions as a powerful adductor and internal rotator of the humerus.

There have been no known cases of isolated pectoralis major atrophy as a result of a nerve lesion. Poland first described a condition in which unilateral absence of the pectoral muscles was evident along with other myocutaneous manifestations occurring on the ipsilateral side of the body, including hand size discrepancies ("Poland's syndrome"). The cause of the disorder is unknown; however, the most common theory involves a disruption of subclavian artery circulation during pregnancy. Patients with unilateral absence of the pectoralis major rarely have functional deficits and their concerns are usually cosmetic in nature [143–145].

Rupture of the pectoralis major tendon is a common occurrence in clinical practice, especially in those who participate in heavy bench pressing activities [145–147]. The patient will generally experience a "popping" sensation followed by pain, swelling, and ecchymosis in the axilla. The swelling rapidly subsides within a few days, leaving a classic "web" deformity in the axilla which can be detected by simple observation of the anterior chest.

Strength testing of the pectoralis major is typically indicated after re-attachment of the ruptured tendon; however, perceived weakness is more likely to be due to pain and guarding rather than true muscular weakness. The muscle is tested by first having the patient forward flex both arms to 90° of elevation with each humerus internally rotated. Alternatively, the test can also be performed with the arms abducted to 90° within the scapular plane. The patient then actively adducts the arms against resistance applied by the examiner (Fig. 3.42). It has been suggested that the upper and lower portion of the muscle can be separately tested by varying the degree of forward elevation [71]; however, this has not been substantiated by any clinical, biomechanical, or electromyographic study to date.

Pectoralis Minor
The pectoralis minor takes origin from the second through the fifth ribs on the anterior chest wall and inserts along the anteromedial aspect of

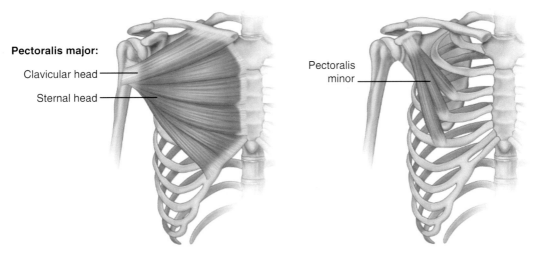

Pectoralis major:

Clavicular head

Sternal head

Pectoralis minor

Fig. 3.41 Illustrations showing the general anatomy of the pectoralis major (sternal and clavicular heads) and pectoralis minor muscles.

Fig. 3.42 Pectoralis major strength testing. With the patient sitting or standing, both arms can either be flexed to 90° or abducted to 90° in the scapular plane with maximal internal rotation. The patient then adducts the arms against resistance provided by the examiner. (From Dodson and Williams III [163]; with permission).

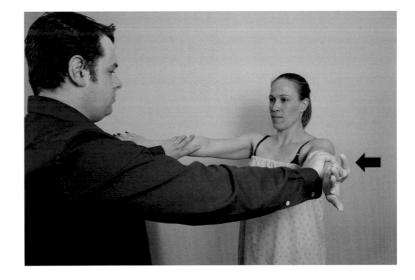

the coracoid process (see Fig. 3.41). The medial pectoral nerve provides motor innervation to the muscle and is derived from the C8 and T1 spinal nerve roots. Reflection of the muscle anteriorly would reveal the brachial plexus and the middle portion of the axillary artery.

Based on the orientation of its fibers, the pectoralis minor has been theorized to primarily cause scapular protraction and internal rotation. However, Diveta et al. [148] found no relationship between the strength of the pectoralis minor and the resting position of the scapula, although the investigators did not evaluate muscle length nor did they perform EMG testing to prove that the pectoralis minor muscle was actually firing during their testing maneuvers. Many researchers believe that the pectoralis minor plays a relatively small role in normal scapular kinematics. This is supported by several case reports in which congenital absence or isolated tearing of the pectoralis minor did not result in significantly disability [149–151]. In addition, pectoralis minor tendon

Fig. 3.43 Pectoralis minor strength testing. With the patient supine, the examiner places their hand on the anterior shoulder and asks the patient to thrust the shoulder forward against resistance. The patient's hands should be raised off the table during the test to prevent increased leverage.

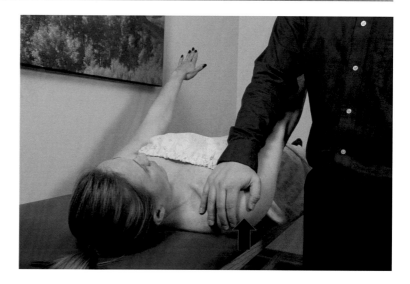

transfers have been performed for irreparable anterosuperior rotator cuff tears [152] and tenotomies have been performed to decompress the thoracic outlet [153, 154] without any apparent effects on scapular motion. On the other hand, tightness of the pectoralis minor has been found to cause scapular malposition and may also be involved with altered scapular motion [155, 156] and subacromial impingement [157–159].

Although isolated lesions of the pectoralis minor are rarely reported, they are probably underdiagnosed as a result of their relatively benign course. In one small case series, Bhatia et al. [160] described an overuse insertional tendinitis of the pectoralis minor in five weightlifters; however, the diagnosis was subjectively assumed after injection near the medial border of the coracoid resulted in symptomatic relief. Other than a case report by Mehallo [150] in 2004, we are unaware of any other cases of isolated pectoralis minor weakness as a result of tearing or neurologic injury. Additionally, there are no EMG studies that have confirmed the utility of any manual muscle test for strength testing of the pectoralis minor muscle.

Although rarely performed with unconfirmed validity, strength evaluation of the pectoralis minor is done with the patient in the supine position. The examiner places one hand on the anterior aspect of the shoulder and asks the patient to thrust the tested shoulder forward against resistance applied by the examiner's hand (Fig. 3.43).

To prevent the patient from obtaining leverage, the patient's ipsilateral hand can be raised away from the table during testing. As with many other examination maneuvers, this test likely does not isolate the pectoralis minor and is probably best used as a screening tool in high-functioning patients with shoulder discomfort.

3.5   Conclusion

The mechanisms involved with shoulder motion are complex and weakness of any of the individual components can result in pain and dysfunction. Although only a few important strength tests should be selected for any given patient to support a diagnosis, these maneuvers can provide important clues to the underlying diagnosis which can help guide the use of provocative tests.

References

1. Gandevia SC, McKenzie DK. Activation of human muscles at short muscle lengths during maximal static efforts. J Physiol. 1988;407:599–613.
2. Gareis H, Solomonow M, Baratta R, Best R, D'Ambrosia R. The isometric length-force models of nine different skeletal muscles. J Biomech. 1992;25(8):903–16.
3. Lieber RL, Boakes JL. Sarcomere length and joint kinematics during torque production in frog hindlimb. Am J Physiol. 1988;254(6 Pt 1): C759–68.

4. Lieber RL, Ljung BO, Fridén J. Intraoperative sarcomere length measurements reveal differential design of human wrist extensor muscles. J Exp Biol. 1997;200(Pt 1):19–25.

5. Powell PL, Roy RR, Kanim P, Bello MA, Edgerton VR. Predictability of skeletal muscle tension from architectural determinations in guinea pig hindlimbs. J Appl Physiol Respir Environ Exerc Physiol. 1984;57(6):1715–21.

6. Hertel R, Ballmer FT, Lombert SM, Gerber C. Lag signs in the diagnosis of rotator cuff rupture. J Shoulder Elbow Surg. 1996;5(4):307–13.

7. Hertel R, Lambert SM, Ballmer FT. The deltoid extension lag sign for diagnosis and grading of axillary nerve palsy. J Shoulder Elbow Surg. 1998;7(2):97–9.

8. Walch G, Boulahia A, Calderone S, Robinson AH. The 'dropping and 'hornblower's' signs in evaluation of rotator-cuff tears. J Bone Joint Surg Br. 1998;80(4):624–8.

9. Lovett RW, Martin EG. Certain aspects of infantile paralysis with a description of a method of muscle testing. JAMA. 1916;66:729–33.

10. Medical Research Council. Aids to the evaluation of peripheral nerve injuries. In: Her Majesty's stationery office. London: Medical Research Council; 1943.

11. Barr AE, Diamond BE, Wade CK, Harashima T, Pecorella WA, Potts CC, Rosenthal H, Fleiss JL, McMahon DJ. Reliability of testing measures in Duchenne or Becker muscular dystrophy. Arch Phys Med Rehabil. 1991;72(5):315–9.

12. Blair L. The role of the physical therapist in the evaluation studies of the poliomyelitis vaccine field trials. Phys Ther Rev. 1955;37(7):437.

13. Florence JM, Pandya S, King WM, Robison JD, Baty J, Miller JP, Schierbecker J, Signore LC. Intrarater reliability of manual muscle test (Medical Research Council scale) grades in Duchenne's muscular dystrophy. Phys Ther. 1992;72(2):115–26.

14. Frese E, Brown M, Norton BJ. Clinical reliability of manual muscle testing. Phys Ther. 1987;67(7):1072–6.

15. Hsieh CY, Phillips RB. Reliability of manual muscle testing with a computerized dynamometer. J Manipulative Physiol Ther. 1990;13(2):72–82.

16. Iddings DM, Smith LK, Spencer WA. Muscle testing: part 2. Reliability in clinical use. Phys Ther Rev. 1961;41:249–56.

17. Jacobs G. Applied kinesiology: an experimental evaluation by double blind methodology. J Manipulative Physiol Ther. 1981;4:141–5.

18. Lawson A, Calderon L. Interexaminer agreement for applied kinesiology manual muscle testing. Percept Mot Skills. 1997;84(2):539–46.

19. Lilienfeld AM, Jacobs M, Willis M. A study of reproducibility of muscle testing and certain other aspects of muscle scoring. Phys Ther Rev. 1954;34:279–89.

20. Perry J, Weiss WB, Burnfield JM, Gronley JK. The supine hip extension manual muscle test: a reliability and validity study. Arch Phys Med Rehabil. 2004;85(8):1345–50.

21. Silver M, McElroy A, Morrow L, Heafner BK. Further standardization of manual muscle test for clinical study: applied in chronic renal disease. Phys Ther. 1970;50:1456–66.

22. Wadsworth CT, Krishnan R, Sear M, Harrold J, Nielsen DH. Intrarater reliability of manual muscle testing and hand-held dynametric muscle testing. Phys Ther. 1987;67(9):1342–7.

23. Cibulka MT, Weissenborn D, Donham M, Rammacher H, Cuppy P, Ross AS. A new manual muscle test for assessing the entire trapezius muscle. Physiother Theory Pract. 2013;29(3):242–8.

24. Kelly BT, Kadrmas WR, Speer KP. The manual muscle examination for rotator cuff strength. An electromyographic investigation. Am J Sports Med. 1996;24(5):581–8.

25. Leggin BG, Neuman RM, Iannotti JP, Williams GR, Thompson EC. Intrarater and interrater reliability of three isometric dynamometers in assessing shoulder strength. J Shoulder Elbow Surg. 1996;5(1):18–24.

26. Bohannon R. Testing isometric limb muscle strength with dynamometers. Phys Rehab Med. 1990;2(2):75–86.

27. Bohannon RW. Research incorporating hand-held dynamometry: publication trends since 1948. Percept Mot Skills. 1998;86(3 Pt 2):1177–8.

28. Bohannon RW. Test-retest reliability of hand-held dynamometry during a single session of strength assessment. Phys Ther. 1986;66(2):206–9.

29. Brooke MH, Griggs RC, Mendell JR, Fenichel JB, Shumate JB, Pellegrino RJ. Clinical trial in Duchenne dystrophy. I. The design of the protocol. Muscle Nerve. 1981;4(3):186–97.

30. Gonnella C, Harmon G, Jacobs M. The role of the physical therapist in the gamma globulin poliomyelitis prevention study. Phys Ther Rev. 1953;33(7):337–45.

31. Aitkens S, Lord J, Bernauer E, Fowler Jr WM, Lieberman JS, Berck P. Relationship of manual muscle testing to objective strength measurements. Muscle Nerve. 1989;12(3):173–7.

32. Pearn J. Two early dynamometers. An historical account of the earliest measurements to study human muscular strength. J Neurol Sci. 1978;37(1–2):127–34.

33. Li RC, Jasiewicz JM, Middleton J, Condie P, Barriskill A, Hebnes H, Purcell B. The development, validity, and reliability of a manual muscle testing device with integrated limb position sensors. Arch Phys Med Rehabil. 2006;87(3):411–7.

34. Abernethy P, Wilson G, Logan P. Strength and power assessment. Issues, controversies and challenges. Sports Med. 1995;19(6):401–17.

35. Farrell M, Richards JG. Analysis of the reliability and validity of the kinetic communicator exercise device. Med Sci Sports Exerc. 1986;18(1):44–9.

36. Knapik JJ, Wright JE, Mawdsley RH, Braun JM. Isokinetic, isometric and isotonic strength relationships. Arch Phys Med Rehabil. 1983;64(2):77–80.

37. Ly LP, Handelsman DJ. Muscle strength and ageing: methodological aspects of isokinetic dynamometry and androgen administration. Clin Exp Pharmacol Physiol. 2002;29(1–2):37–47.

38. Verdijk LB, van Loon L, Meijer K, Savelberg HH. One-repetition maximum strength test represents a valid means to assess leg strength in vivo in humans. J Sports Sci. 2009;27(1):59–68.

39. Burnham RS, Bell G, Olenik L, Reid DC. Shoulder abduction strength measurement in football players: reliability and validity of two field tests. Clin J Sport Med. 1995;5(2):90–4.

40. Dolny DG, Collins MG, Wilson T, Germann ML, Davis HP. Validity of lower extremity strength and power utilizing a new closed chain dynamometer. Med Sci Sports Exerc. 2001;33(1):171–5.

41. Holm I, Hammer S, Larsen S, Nordsletten L, Steen H. Can a regular leg extension bench be used in testing deficits of the quadriceps muscle during rehabilitation. Scand J Med Sci Sports. 1995;5(1):29–35.

42. Surburg PR, Suomi R, Poppy WK. Validity and reliability of a hand-held dynamometer with two populations. J Orthop Sports Phys Ther. 1992;16(5):229–34.

43. Stark T, Walker B, Phillips JK, Fejer R, Beck R. Hand-held dynamometry correlation with the gold standard isokinetic dynamometry: a systematic review. PM R. 2011;3(5):472–9.

44. Reinking MF, Bockrath-Pugliese K, Worrell T, Kegerreis RL, Miller-Sayers K, Farr J. Assessment of quadriceps muscle performance by hand-held, isometric, and isokinetic dynamometry in patients with knee dysfunction. J Orthop Sports Phys Ther. 1996;24(3):154–9.

45. Bohannon RW, Andrews AW. Accuracy of spring and strain gauge hand-held dynamometers. J Orthop Sports Phys Ther. 1989;10(8):323–5.

46. Hayes JM, Zehr DJ. Traumatic muscle avulsion causing winging of the scapula. J Bone Joint Surg Am. 1981;63(3):495–7.

47. Hosking JP, Bhat US, Dubowitz V, Edwards RH. Measurements of muscle strength and performance in children with normal and diseased muscle. Arch Dis Child. 1976;51(12):957–63.

48. Agre JC, Magness JL, Hull SZ, Wright TL, Baxter R, Patterson R, Stradel L. Strength testing with a portable dynamometer: reliability for upper and lower extremities. Arch Phys Med Rehabil. 1987;68(7):454–8.

49. Brinkmann JR. Comparison of a hand-held and fixed dynamometer in measuring strength of patients with neuromuscular disease. J Orthop Sports Phys Ther. 1994;19(2):100–4.

50. Byl NN, Richards S, Asturias J. Intrarater and interrater reliability of strength measurements of the biceps and deltoid using a hand held dynamometer. J Orthop Sports Phys Ther. 1988;9(12):399–405.

51. Wikhom JB, Bohannon RW. Hand-held dynamometer measurements: tester strength makes a difference. J Orthop Sports Phys Ther. 1991;13(4):191–8.

52. Kolber MJ, Beekhuizen K, Cheng MS, Fiebert IM. The reliability of hand-held dynamometry in measuring isometric strength of the shoulder internal and external rotator musculature using a stabilization device. Physiother Theory Pract. 2007;23(2):119–24.

53. Kollock Jr RO, Onate JA, Van Lunen B. The reliability of portable fixed dynamometry during hip and knee strength assessments. J Athl Train. 2010;45(4):349–56.

54. Scott DA, Bond EQ, Sisto SA, Nadler SF. The intra- and interrater reliability of hip muscle strength assessments using a handheld versus a portable dynamometer anchoring station. Arch Phys Med Rehabil. 2004;85(4):598–603.

55. Toonstra J, Mattacola CG. Test-retest reliability and validity of isometric knee-flexion and -extension measurement using 3 methods of assessing muscle strength. J Sport Rehabil 2013;Technical Notes(7). pii: 2012–0017.

56. Burden A, Bartlett R. Normalisation of EMG amplitude: an evaluation and comparison of old and new methods. Med Eng Phys. 1999;21(4):247–57.

57. Burden A. How should we normalize electromyographs obtained from healthy participants? What we have learned from over 25 years of research. J Electromyogr Kinesiol. 2010;20(6):1023–35.

58. Hunter AM, St Clair Gibson A, Lambert M, Noakes TD. Electromyographic (EMG) normalization method for cycle fatigue protocol. Med Sci Sports Exerc. 2002;34(5):857–61.

59. Clark BC, Cook SB, Ploutz-Snyder LL. Reliability of techniques to assess human neuromuscular function in vivo. J Electromyogr Kinesiol. 2007;17(1):90–101.

60. Warth RJ, Spiegl UJ, Millett PJ. Scapulothoracic bursitis and snapping scapula syndrome: a critical review of current evidence. Am J Sports Med. 2014;43:236–45.

61. Lindman R, Eriksson A, Thornell LE. Fiber type composition of the human female trapezius muscle: enzyme-histochemical characteristics. Am J Anat. 1991;190(4):385–92.

62. Lindman R, Eriksson A, Thornell LE. Fiber type composition of the human male trapezius muscle: enzyme-histochemical characteristics. Am J Anat. 1990;189(3):236–44.

63. Inman VT, Saunders JB, Abbott LC. Observations of the function of the shoulder joint. J Bone Joint Surg. 1944;26A:1–31.

64. Johnson GR, Spalding D, Nowitzke A, Bogduk N. Modelling the muscles of the scapula morphometric and coordinate data and functional implications. J Biomech. 1996;29(8):1039–51.

65. Schickendantz MS, Ho CP, Keppler L, Shaw MD. MR imaging of the thrower's shoulder. Internal impingement, latissimus dorsi/subscapularis strains, and related injuries. Magn Reson Imaging Clin N Am. 1999;7(1):39–49.

66. Kibler WB, Sciascia A, Uhl T. Medial scapular muscle detachment: clinical presentation and surgical treatment. J Shoulder Elbow Surg. 2013;23(1):58–67.

67. Kibler WB. The role of the scapula in athletic shoulder function. Am J Sports Med. 1998;26(2):325–37.
68. Mottram SL. Dynamic stability of the scapula. Man Ther. 1997;2(3):123–31.
69. Wadsworth DJ, Bullock-Saxton JE. Recruitment pattern of the scapula rotator muscles in freestyle swimmers with subacromial impingement. Int J Sports Med. 1997;18(8):618–24.
70. Ruwe PA, Pink M, Jobe FW, Perry J, Scovazzo ML. The normal and the painful shoulders during the breaststroke. Electromyographic and cinematographic analysis of twelve muscles. Am J Sports Med. 1994;22(6):789–96.
71. McFarland EG. Examination of the shoulder: the complete guide. New York: Thieme Medical Publishers, Inc; 2006.
72. Ekstrom RA, Soderberg GL, Donatelli RA. Normalization procedures using maximum voluntary isometric contractions for the serratus anterior and trapezius muscles during surface EMG analysis. J Electromyogr Kinesiol. 2005;15(4):418–28.
73. Ekstrom RA, Donatelli RA, Soderberg GL. Surface electromyographic analysis of exercises for the trapezius and serratus anterior muscles. J Orthop Sports Phys Ther. 2003;33(5):247–58.
74. Moseley Jr JB, Jobe FW, Pink M, Perry J, Tibone J. EMG analysis of the scapula muscles during a shoulder rehabilitation program. Am J Sports Med. 1992;20(2):128–34.
75. DePalma AF. Origin and comparative anatomy of the pectoral limb. In: DePalma AF, editor. Surgery of the shoulder. Philadelphia, PA: Lippincott Williams & Wilkins; 1950. p. 1–14.
76. Smith J, Padgett DJ, Kaufman KR, Harrington SP, An KN, Irby SE. Rhomboid muscle electromyography activity during 3 different manual muscle tests. Arch Phys Med Rehabil. 2004;85(6):987–92.
77. Park SY, Yoo WG. Activation of the serratus anterior and upper trapezius in a population with winged and tipped scapulae during push-up-plus and diagonal shoulder-elevation. J Back Musculoskelet Rehabil 2014 [Epub ahead of print].
78. Celik D, Sirmen B, Demirhan M. The relationship of muscle strength and pain in subacromial impingement syndrome. Acta Orthop Traumatol Turc. 2011;45(2):79–84.
79. Pink M, Jobe FW, Perry J, Browne A, Scovazzo ML, Kerrigan J. The painful shoulder during the butterfly stroke. An electromyographic and cinematographic analysis of twelve muscles. Clin Orthop Relat Res. 1993;288:60–72.
80. Pink M, Jobe FW, Perry J, Kerrigan J, Browne A, Scovazzo ML. The normal shoulder during the butterfly swim stroke. An electromyographic and cinematographic analysis of twelve muscles. Clin Orthop Relat Res. 1993;288:48–59.
81. Pink M, Perry J, Browne A, Scovazzo ML, Kerrigan J. The normal shoulder during freestyle swimming. An electromyographic and cinematographic analysis of twelve muscles. Am J Sports Med. 1991;19(6):569–76.
82. Scovazzo ML, Browne A, Pink M, Jobe FW, Kerrigan J. The painful shoulder during freestyle swimming. An electromyographic cinematographic analysis of twelve muscles. Am J Sports Med. 1991;19(6):577–82.
83. Glousman R. Electromyographic analysis and its role in the athletic shoulder. Clin Orthop Relat Res. 1993;288:27–34.
84. Burkhart SS, Morgan CD, Kibler WB. The disabled throwing shoulder: spectrum of pathology Part III: the SICK scapula, scapular dyskinesis, the kinetic chain, and rehabilitation. Arthroscopy. 2003;19(6):641–61.
85. Pouliart N, Gagey N. Significance of the latissimus dorsi for shoulder instability. II. Its influence on dislocation behavior in a sequential cutting protocol of the glenohumeral capsule. Clin Anat. 2005;18(7):500–9.
86. Pouliart N, Gagey N. Significance of the latissimus dorsi for shoulder instability. I. Variations in its anatomy around the humerus and scapula. Clin Anat. 2005;18(7):493–9.
87. Schachter AK, McHugh MP, Tyler TF, Kreminic IJ, Orishimo KF, Johnson C, Ben-Avi S, Nicholas SJ. Electromyographic activity of selected scapular stabilizers during glenohumeral internal and external rotation contractions. J Shoulder Elbow Surg. 2010;19(6):884–90.
88. Laudner KG, Williams JG. The relationship between latissimus dorsi stiffness and altered scapular kinematics among asymptomatic collegiate swimmers. Phys Ther Sport. 2013;14(1):50–3.
89. Park SY, Yoo WG. Comparison of exercises inducing maximum voluntary isometric contraction for the latissimus dorsi using surface electromyography. J Electromyogr Kinesiol. 2013;23(5):1106–10.
90. Nagda SH, Cohen SB, Noonan TJ, Raasch WG, Ciccotti MG, Yocum LA. Management and outcomes of latissimus dorsi and teres major injuries in professional baseball pitchers. Am J Sports Med. 2011;39(10):2181–6.
91. Nobuhara K. The shoulder: its function and clinical aspects, vol. 1. Singapore: World Scientific Publishing; 2001.
92. Scheving LE, Pauly JE. An electromyographic study of some muscles acting on the upper extremity of man. Anat Rec. 1959;135:239–45.
93. Schickendantz MS, Kaar SG, Meister K, Lund P, Beverley L. Latissimus dorsi and teres major tears in professional baseball pitchers: a case series. Am J Sports Med. 2009;37(10):2016–20.
94. Curtis AS, Burbank KM, Tierney JJ, Scheller AD, Curran AR. The insertional footprint of the rotator cuff: an anatomic study. Arthroscopy 2006;22(6):609.e1.
95. Dugas JR, Campbell DA, Warren RR, Robie BH, Millett PJ. Anatomy and dimensions of rotator cuff insertions. J Shoulder Elbow Surg. 2002;11(5): 498–503.
96. Minagawa H, Itoi E, Konno N, Kido T, Sano A, Urayama M, Sato K. Humeral attachment of the supraspinatus and infraspinatus tendons: an anatomic study. Arthroscopy. 1998;14(3):302–6.

97. Mochizuki T, Sugaya H, Uomizu M, Maeda K, Matsuki K, Sekiya I, Muneta T, Akita K. Humeral insertion of the supraspinatus and infraspinatus. New anatomic findings regarding the footprint of the rotator cuff. J Bone Joint Surg Am. 2008;90(5): 962–9.

98. Roh MS, Wang VM, April EW, Pollock RG, Bigliani LU, Flatow EL. Anterior and posterior musculotendinous anatomy of the supraspinatus. J Shoulder Elbow Surg. 2000;9(5):436–40.

99. Ruotolo C, Fow JE, Nottage WM. The supraspinatus footprint: an anatomic study of the supraspinatus insertion. Arthroscopy. 2004;20(3):246–9.

100. Volk AG, Vangsness Jr CT. An anatomic study of the supraspinatus muscle and tendon. Clin Orthop Relat Res. 2001;384:280–5.

101. Jobe FW. Operative techniques in upper extremity sports injuries. St. Louis: Mosby; 1996.

102. Blackburn TA, McLeod WD, White B, Wofford L. EMG analysis of posterior rotator cuff exercise. Athl Train. 1990;25(1):40–5.

103. Malanga GA, Jenp YN, Growney EW, An KN. EMG analysis of shoulder positioning in testing and strengthening of the supraspinatus. Med Sci Sports Exerc. 1996;28(6):661–4.

104. Colachis Jr SC, Strohm BR, Brechner VL. Effects of axillary nerve block on muscle force in the upper extremity. Arch Phys Med Rehabil. 1969;50(11): 647–54.

105. Colachis Jr SC, Strohm BR. Effect of suprascapular and axillary nerve blocks on muscle force in upper extremity. Arch Phys Med Rehabil. 1971;52(1): 22–9.

106. Burkhart SS. Arthroscopic treatment of massive rotator cuff tears: clinical results and biomechanical rationale. Clin Orthop Relat Res. 1991;267:45–56.

107. Lajtai G, Wieser K, Ofner M, Raimann G, Aitzetmüller G, Jost B. Electromyography and nerve conduction velocity for the evaluation of the infraspinatus muscle and the suprascapular nerve in professional beach volleyball players. Am J Sports Med. 2012;40(10):2303–8.

108. Niemann A, Juzeszyn S, Kahanov L, E Eberman L. Suprascapular neuropathy in a collegiate baseball player. Asian J Sports Med 2013;4(1):L76-81.

109. Kolbe AB, Collins MS, Sperling JW. Severe atrophy and fatty degeneration of the infraspinatus muscle due to isolated infraspinatus tendon tear. Skeletal Radiol. 2012;41(1):107–10.

110. Beeler S, Ek ET, Gerber C. A comparative analysis of fatty infiltration and muscle atrophy in patients with chronic rotator cuff tears and suprascapular neuropathy. J Shoulder Elbow Surg. 2013;22(11): 1537–46.

111. Dramis A, Pimpalnerkar A. Suprascapular neuropathy in volleyball players. Acta Orthop Belg. 2005;71(3):269–72.

112. Ferretti A, Cerullo G, Russo G. Suprascapular neuropathy in volleyball players. J Bone Joint Surg Am. 1987;69(2):260–3.

113. Ferretti A, De Carli A, Fontana M. Injury of the suprascapular nerve at the spinoglenoid notch. The natural history of infraspinatus atrophy in volleyball players. Am J Sports Med. 1998;26(6):759–63.

114. Sandow MJ, Ilic J. Suprascapular nerve rotator cuff compression syndrome in volleyball players. J Shoulder Elbow Surg. 1998;7(5):516–21.

115. Ringel SP, Treihaft M, Carry M, Fisher R, Jacobs P. Suprascapular neuropathy in pitchers. Am J Sports Med. 1990;18(1):80–6.

116. Smith AN. Suprascapular neuropathy in a collegiate pitcher. J Athl Train. 1995;30(1):43–6.

117. Greis PE, Kuhn JE, Schultheis J, Hintermeister R, Hawkins R. Validation of the lift-off test and analysis of subscapularis activity during maximal internal rotation. Am J Sports Med. 1996;24(5): 589–93.

118. Chang YW, Hughes RE, Su FC, Itoi E, An KN. Prediction of muscle force involved in shoulder internal rotation. J Shoulder Elbow Surg. 2000;9(3): 188–95.

119. Suenaga N, Minami A, Fujisawa H. Electromyographic analysis of internal rotational motion of the shoulder in various arm positions. J Shoulder Elbow Surg. 2003;12(5):501–5.

120. Jenp YN, Malanga GA, Growney ES, An KN. Activation of the rotator cuff in generating isometric shoulder rotation torque. Am J Sports Med. 1996;24(4):477–85.

121. Stefko JM, Jobe FW, VanderWilde RS, Carden E, Pink M. Electromyographic and nerve block analysis of the subscapularis liftoff test. J Shoulder Elbow Surg. 1997;6(4):347–55.

122. Gerber C, Krushell RJ. Isolated rupture of the tendon of the subscapularis muscle. Clinical features in 16 cases. J Bone Joint Surg Br. 1991;73(3):389–94.

123. Millett PJ, Schoenahl JY, Allen MJ, Motta T, Gaskill TR. An association between the inferior humeral head osteophyte and teres minor fatty infiltration: evidence for axillary nerve entrapment in glenohumeral osteoarthritis. J Shoulder Elbow Surg. 2013; 22(2):215–21.

124. Iamsaard S, Thunyaharn N, Chaisiwamongkol K, Boonruangsri P, Uabundit N, Hipkaeo W. Variant insertion of the teres major muscle. Anat Cell Biol. 2012;45(3):211–3.

125. Pearl ML, Perry J, Torburn L, Gordon LH. An electromyographic analysis of the shoulder during cones and planes of arm motion. Clin Orthop Relat Res. 1992;284:116–27.

126. Campbell ST, Ecklund KJ, Chu EH, McGarry MH, Gupta R, Lee TQ. The role of pectoralis major and latissimus dorsi muscles in a biomechanical model of massive rotator cuff tear. J Shoulder Elbow Surg. 2014;23:1136–42.

127. Henseler JF, Nagels J, van der Zwaal P, Nelissen RG. Teres major tendon transfer for patients with massive irreparable posterosuperior rotator cuff tears: short-term clinical results. Bone Joint J. 2013; 95-B(4):523–9.

128. Omid R, Lee B. Tendon transfers for irreparable rotator cuff tears. J Am Acad Orthop Surg. 2013;21(8):492–501.
129. Villacis D, Merriman J, Wong K, Rick Hatch 3rd GF. Latissimus dorsi tendon transfer for irreparable rotator cuff tears: a modified technique using arthroscopy. Arthrosc Tech. 2013;2(1):e27–30.
130. Grosclaude M, Najihi N, Lädermann A, Menetrey J, Ziltener JL. Teres major muscle tear in two professional ice hockey players: case study and literature review. Orthop Traumatol Surg Res. 2012;98(1):122–5.
131. Maldjian C, Adam R, Oxberry B, Chew F, Kelly J. Isolated tear of the teres major: a waterskiing injury. J Comput Assist Tomogr. 2000;24(4):594–5.
132. Lee SB, An KN. Dynamic glenohumeral stability provided by three heads of the deltoid muscle. Clin Orthop Relat Res. 2002;400:40–7.
133. Yanagawa T, Goodwin CJ, Shelburne KB, Giphart JE, Torry MR, Pandy MG. Contributions of the individual muscles of the shoulder to glenohumeral joint stability during abduction. J Biomech Eng. 2008;130(2):021024.
134. Bertelli JA, Ghizoni MF. Abduction in internal rotation: a test for the diagnosis of axillary nerve palsy. J Hand Surg Am. 2011;36(12):2017–23.
135. Fujihara Y, Doi K, Dodakundi C, Hattori Y, Sakamoto S, Takagi T. Simple clinical test to detect deltoid muscle dysfunction causing weakness of abduction–"akimbo" test. J Reconstr Microsurg. 2012;28(6):375. -379.
136. Dirim B, Brouha SS, Pretterklieber ML, Wolff KS, Frank A, Pathria MN, Chung CB. Terminal bifurcation of the biceps brachii muscle and tendon: anatomic considerations and clinical implications. AJR Am J Roentgenol. 2008;191(6):W248–55.
137. Kervancioglu P, Orhan M. An anatomical study on the three-headed biceps brachii in human fetuses, and clinical relevance. Folia Morphol (Warsz). 2011;70(2):116–20.
138. Lee SE, Jung C, Ahn KY, Nam KI. Bilateral asymmetric supernumerary heads of biceps brachii. Anat Cell Biol. 2011;44(3):238–40.
139. Poudel PP, Bhattarai C. Study on the supernumerary heads of the biceps brachii muscle in Nepalese. Nepal Med Coll J. 2009;11(2):96–8.
140. Logan PM, Janzen D, Connell DG. Tear of the distal biceps tendon presenting as an antecubital mass: magnetic resonance imaging appearances. Can Assoc Radiol J. 1996;47(5):342–6.
141. Tantisricharoenkul G, Tan EW, Fayad LM, McCarthy EF, McFarland EG. Malignant soft tissue tumors of the biceps muscle mistaken for proximal biceps tendon rupture. Orthopedics. 2012;35(10):e1548–52.
142. Bennett GE. Elbow and shoulder lesions of baseball players. Am J Surg. 1959;98:484–92.
143. Huemer GM, Puelzl P, Schoeller T. Breast and chest wall reconstruction with the transverse musculocutaneous gracilis flap in Poland syndrome. Plast Reconstr Surg. 2012;130(4):779–83.
144. La Marca S, Delay E, Toussoun G, Ho Quoc C, Sinna R. [Treatment of Poland syndrome thorax deformity with the lipomodeling technique: about ten cases]. Ann Chir Plast Esthet 2013;58(1):60–8.
145. Nishibayashi A, Tomita K, Yano K, Hosokawa K. Correction of complex chest wall deformity in Poland's syndrome using a modified Nuss procedure. J Plast Reconstr Aesthet Surg. 2013;66(2):e53–5.
146. Hasegawa K, Schofer JM. Rupture of the pectoralis major: a case report and review. J Emerg Med. 2010;38(2):196–200.
147. Jones MW, Matthews JP. Rupture of the pectoralis major in weight lifters: a case report and review of the literature. Injury. 1988;19(3):219.
148. DiVeta J, Walker ML, Skibinski B. Relationship between performance of selected scapular muscles and scapular abduction in standing subjects. Phys Ther. 1990;70(8):470–9.
149. Boyd S. Congenital absence of chondro-sternal portion of right pectoralis major and the greater part of pectoralis minor. Proc R Soc Med 1911;4(Clin Sect):84–5.
150. Mehallo CJ. Isolated tear of the pectoralis minor. Clin J Sports Med. 2004;14(4):245–56.
151. Mysnyk MC, Johnson DE. Congenital absence of the pectoralis muscles in two collegiate wrestling champions. Clin Orthop Relat Res. 1991;265:183–6.
152. Paladini P, Campi F, Merolla G, Pellegrini A, Porcellini G. Pectoralis minor tendon transfer for irreparable anterosuperior cuff tears. J Shoulder Elbow Surg. 2013;22(6):e1–5.
153. Sanders RJ, Rao NM. The forgotten pectoralis minor syndrome: 100 operations for pectoralis minor syndrome alone or accompanied by neurogenic thoracic outlet syndrome. Ann Vasc Surg. 2010;24(6):701–8.
154. Vemuri C, Wittenberg AM, Caputo FJ, Earley JA, Driskill MR, Rastogi R, Emery VB, Thompson RW. Early effectiveness of isolated pectoralis minor tenotomy in selected patients with neurogenic thoracic outlet syndrome. J Vasc Surg. 2013;57(5):1345–52.
155. Borstad JD, Ludewig PM. The effect of long versus short pectoralis minor resting length on scapular kinematics in healthy individuals. J Orthop Sports Phys Ther. 2005;35(4):227–38.
156. Muraki T, Aoki M, Izumi T, Fujii M, Hidaka E, Miyamoto S. Lengthening of the pectoralis minor muscle during passive shoulder motions and stretching techniques: a cadaveric biomechanical study. Phys Ther. 2009;89(4):333–41.
157. Hébert LJ, Moffet H, McFadyen BJ, Dionne CE. Scapular behavior in shoulder impingement syndrome. Arch Phys Med Rehabil. 2002;83(1):60–9.
158. Ludewig PM, Cook TM. Alterations in shoulder kinematics and associated muscle activity in people with symptoms of shoulder impingement. Phys Ther. 2000;80(3):276–91.

159. Lukasiewicz AC, McClure P, Michener L, Pratt N, Sennett B. Comparison of 3-dimensional scapular position and orientation between subjects with and without shoulder impingement. J Orthop Sports Phys Ther. 1999;29(10):574–83.

160. Bhatia DN, de Beer JF, van Rooyen KS, Lam F, du Toit DF. The "bench-presser's shoulder": an overuse insertional tendinopathy of the pectoralis minor muscle. Br J Sports Med. 2007; 41(8):e11.

161. Ribeiro F, Oliveira J. Factors influencing proprioception: what do they reveal? In: Klika V, editor. Biomechanics in applications. InTech, 2011. doi:10.5772/20335. ISBN: 978-953-307-969-1. Available from: http://www.intechopen.com/books/ biomechanics-in-applications/factors-influencing-proprioception-what-do-they-reveal.

162. Spiegl UJ, Warth RJ, Millett PJ. Symptomatic internal impingement of the shoulder in overhead athletes. Sports Med Arthrosc. 2014;22(2):120–9.

163. Dodson CC, Williams III RJ. Traumatic shoulder muscle ruptures. In: Johnson DL, Mair SD, editors. Clinical sports medicine. Philadelphia: Elsevier; 2006. Chapter 30.

Rotator Cuff Disorders

4

4.1 Introduction

Rotator cuff disease ranks among the most common musculoskeletal disorders to be encountered in clinical practice. As a result, we have witnessed a rapid evolution in diagnostic methods and treatment options for the entire spectrum of rotator cuff disorders over the past few decades.

The derangement of normal anatomy and subsequent rotator cuff impingement is often cited as the primary cause for rotator cuff disease. However, the undersurface of the coracoacromial arch may not always be the culprit in this complex array of syndromes. Traumatic events, repetitive microtrauma, and glenohumeral instability may also be causative in a large proportion of patients. These factors, among others, are important to consider when evaluating the patient with a suspected rotator cuff lesion.

Therefore, proficiency in the physical diagnosis of various rotator cuff lesions requires a solid differential diagnosis, an appreciation of normal anatomy and biomechanics and the awareness that surrounding structures involved with normal function may also contribute to pathologic conditions. This is important not only for the initial examination by the treating physician, but also for the teams of individuals who care for these patients.

4.2 Anatomy and Biomechanics

The rotator cuff is often conceptualized as being composed of four separate muscles, tendons, and insertion sites that each has its designated functions. However, in reality, although each muscle belly arises from different areas of the scapular body, their tendons converge and coalesce to form a single, continuous tendon sheet that inserts upon the greater and lesser tuberosities of the proximal humerus (Fig. 4.1). This structural configuration suggests that the individual muscles of the rotator cuff work simultaneously and in synchrony to achieve its primary function—to dynamically stabilize and compress the humeral head within the glenoid fossa [2].

Maintenance of a stable fulcrum requires balanced axial and coronal plane force couples (Fig. 4.2) [3, 4]. This concept, initially developed by Burkhart [4] in 1991, is produced by the strategic anatomic positioning of the muscles around the shoulder. Specifically, the combined actions of the anterior cuff (i.e., the subscapularis) and the posterior cuff (i.e., the infraspinatus) work to compress the humeral head within the glenoid fossa due to their parallel force vectors in the axial plane. In the coronal plane, contraction of each rotator cuff muscle and the deltoid muscle also generates a net force vector that drives the humeral head medially against the glenoid.

R.J. Warth and P.J. Millett, *Physical Examination of the Shoulder: An Evidence-Based Approach*,
DOI 10.1007/978-1-4939-2593-3_4, © Springer Science+Business Media New York 2015

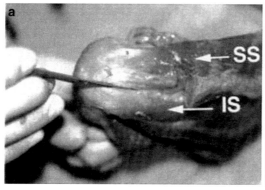
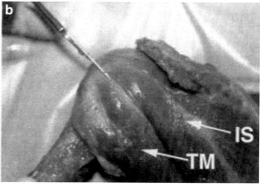

Fig. 4.1 Cadaveric dissection photographs demonstrating the coalescence of the rotator cuff tendons as they approach their respective insertion sites on the humerus. (**a**) View from posterosuperiorly showing the approximate interval between the supraspinatus (SS) and the infraspinatus (IS). (**b**) View from posteriorly showing the approximately interval between the infraspinatus (IS) and teres minor (TM). (From Dugas et al. [1]; with permission).

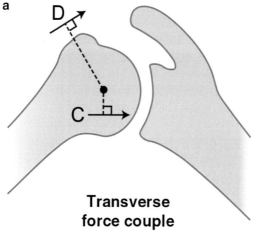
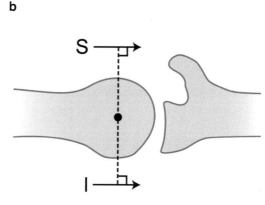

Fig. 4.2 Illustration highlighting the important force couples that help maintain concavity compression and overall glenohumeral stability. (**a**) The combined actions of the deltoid muscle (D) and the rotator cuff (C) make up the transverse plane force couple and pull the humeral head medially towards the glenoid fossa. (**b**) The combined actions of the subscapularis (S) and the infraspinatus (I) make up the axial plane force couple and also work to drive the humeral head medially towards the glenoid fossa.

Disruption of any of these force couples, as in the case of a rotator cuff tear or deltoid weakness, can produce disordered shoulder function through a variety of mechanisms. This concept led to the biomechanical principle of concavity compression, described by Lippitt and Matsen [5] in 1993, in which the balanced, parallel force couples generated by the rotator cuff and deltoid compress the convex humeral head into the concave glenoid fossa thereby enhancing glenohumeral stability in the mid-ranges of motion. In addition to providing a stable fulcrum for motion, balanced force couples (with resulting concavity compression) improve glenohumeral stability by increasing the force and degree of humeral angulation required for the humeral head to translate over the glenoid rim in any direction (i.e., an increased balance stability angle, as discussed in Chap. 6). It is easy to imagine that disruption of axial or coronal plane force couples would result in dysfunction of the concavity compression mechanism leading to scapular dyskinesis and

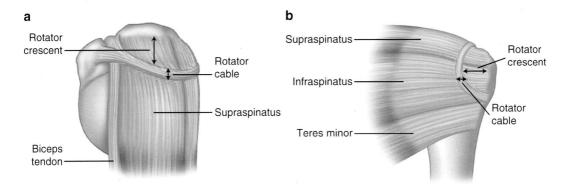

Fig. 4.3 (**a**) Superior and (**b**) posterior view illustrating the position of the rotator cable. The rotator cable is a thickened area of the rotator cuff that provides a path for force dispersion which helps to prevent tension overload within the rotator crescent (the area of tendon surrounded by the rotator cable).

subsequent shoulder discomfort (see Chap. 9 for more information on scapular dyskinesis and its relationship with rotator cuff tears).

The rotator cable, described by Burkhart [3] in 1993 as a part of the "suspension bridge model," is a thickened area of tendon that extends across the supraspinatus and infraspinatus tendons which biomechanically allows their respective forces of contraction to disperse along the length of the cable, eventually concentrating at its anterior and posterior insertion sites (Fig. 4.3). The rotator cable surrounds a crescent-shaped area of tendon (i.e., the rotator crescent) that is somewhat protected from the strong forces produced by the supraspinatus and infraspinatus tendons as a result of the function of the rotator cable. The force couple principle in combination with the function of the rotator cable may provide an explanation as to why some patients are able to maintain adequate shoulder function despite the presence of a large full-thickness supraspinatus tear. However, recent evidence suggests that the load-sharing capability of the rotator cuff is diminished in the presence of a partial- or full-thickness tear which subsequently promotes tear extension [6, 7]. In other words, the defect in the cuff tendon decreases the available area required to disperse normal tensile forces produced by muscle contraction. Because these normal contraction forces must be transmitted (and redirected) through a smaller area of intact tendon, the magnitude of stress concentration along the margins of the cuff tear increases exponentially as the size of the tear increases.

Anterior or posterior extension of a rotator cuff tear can also occur as a result of the disruption of balanced force couples. A study by Hughes and An [8] found that normal supraspinatus tendons exerted a maximum force of approximately 175 N whereas normal infraspinatus tendons exerted a maximum force of greater than 900 N. This has important implications for the development and progression of rotator cuff tears—posterior extension of a tear into the infraspinatus tendon dramatically increases the force applied to the remaining intact tendon sheet which can accelerate tear progression. Because the force exerted by the infraspinatus must be similar to that of the subscapularis to maintain balanced force couples, this concept of tear extension can also be applied anteriorly into the subscapularis muscle. Thus, anterior or posterior extension of a rotator cuff tear into the subscapularis and/or the infraspinatus tendons, respectively, disrupts the balance of native force couples which also accelerates tear progression. Longitudinal (or medial) tear extension of the supraspinatus with or without retraction can also disrupt glenohumeral kinematics; however, the pathomechanism typically involves proximal humeral head migration, highlighting the importance of the rotator cuff as a dynamic depressor of the humeral head (Fig. 4.4).

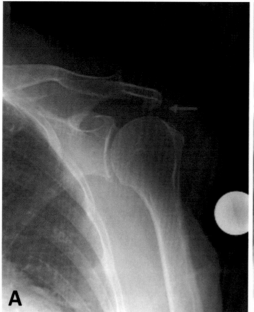
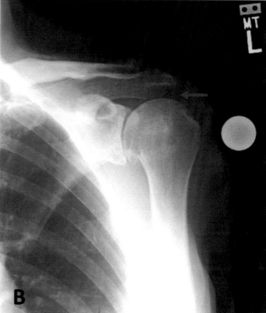

Fig. 4.4 (**a**) Anteroposterior (AP) radiograph demonstrating a normal acromiohumeral distance (*red arrow*) in a patient with an intact rotator cuff. (**b**) AP radiograph of a patient with a massive rotator cuff tear. Proximal migration of the humerus and a subsequent decrease in the acromiohumeral distance (*red arrow*) can be seen.

4.3 Subacromial Impingement

Subacromial impingement is one of the most common causes of shoulder pain encountered in clinical practice. In the past, some authors believed impingement was the result of extrinsic factors, citing various potential sources of external cuff compression [9–11]. Others believed the disorder was related to intrinsic cuff degeneration, leading to cuff weakness and proximal humeral migration followed by cuff abrasion under the acromion [12]. However, recent thinking suggests that subacromial impingement is likely multifactorial involving a combination of both intrinsic and extrinsic factors that ultimately lead to rotator cuff disease.

4.3.1 Pathogenesis Involving Extrinsic Factors

Neer [10] originally described subacromial impingement as the repeated contact between the greater tuberosity and the undersurface of the acromion and coracoacromial ligament (Figs. 4.5 and 4.6). He hypothesized that this repetitive mechanical impingement led to the development of proliferative anterolateral acromial spurs. He subsequently dissected 100 cadaveric shoulders and again revealed these traction spurs on the anterolateral acromion. With this finding, he proposed that anterior acromioplasty should be performed to prevent impingement and subsequent bursitis and rotator cuff disease. Later, realizing that subacromial impingement likely involves a continuum of disease processes, Neer [10] described three basic stages in the development of impingement syndrome. Stage I of impingement, occurring asymptomatically in patients younger than 25 years of age, involves subacromial edema, hemorrhage, and bursitis. Between the ages of 25 and 40, continued impingement results in rotator cuff fibrosis and tendinitis, eliminating the normal lubricating effect of the subacromial bursa. Beyond the age of 40 years, continued impingement becomes more symptomatic with the development of acromial spurs along with partial- and full-thickness rotator cuff tears.

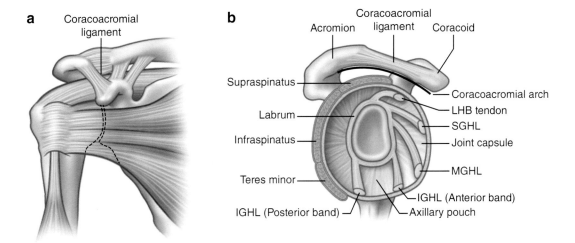

Fig. 4.5 (**a**) Anterior view of the coracoacromial ligament with the rotator cuff musculature passing closely beneath. (**b**) Sagittal view of the coracoacromial arch which is made up of the anterolateral acromion, coracoacromial ligament, and the posterior aspect of the coracoid. With the humeral head removed, the rotator cuff musculature can be seen traveling closely beneath the coracoacromial arch.

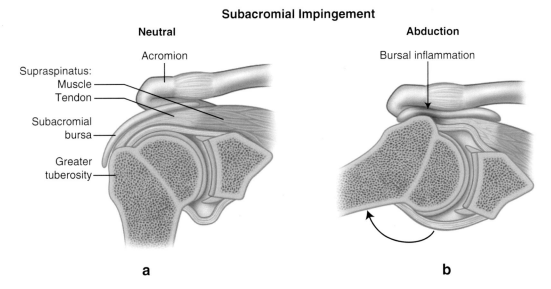

Fig. 4.6 (**a**) Anteroposterior (AP) cross-section view of the shoulder illustrating the position of the supraspinatus muscle-tendon unit and the subacromial bursa relative to the inferior acromion when the humerus is in a neutral resting position. (**b**) When the humerus is elevated, the supraspinatus and subacromial bursa can make contact with the undersurface of the acromion, often resulting in rotator cuff pathology with impingement-like symptoms.

Neer's description of the stages of impingement syndrome is one of the most popular pathomechanistic explanations behind the development of chronic rotator cuff disease. While there are several studies that support this mechanism [11, 13, 14], the precise etiology and location of subacromial impingement is debatable.

Fig. 4.7 Axillary radiograph demonstrating os acromiale (*yellow arrow*). This patient presented to our clinic with impingement-like symptoms.

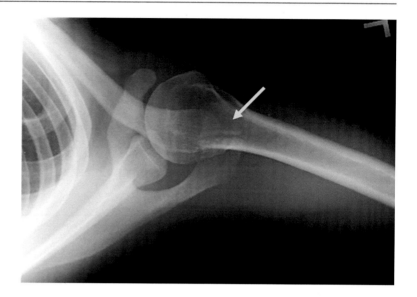

4.3.1.1 Coracoacromial Ligament

The coracoacromial ligament originates from the distal-lateral extension of the coracoid process and travels posterosuperiorly to insert upon the anterolateral margin of the acromion [15, 16]. As part of the coracoacromial arch, this ligament is commonly described as being involved with rotator cuff impingement lesions due to the proximity of the cuff tendons that pass closely beneath, especially as the arm is elevated. The coracoacromial ligament has a number of anatomic variations [17–19]; however, only those variations that involve a distinct anterolateral and posteromedial bundle are likely to be related to rotator cuff impingement and subsequent tearing. In a cadaveric study, Fremery et al. [20] found that shoulders with rotator cuff tears and clinical evidence of impingement had stronger, thicker anterolateral bands compared to shoulders with unrelated issues. Evidence of traction spur formation within the anterolateral band has also been found which further implicates its involvement with the development of impingement [21]. Chambler et al. [22] suggested that arm abduction results in increased tension of the coracoacromial ligament which may provide an explanation for the development of traction spurs in these patients. A more recent cadaveric study by Yamamoto et al. [23] found that the superior cuff made contact with and, in fact, generated increased tension through the coracoacromial ligament during range of motion testing in a series of normal, healthy shoulders. This finding may provide at least one possible explanation behind the development of traction-type spurs on the anterolateral acromion with advancing age, potentially leading to extrinsic compression of the superior cuff tendons. However, whether or not the thickness of the anterolateral band is a cause or effect of rotator cuff disease has not been elucidated.

4.3.1.2 Os Acromiale

The acromion is also subject to developmental abnormalities as a result of failed fusion of secondary ossification centers. This failed fusion results in a defect known as an "os acromiale" and occurs in approximately 8 % of the population where 1/3 of these individuals are affected bilaterally [24]. Os acromiale is a mobile accessory ossicle that, when unstable and pulled inferiorly by contraction of the deltoid with arm elevation, has been associated with the development of identifiable impingement lesions and pain at the top of the shoulder (Fig. 4.7). However, this relationship has been refuted on several occasions [25–29]. In addition, surgical treatment strategies for os acromiale that involve increasing the volume of the subacromial space has not resulted in an improvement in clinical outcomes [26]. Further study is therefore needed to clarify the effects of os acromiale on normal rotator cuff tendons.

Fig. 4.8 Illustration of the three types of acromial morphologies as described by Bigliani et al. [30]. Type I: Flat acromion. Type II: Curved acromion. Type III: Hooked acromion. Patients with a type III hooked acromion may have an increased propensity to develop subacromial impingement and rotator cuff disease.

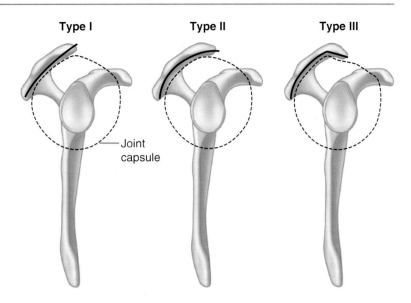

4.3.1.3 Acromial Morphology and Glenoid Version

The anterior aspect of the acromion may, in itself, be a potential site of rotator cuff abrasion and subsequent tearing regardless of the presence or absence of space-occupying traction spurs associated with the coracoacromial ligament. In 1991, Bigliani et al. [30] described the three most common acromial morphologies as flat (type I), curved (type II), and hooked (type III), citing the hooked acromion as most relevant to the development of subacromial impingement (Fig. 4.8). In a cadaveric study, Flatow et al. [13] demonstrated that the type III acromion has an increased propensity to make contact with the rotator cuff tendons when compared to the other acromial morphologies that were previously described by Bigliani et al. [30]. Wang et al. [31] found that acromial morphology influenced the success of conservative management for rotator cuff tears. In their study, the majority of patients with either a type I or II acromion responded favorably to conservative management. In contrast, more than half of those patients with a type III acromion failed nonoperative treatment and required subsequent surgical intervention. Unfortunately, these authors did not report their findings at the time of surgery. In another study, Gill et al. [14] found that acromial morphology was an independent factor associated with the development of

rotator cuff pathology using multivariate logistic regression analysis. Additionally, Natsis et al. [32] found a statistically significant increase in the rate of anterolateral acromial spur formation in those with a type III acromion. They concluded that a type III acromion with anterolateral spur formation was contributing factor associated with the development of rotator cuff impingement and tearing. In 2012, Hamid et al. [33] arrived at similar conclusions. However, despite these results, there are also a number of studies that refute the oft-cited correlation between the type III acromion and the development or progression of rotator cuff tears [17, 31, 34–38]. As a result of this conflicting data, further study is needed to determine if acromial morphology, as described by Bigliani et al [30], is truly associated with the development of symptomatic subacromial impingement and rotator cuff tears.

More recently, other acromial morphologies have been also been described—namely, the convex acromion (type IV; as described by Vanarthos and Monu [39] as an addendum to the original classification system developed by Bigliani et al. [30] Fig. 4.9) and the keeled acromion (originally described by Tucker and Snyder [41] Fig. 4.10). While the type IV acromion has not been implicated as an anatomic factor associated with rotator cuff disease, the keeled acromion may be involved to some extent. The keeled acromion,

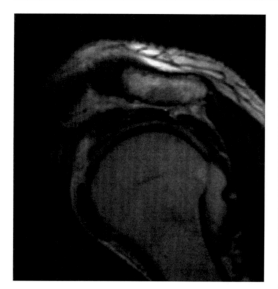

Fig. 4.9 Magnetic resonance image (MRI) demonstrating a type IV convex acromion as described by Vanarthos and Monu [39]. Although a common variant, this acromial morphology has not been associated with rotator cuff disease in the literature. (From Sanders and Miller [40]; with permission).

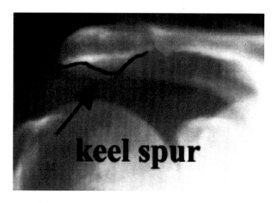

Fig. 4.10 Anteroposterior (AP) radiograph demonstrating a keeled acromion as described by Tucker and Snyder [41]. This acromial morphology may have some involvement in the development of subacromial impingement, although further study is needed to substantiate this claim (From Tucker and Snyder [41]; with permission).

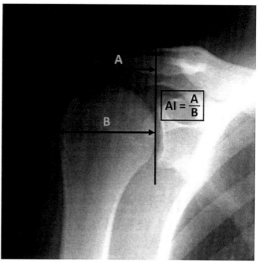

Fig. 4.11 True anteroposterior (AP) radiograph demonstrating measurement of the acromial index. A first line is drawn connecting the superior and inferior rims of the glenoid and extended superiorly such that the line completely crosses the acromion. A second line is drawn vertically that corresponds with the most lateral extent of the acromion. The distance between the first line and the second line is labeled "A." A third line is drawn vertically that corresponds with the most lateral extent of the greater tuberosity. The distance between this third line and the first line is labeled "B." The ratio of A/B is equal to the acromial index. Theories exist that rationalize both increased and decreased acromial indices with rotator cuff disease; however, further study is needed to elucidate the precise role of the acromion in the development of rotator cuff disease.

which was described as a central spur (or convexity) located on the undersurface of the acromion, was significantly associated with the presence of both partial- (bursal-sided) and full-thickness rotator cuff tears in the original study published by Tucker and Snyder [41]. Several recent studies have also suggested that a steep acromial slope may be another factor associated with the development of impingement lesions [34, 42–44]; however, further study needs to be conducted to substantiate these claims.

Excessive lateral extension of the acromion, which is best quantified through calculation of the acromial index (Fig. 4.11), has also been reported as a potential contributor to the development of rotator cuff impingement and tearing. Some investigators report that decreased coverage of the humeral head by the acromion (i.e., a decreased acromial index) may allow the humeral head to utilize the anterolateral acromion as a fulcrum or lever to aid in glenohumeral elevation, possibly causing abrasion of the cuff tendons and subsequent rotator cuff tearing [45, 46]. Nyffeler et al. [47] suggested that a large acromial index may result in a more superiorly directed force vector produced by the middle fibers of the deltoid, potentially leading to superior migration of the humeral head which, in turn, decreases the available space for the cuff tendons to pass beneath the acromion. This theory has been partially validated since other more recent studies have found statistically significant associations between increased acromial indices and the presence of rotator cuff tears [31, 33, 34, 47–50]. Although the acromial index appears to play some role in the development of rotator cuff disease, additional studies are needed to fully elucidate the exact pathomechanisms behind this phenomenon.

Inclination of the glenoid in the coronal plane has also been associated with the development of rotator cuff tears on several occasions [51–53]. Tétrault et al. [52] performed measurements using magnetic resonance imaging (MRI) to determine the orientation of the supraspinatus muscle fibers relative to the glenoid surface. In that study, the mean angle formed between the supraspinatus tendon and the glenoid surface was approximately 80° in the coronal plane. The authors suggested that a decrease in this angle (i.e., increased upward tilt of the glenoid) may result in a more vertically oriented force vector produced by the supraspinatus, thus preferentially pulling the humeral head superiorly [52]. If this theoretical mechanism is factually correct, the supraspinatus tendon could then make contact with the acromion, possibly leading to the cascade of events commonly associated with rotator cuff disease. A similar mechanism may occur when considering glenoid anteversion and retroversion in which tearing of the subscapularis and infraspinatus is observed, respectively [52]. Although at least one study found that surgically decreasing the glenoid inclination angle may decrease the measured amount of superior humeral head translation with passive abduction [49], none of the more recent imaging studies have shown significant associations between any type or degree of glenoid version and the presence of rotator cuff lesions, regardless of location of the tear or the tendon involved [54, 55].

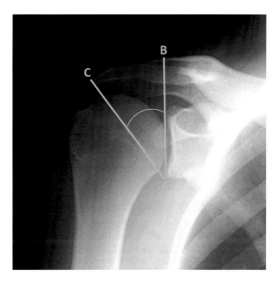

Fig. 4.12 True anteroposterior (AP) radiograph demonstrating measurement of the critical shoulder angle. Line "AB" is first drawn, which connects the most lateral points of the superior and inferior glenoid rim. Line "AC" is then drawn, which connects the previously drawn point "A" to the most lateral point of the acromion (designated as point "C"). The angle formed between lines "AB" and "AC" represents the critical shoulder angle. According to Moor et al. [57] an angle of less than 30° increases the risk for osteoarthritis whereas an angle of greater than 35° increases the risk for degenerative rotator cuff tears.

The critical shoulder angle (CSA) (recently described by Gerber et al. [56] and Moor et al. [57, 58]) is another radiographic measurement purported to have an association with rotator cuff tears or osteoarthritis. The CSA is obtained from true anteroposterior (AP) radiographs and takes into account both the acromial index and the degree of glenoid inclination in the scapular plane (Fig. 4.12). The original developers of this measurement have suggested that the CSA may have an ability to predict the future development of degenerative rotator cuff tears (when the CSA > 35°) and glenohumeral osteoarthritis (when the CSA < 30°). However, a well-designed prospective study would be needed to confirm these claims given the current lack of conclusive clinical data suggesting any association between either the acromial index or glenoid inclination and any shoulder pathology.

4.3.2 Pathogenesis Involving Intrinsic Factors

While extrinsic factors probably have some role in the development of subacromial impingement, many authors believe that the initiation and progression of rotator cuff disease primarily occurs as a result of intrinsic cuff degeneration. They argue that degenerative changes and/or traumatic injuries weaken the contractile strength of supraspinatus muscle which predictably leads to superior humeral head migration and cuff impingement beneath the acromion with humeral elevation. Spurring of the anterolateral acromion and erosion of the greater tuberosity are then observed (due to repeated reciprocal contact) along with rotator cuff degeneration.

The deterioration of tendon quality due to advanced age is often implicated as one of the primary causes of rotator cuff weakness, potentially resulting in proximal humeral head migration, subsequent bursal irritation and cuff tendinopathy. While the incidence and severity of rotator cuff disease has been found to increase with age on several occasions, Ogata and Uhthoff [59] found that acromial osteophytes were not always present in older patients. Further, those who did have acromial osteophytes actually had articular-sided partial-thickness rotator cuff tears (as opposed to bursal-sided tears). However, a more recent study identified the presence of anterolateral acromial spurs as an independent risk factor for the development of rotator cuff disease [33]. Further research is needed to identify and elucidate the roles of mechanical compression and intrinsic tendon degeneration on the progression of rotator cuff disease.

The tenuous microvascular blood supply to the supraspinatus and infraspinatus tendons has also been suggested as a possible intrinsic factor related to the development and progression of certain rotator cuff tears [12, 35, 60–65]. Lohr and Uhthoff [12] identified an area along the edges of supraspinatus tears in which no vessels were present, suggesting that spontaneous healing of a torn rotator cuff tendon is probably not feasible without surgical intervention. Ling et al. [63] studied the vascular supply of the supraspinatus tendon in 22 adults

using scanning electron microscopy. They described a hypovascular zone on the surface of the supraspinatus tendon, confirming the findings that had been reported by others (Fig. 4.13) [62, 64, 65]. More recently, Brooks et al. [35] found that both the supraspinatus and infraspinatus tendons were hypovascular in the most distal 15 mm of their respective insertion sites on the greater tuberosity. This area of the insertional footprint, termed the "critical zone" by Moseley and Goldie [64] in 1963, may have an increased propensity to develop partial- or full-thickness rotator cuff tears as a result of poor tendon nutrition and a limited capacity for spontaneous healing. Although several studies have revealed evidence of apoptosis and hypoxia in rotator cuff tendons with visible tears and impingement lesions [18, 66–68], some authors believe these findings are the *result* of cuff degeneration rather than the *cause* of cuff degeneration [69].

4.3.3 Physical Examination

Numerous studies have evaluated the utility of physical examination tests to reliably identify subacromial impingement. The Neer impingement sign [10], Hawkins–Kennedy test [70], and the painful arc sign [71] are the most useful and most widely utilized tests for the detection of subacromial impingement. Tenderness to palpation at the location of Codman's point (described below) may also suggest rotator cuff impingement. Because pathologies other than impingement can produce impingement-like signs and symptoms during the physical examination, sensitivity and specificity data for these tests are variable [72–78]. Therefore, consideration of all available information, including other clinical tests and historical features, is necessary to synthesize an accurate physical diagnosis in every patient. When the diagnosis is in question, it is often useful to inject a local anesthetic into the subacromial space before repeating each test. This method is typically used to identify whether the patient's subjective weakness is primarily due to guarding or due to actual muscle weakness. The relief of impingement-like signs and symptoms

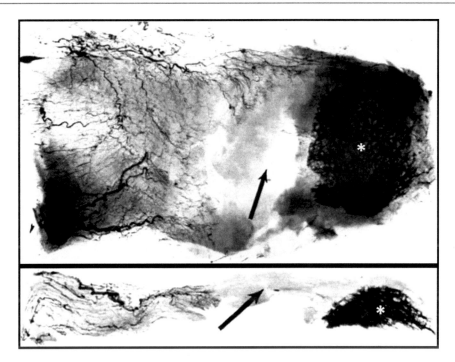

Fig. 4.13 (**a**) Axial slide showing the microvascular pattern of the supraspinatus tendon. (**b**) Coronal slide showing the microvascular pattern of the supraspinatus tendon. *Arrows* correspond to the region of avascularity and *asterisks* indicate the location of the supraspinatus footprint on the greater tuberosity. (From [65] with permission).

that were present before the injection usually confirms the diagnosis. This technique is usually referred to as the Neer impingement *test* which should not be confused with the Neer impingement *sign* (described below).

4.3.3.1 Neer Impingement Sign

The Neer impingement sign, first described by Neer [10] in 1972, is elicited by passive and maximal forward elevation of the humerus and stabilization of the scapula with the examiner's contralateral hand (Fig. 4.14). Stabilization of the scapula is essential to maximize the utility of the test since upward rotation of the scapula (and therefore the acromion) with forward elevation will decrease the likelihood of reproducing cuff impingement under the acromion. Reproduction of the patient's symptoms is indicative of a positive test. Several investigators have evaluated the clinical efficacy of the Neer impingement sign in its ability to accurately diagnose subacromial impingement (Table 4.1) [72, 73, 75, 76, 78, 80].

Both Fodor et al. [73] and Kelly et al. [79] used ultrasonic evaluation to determine the sensitivity and specificity of the Neer sign in the diagnosis of subacromial impingement. Interestingly, although each study reported similar sensitivity values, their specificity values were divergent (95 % and 10 %, respectively). These results highlight the significant variability that may exist in the performance and interpretation of physical examination findings, specifically with regard to subacromial impingement syndrome. Nevertheless, Hegedus et al. [81] attempted to account for various confounding factors and study quality in a recent meta-analysis. In that study, the overall calculated sensitivity of the Neer impingement sign was 72 % while its overall specificity was approximately 60 %. Clearly, this maneuver is not adequate to diagnose subacromial impingement in isolation; however, combination of its results with those obtained from the Hawkins–Kennedy test and the painful arc sign (described below) are likely to improve diagnostic accuracy.

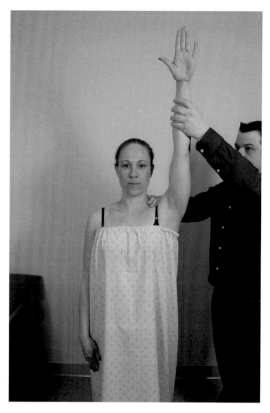

Fig. 4.14 Neer impingement sign. The examiner stabilizes the scapula with one hand and uses the other hand to passively forward-flex the humerus to a point of maximal elevation. Reproduction of the patient's symptoms with this maneuver may suggest the presence of subacromial impingement.

4.3.3.2 Hawkins–Kennedy Test

The Hawkins–Kennedy test [70] was first described in 1980; however, it was not originally thought to be as reliable or reproducible as the Neer impingement sign. A positive Hawkins–Kennedy test is the result of greater tuberosity contact on the undersurface of the coracoacromial ligament that is thought to reproduce symptoms related to subacromial impingement. To perform this test, the shoulder is brought to 90° of abduction in the scapular plane with the elbow also flexed 90°. From this position, the humerus is slowly and maximally internally rotated (Fig. 4.15). Reproduction of the patient's symptoms (typically pain over the anterior shoulder) is deemed a positive test and may be indicative of superior cuff impingement. Numerous studies have evaluated the efficacy of the Hawkins–Kennedy test in its ability to diagnose subacromial impingement with variable results (Table 4.2) [72–76, 78, 80, 82]. The meta-analysis by Hegedus et al. [81] reported similar overall sensitivities and specificities for both the Neer impingement sign and the Hawkins–Kennedy tests.

4.3.3.3 Painful Arc Sign

The painful arc sign [71] is elicited with resisted abduction of the shoulder in the scapular plane (20–30° of forward angulation) with the elbow

Table 4.1 Diagnostic efficacy of the Neer impingement sign in isolation

Diagnostic efficacy of the Neer impingement sign in isolation							
Investigators	Maneuver	Pathology	Standard	LR+	LR−	Sensitivity (%)	Specificity (%)
Silva et al. [78]	Neer	SIS	MRI	0.98	1.1	68	30
Fodor et al. [73]	Neer	SIS	Ultrasound	10.8	0.48	54	95
Michener et al. [76]	Neer	SIS	Arthroscopy	1.76	0.35	81	54
Kelly et al. [79]	Neer	SIS	Ultrasound	0.62	3.80	62	10
Chew et al. [72]	Neer	SIS	Ultrasound	1.60	0.60	64	61
Toprak et al. [80]	Neer	SIS	Ultrasound	1.67	0.38	80	52

SIS subacromial impingement syndrome, *LR* likelihood ratio

Fig. 4.15 Hawkins–Kennedy test. The examiner passively abducts the humerus in the scapular plane to approximately 90° with the elbow also flexed to 90°. The examiner then internally rotates the humerus which is thought to induce impingement between the greater tuberosity and the undersurface of the acromion. Reproduction of the patient's symptoms with this test may be suggestive of subacromial impingement.

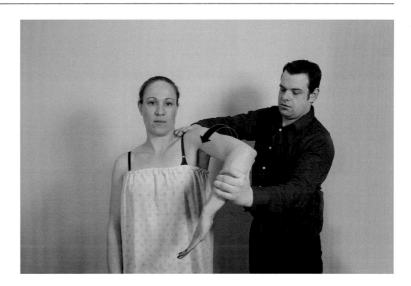

Table 4.2 Diagnostic efficacy of the Hawkins–Kennedy test in isolation

Diagnostic efficacy of the Hawkins–Kennedy test in isolation

Investigators	Maneuver	Pathology	Standard	LR+	LR−	Sensitivity (%)	Specificity (%)
Silva et al. [78]	H–K	SIS	MRI	1.23	0.65	74	40
Fodor et al. [73]	H–K	SIS	Ultrasound	6.50	0.31	72	89
Michener et al. [76]	H–K	SIS	Arthroscopy	1.63	0.61	63	62
Kelly et al. [79]	H–K	SIS	Ultrasound	1.48	0.52	74	50
Chew et al. [72]	H–K	SIS	Ultrasound	1.30	0.40	87	32
Salaffi et al. [77]	H–K	SIS	Ultrasound	2.50	0.51	64	71
Fowler et al. [74]	H–K	SIS	Arthroscopy	2.10	1.60	58	72
Toprak et al. [80]	H–K	SIS	Ultrasound	1.26	0.70	67	47

SIS subacromial impingement syndrome, *H–K* Hawkins–Kennedy, *LR* likelihood ratio

in full extension (Fig. 4.16). Pain with this maneuver is another possible indicator of subacromial impingement, especially when used in combination with the tests described above. Although this test is not very sensitive in isolation, it does boast a modest specificity as reported by Hegedus et al. [81] (Table 4.3). Therefore, since both the Neer impingement sign and the Hawkins–Kennedy test each has low specificity values, addition of the painful arc sign (which has a higher reported specificity) may improve overall diagnostic accuracy when all three maneuvers are used in a composite exam to diagnose subacromial impingement.

4.4 Subcoracoid Impingement

Subcoracoid impingement is a potential cause for anterior shoulder pain as a result of compression of the subscapularis between the posterolateral edge of the coracoid process and the lesser tuberosity of the humerus [83–86]. In contrast to subacromial impingement which likely involves a multitude of intrinsic and extrinsic factors, most authors agree that many subscapularis tears associated with a narrowed coracohumeral interval (i.e., the distance between the coracoid tip to the crest of the lesser tuberosity measured by

Fig. 4.16 Painful arc sign. In this test, the patient attempts to abduct the humerus within the scapular plane against resistance provided by the examiner. Weakness or pain with this maneuver may indicate the presence of subacromial impingement, although other tests are needed to confirm this finding. In this image, both arms are tested simultaneously which may be more sensitive for the detection of more subtle pathology.

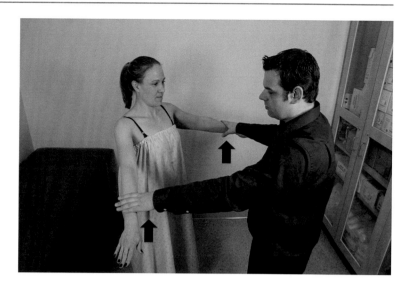

Table 4.3 Diagnostic efficacy of the painful arc sign in isolation

Diagnostic efficacy of the painful arc sign in isolation							
Investigators	Maneuver	Pathology	Standard	LR+	LR−	Sensitivity (%)	Specificity (%)
Fodor et al. [73]	Painful arc	SIS	Ultrasound	3.40	0.41	67	80
Michener et al. [76]	Painful arc	SIS	Arthroscopy	2.25	0.38	75	67
Kelly et al. [79]	Painful arc	SIS	Ultrasound	0.59	1.40	49	33
Chew et al. [72]	Painful arc	SIS	Ultrasound	3.70	0.40	71	81

SIS subacromial impingement syndrome, *LR* likelihood ratio

axial MRI scans) are most likely caused by external tendon compression (Fig. 4.17) [86, 88].

4.4.1 Pathogenesis

In 1909, Goldthwait [89] first described the concept of subcoracoid impingement as it related to anterior shoulder pain. Many years later, Gerber et al. [85] first described the surgical management of coracoid impingement and noted that the coracoid process was potentially involved with pathology of the anterosuperior cuff tendons (subscapularis tendon and the anterior portion of the supraspinatus tendon), subcoracoid bursa, and the long head of the biceps tendon.

Subcoracoid impingement can have primary, secondary, or idiopathic causes. Although primary subcoracoid impingement has been relatively understudied, it probably involves multiple

intrinsic and extrinsic factors that lead to a narrowed coracohumeral interval. There are numerous potential secondary causes for subcoracoid impingement. Malunited fractures of the glenoid neck, proximal humerus, glenoid or coracoid can impinge upon the subscapularis muscle, thus resulting in anterior shoulder pain [85]. Importantly, patients with anterior glenohumeral instability (discussed in Chap. 6) may also present with subcoracoid impingement due to increased anterior translation of the humerus which subsequently narrows the coracohumeral interval. Iatrogenic causes can include any type of anterior shoulder surgery, potentially causing the formation of subcoracoid adhesions and a functionally narrowed coracohumeral interval. Idiopathic causes may include ganglion cysts, congenitally malformed coracoid processes or subscapularis calcifications.

Recently, several studies have described the various morphologic characteristics of the coracoid and their potential roles in the development

a

b

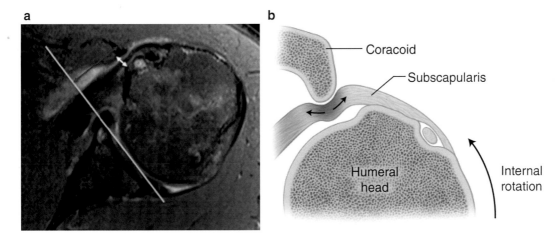

Fig. 4.17 (**a**) Axial MRI slice demonstrating measurement of the coracoid index and the coracohumeral interval with the humerus internally rotated. The *white line* connects the anterior and posterior glenoid rim. The *double-headed red arrow* lies perpendicular to the *white line* and travels to the most lateral tip of the coracoid process. The distance traveled by the *red arrow* represents the coracoid index. The *double-headed white arrow* represents the distance between the lesser tuberosity and the most posterior aspect of the coracoid process. The distanced traveled by the *white arrow* represents the coracohumeral interval. (**b**) Illustration depicting the mechanism of impingement between the lesser tuberosity and the posterior aspect of the coracoid. When the humerus is internally rotated, the coracoid induces a "roller wringer" effect on the subscapularis tendon which induces stretching and tearing of the tendon when the coracohumeral interval is narrowed [87].

of subscapularis impingement and anterior shoulder pain [28, 90–93]. Bhatia et al. [90] found that the posterolateral edge of the coracoid was involved with anterosuperior cuff impingement. Richards et al. [88] found that a narrowed coracohumeral interval was significantly associated with subscapularis pathology. More specifically, those patients without subscapularis pathology had a coracohumeral interval of 10±1.3 mm while those with subscapularis pathology had a coracohumeral interval of 5±1.7 mm ($p<0.0001$). Similarly, a sonographic study by Tracy et al. [94] found that asymptomatic patients had an interval of 12.2±2.5 mm while patients with clinical evidence of subcoracoid impingement had an interval of 7.9±1.4 mm. Ferreira Neto et al. [95] found that women have a smaller coracohumeral interval compared to men when the arm was internally rotated, suggesting that subcoracoid impingement of the subscapularis may be more likely in female patients. Despite this evidence, the instigating factor involved in the development of anterosuperior cuff pathology in patients with a narrowed coracohumeral interval has yet to be completely elucidated.

4.4.2 Physical Examination

Patients with subcoracoid impingement typically complain of dull pain (rarely, a sharp pain) over the anterior aspect of the shoulder. This pain may radiate distally along the brachium if the long head of the biceps tendon is involved. Although patients typically present with a full range of motion, they typically present with pain over the coracoid that is exacerbated by forward flexion, internal rotation, and cross-body adduction. Because this entity has not been studied extensively, it remains a diagnosis of exclusion when all other causes of anterior shoulder pain have been ruled out. Despite the lack of literature on the subject, it is important to remember that subcoracoid impingement may be the result of disordered scapular mechanics. Thus, it is critically important to evaluate the scapula in patients suspected of having subcoracoid impingement (physical evaluation of the scapula is discussed in Chap. 9). In the setting of a normal scapular exam, the subcoracoid impingement test may be an important tool in the diagnosis of subcoracoid impingement.

4.4.2.1 Subcoracoid Impingement Test

The subcoracoid impingement test, which is a modified version of the Hawkins–Kennedy test, is useful to perform in any patient with shoulder discomfort, especially anteriorly. The test is performed by placing the patient's arm in 90° of forward flexion, submaximal internal rotation and 90° of elbow flexion. From this position, the patient's arm is progressively adducted and internally rotated. As the arm is adducted and internally rotated, the patient with subcoracoid impingement will complain of a dull anterior shoulder pain (Fig. 4.18). Because this maneuver

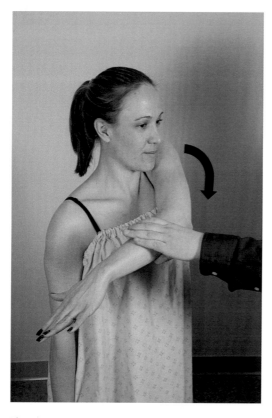

Fig. 4.18 Subcoracoid impingement test. The examiner passively abducts to humerus to 90°, maximally internally rotates the humerus and flexes the elbow to 90°. From this position, the examiner passively adducts the shoulder across the chest. When resistance is felt, it is sometimes useful to gently force the humerus into a greater degree of adduction, especially in cases where the test is inconclusive. The test is positive for subcoracoid impingement when a dull anterior shoulder pain is elicited. Note that pain over the acromioclavicular (AC) joint with this test is not considered a positive test, but may indicate the presence of AC joint pathology.

is similar to the cross-body adduction test for acromioclavicular (AC) joint pathology, it is important to note the precise location and quality of the pain that is generated by the test (i.e., pain at the top of the shoulder is more likely associated with AC joint pathology; see Chap. 7 for further details). Although this test has not been fully evaluated in the literature, we have found the test useful to identify patients with chronic lesions involving the subscapularis tendon. Because the subscapularis muscle makes a significant contribution to the bicipital sheath, testing for pathology of the long head of the biceps tendon is also indicated when subcoracoid impingement is suspected (physical examination of the long head of the biceps tendon is discussed in Chap. 5).

4.5 Symptomatic Internal Impingement

The term "internal impingement" refers to a normal physiologic occurrence where the greater tuberosity makes contact with the posterosuperior glenoid labrum when the humerus is abducted and externally rotated. Although its primary function may involve the prevention of hyperexternal rotation and maintenance of stability, repeated episodes of this impingement (which often occurs with repeated overhead activities such as throwing) may lead to posterosuperior labral tears and posterosuperior rotator cuff tears which eventually become symptomatic. In essence, the posterosuperior labrum and rotator cuff become pinched between the greater tuberosity and the bony glenoid rim leading to posterior shoulder pain (due to pathology of the posterosuperior labrum and rotator cuff) especially when the humerus is abducted and externally rotated (Fig. 4.19) [96–100].

4.6 Rotator Cuff Tears

Accurate physical evaluation of the patient with a rotator cuff tear depends on the ability of the clinician to decipher the primary cause of the tear which is most often obtained from the patient history and initial strength examination.

Fig. 4.19 Illustration of
the pathomechanism
behind symptomatic
internal impingement.
Hyperabduction and
external rotation may pinch
the posterosuperior cuff
between the greater
tuberosity and the glenoid,
possibly leading to
articular-sided posterosuperior rotator cuff tears and
tearing of the posterosuperior glenoid labrum.

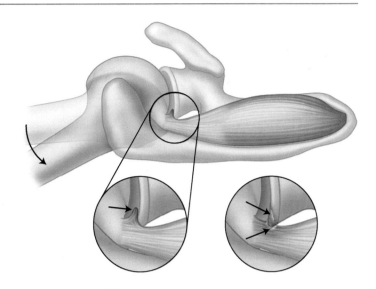

4.6.1   Pathogenesis

The different etiologies of rotator cuff tears are
most often multifactorial, ranging from acute
traumatic injuries to the three main types of
mechanical impingement, namely the "classic"
subacromial impingement, subcoracoid impingement, and internal impingement in throwing athletes that can each progress rotator cuff tearing.
In acute injuries, patients will typically recall the
specific events leading to their shoulder pain,
weakness, and dysfunction. Other, more chronic
lesions, however, may be more difficult to
recognize. Although each type of impingement
involves a chronic process, many patients are
asymptomatic until the tear has reached sufficient
size and/or has resulted in altered glenohumeral
kinematics. As such, it is thought that previously
asymptomatic rotator cuff lesions may progress
to larger, full-thickness tears especially in patients
with altered tendon biology [12, 101]. Without
treatment, small tears with intact glenohumeral
mechanics can progress to larger tears, leading to
weakness and unbalanced force couples and, subsequently, increased shoulder pain and dysfunction [102, 103].

As discussed above, subacromial impingement involves a combination of intrinsic factors
(e.g., poor microvascularity [12, 35, 60–65] and
tendon quality [59]) and extrinsic factors

(e.g., abrasion of tendons beneath the
coracoacromial arch [10, 14, 20, 30, 32, 33]) that
lead to the insidious onset of pain especially at
night and/or with overhead activities. As the cuff
tear develops and increases in size, pain and
weakness become the predominant features. Pain
and weakness become worse as the tear extends
to involve other tendons, such as those of the
infraspinatus (posterosuperior tear) or subscapularis (anterosuperior tear). Left untreated, pain
will often diminish and the patient will complain
of weakness as the primary symptom [104].

Subcoracoid impingement (also discussed
above) is thought to result from a narrowed coracohumeral interval and presents with an insidious onset of dull pain over the anterior aspect of
the shoulder in positions of adduction and internal rotation [83–86]. Similar to subacromial
impingement, the progression of small, structural lesions of the subscapularis can lead to
large, full-thickness tears resulting in progressive pain, dysfunction and, in some cases, anterior instability [10].

Symptomatic internal impingement occurs as
a result of repetitive hyperabduction and external
rotation which leads to posterosuperior articular-
sided rotator cuff tears and labral lesions (see
Fig. 4.19) [86, 99, 100]. These patients may also
report a gradual decrease in throwing performance such as a decline in throwing accuracy and

velocity. Scapular dyskinesis and the SICK scapula syndrome is another predominant feature in throwing athletes who may progress to symptomatic internal impingement [60].

4.6.2 Physical Examination

The possibility of a rotator cuff tear should be strongly suspected in patients older than 60 years of age, those with night pain and those with clinical weakness as detected by the general strength survey. Specifically, strength deficits in internal or external rotation (with the arm both at the side and at 90° of abduction) and/or abduction should direct the clinician to specifically evaluate rotator cuff strength. Although the presence of pain can lead to guarding and the impression of weakness, the sources of pain and weakness must be ascertained to arrive at the correct diagnosis.

4.6.2.1 Supraspinatus

Supraspinatus tendon tears are initially suspected during the initial survey as a result of specific historical findings and the presence of pain and/or weakness with glenohumeral abduction. Furthermore, since painful impingement of the rotator cuff may progress to partial- or full-thickness tears, positive impingement signs may also be present in patients with weakness associated with a rotator cuff tear. Further, since patients with suspected impingement in the absence of a rotator cuff tear are managed differently from those with a concomitant tear, it is essential to rule out the presence of a tear in those with positive impingement signs to avoid unnecessary surgery.

Rent Test

The rent test is a method of trans-deltoid palpation first described by Codman [105] in 1934 that may have some utility in the detection of supraspinatus tendon defects. When performed correctly, Codman suggested that clinicians could locate a point of tenderness and detect a sensation "crepitus" underneath their fingers which would therefore suggest the presence of a rotator cuff tear (Fig. 4.20). Specifically, a gap (or "sulcus"

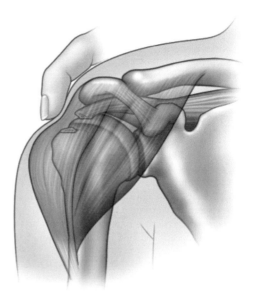

Fig. 4.20 Illustration depicting the "sulcus" [101] which may be palpated while performing the rent test.

[101]) could be felt between the edges of the torn tendon as the humerus was internally and externally rotated during palpation. To perform this test, the examiner stands to the side of the seated patient. With the arms initially at the side, the examiner palpates the area just beneath the anterolateral acromion and lateral to the coracoacromial ligament which also corresponds to an anatomically thin area of the deltoid, possibly facilitating the detection of a tendon defect [106]. When the arm is at the side, this location is referred to as "Codman's point" where the anterior supraspinatus tendon inserts on the greater tuberosity. During palpation, the patient's arm is simultaneously moved through a range of motion, generally involving a combination of slight abduction and extension along with internal and external rotation (Fig. 4.21). At approximately 10° of internal rotation, the examiner can identify the bicipital sheath and the lesser tuberosity, thus providing information regarding spatial orientation [17, 106]. Extension of the shoulder may allow additional palpation of the anterior infraspinatus.

Although many years have passed since its original description, only a few studies have evaluated the diagnostic utility of this test for the

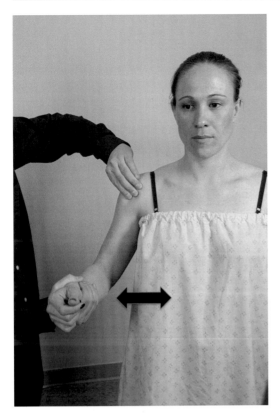

Fig. 4.21 Rent test. While holding the patient's forearm with one hand, the examiner palpates the region just inferior to the anterolateral aspect of the acromion (i.e., Codman's point). With the humerus slightly abducted and extended, the patient's arm is internally and externally rotated while the examiner simultaneously palpates the supraspinatus. A positive test occurs when a sulcus is felt by the examiner regardless of the presence of pain.

detection of rotator cuff tears. Lyons and Tomlinson [107] calculated a sensitivity of 91 % and a specificity of 75 % after performing the test during strength testing in a series of 45 patients. Wolf and Agrawal [101] calculated a sensitivity of 96 and 97 % when test results were compared with MRI and surgical findings; however, all 109 patients in this study had a previous diagnosis of subacromial impingement. Ponce et al. [106] performed the examination in 63 patients who presented with shoulder pain and compared the results to a standardized MRI sequence. Their results suggest that the rent test was more valuable in the detection of full-thickness tears when compared to any of the partial-thickness tears. In addition, sensitivity and specificity values

appeared to increase with increasing patient age: sensitivities were >75 % and specificities approached 100 % for patients older than 55 years of age whereas the test was less predictive in younger patients (sensitivity of 43 % and specificity of 70 %).

Jobe Test

The Jobe test [19] is often performed to elicit weakness as a result of supraspinatus tearing. To perform the test, the arms are passively placed in 90° of abduction in the scapular plane with the thumbs pointed downward (i.e., the "empty can" position; Fig. 4.22). From this position, the examiner places their hands on the top of the patient's forearms and applies a downward pressure while the patient resists. A positive test occurs when asymmetric weakness occurs in the affected shoulder. Although this test isolates the supraspinatus muscle-tendon unit, clinical weakness can be simulated by the presence of significant pain. To alleviate some of this pain and to more directly evaluate supraspinatus strength, the test can be repeated with the thumbs pointed upward (i.e., the "full can" position [108]; Fig. 4.23). This maneuver is thought to position the greater tuberosity away from the coracoacromial arch and may therefore decrease the pain associated with mechanical cuff impingement.

Drop Arm Sign

In some patients with massive supraspinatus tears, the patient may be unable to hold the arm abducted against the force of gravity as the arm drops back to the patient's side. This is called "drop arm sign" (not to be confused with the "drop sign," as discussed below) and is indicative of a large supraspinatus/infraspinatus tear (Fig. 4.24). Although sensitivity and specificity data for the Jobe test and drop arm sign are modest, the combination of both maneuvers is thought to improve diagnostic accuracy (Table 4.4).

4.6.2.2 Infraspinatus

The identification of an external rotation deficit (infraspinatus/teres minor tear) is initially found during the general strength survey with the resisted external rotation maneuvers. However,

Fig. 4.22 Jobe test in the "empty can" position. In this test, both arms are placed in approximately 90° of abduction within the scapular plane and maximally internally rotated (thumbs pointed *downward*). The patient then attempts to further abduct the humerus against resistance applied by the examiner. A positive test occurs when asymmetric weakness occurs involving the affected shoulder.

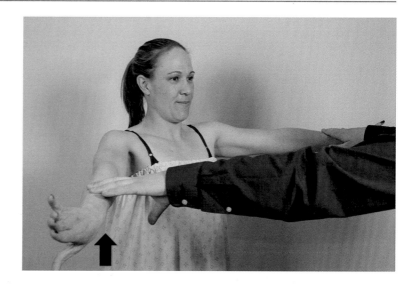

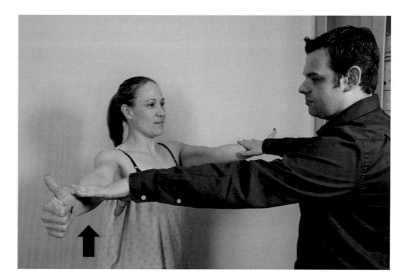

Fig. 4.23 Jobe test in the "full can" position. Both arms are placed in approximately 90° of abduction within the scapular plane and externally rotated (thumbs pointed *upward*). The patient then attempts to further abduct the humerus against resistance applied by the examiner.

A positive test occurs when asymmetric weakness occurs involving the affected shoulder. This variation of the Jobe test is thought to reduce the pain associated with supraspinatus impingement and may be more sensitive to actual weakness rather than guarding due to impingement.

this finding is often subtle or masked by significant pain. The external rotation lag sign is an effective alternative that eliminates the effect of pain on external rotation function.

External Rotation Lag Sign

To elicit the external rotation lag sign, the arm is kept at the patient's side and the elbow is flexed 90°. From this position, the humerus is passively placed in 20–30° of external rotation. A positive external rotation lag sign occurs when the patient is unable to hold this externally rotated position (estimate the amount of internal rotation that occurs, corresponding to degrees of lag; Fig. 4.25). Given recent evidence that the supraspinatus may contribute up to 20 % of the total contraction strength detected when this test is performed in normal shoulders [114], this clinical

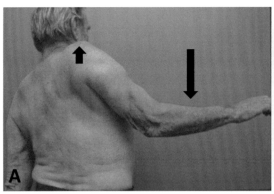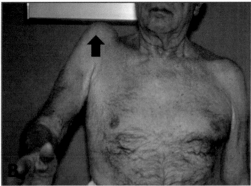

Fig. 4.24 (**a**) Clinical photograph demonstrating the drop arm sign in which the patient is unable to hold the humerus in an abducted position. Notice that the shoulder also "shrugs" in an attempt to compensate for rotator cuff weakness. (**b**) Clinical photograph demonstrating antero-superior escape of the humeral head due to a massive rota- tor cuff tear and coracoacromial ligament rupture. This image highlights the stabilizing effect of the supraspinatus which, in normal individuals, prevents superior humeral head migration. *Source*: Defranco MJ, Walch G. Current issues in reverse total shoulder arthroplasty. J Musculoskel Med 2011;28:85–94.

Table 4.4 Diagnostic efficacies of the Jobe test and the drop arm sign in the detection of supraspinatus tears

Diagnostic efficacy of the Jobe test and drop arm sign							
Investigators	Maneuver	Pathology	Standard	LR+	LR−	Sensitivity (%)	Specificity (%)
Itoi et al. [109]	Empty can	FTT	Arthroscopy	1.75	0.30	87	43
Kim et al. [110]	Empty can	FTT/PTT	MRI/arthroscopy	2.62	0.34	76	71
Itoi et al. [109]	Full can	FT	Arthroscopy	1.77	0.32	83	53
Kim et al. [110]	Full can	FTT/PTT	MRI/arthroscopy	2.41	0.34	77	32
Bak et al. [111]	Drop arm	FT	Ultrasound	2.41	0.71	41	83
Miller et al. [112]	Drop arm	FTPST	Ultrasound	3.20	0.30	73	77

FTT full-thickness tear, *PTT* partial-thickness tear, *FTPST* full-thickness posterosuperior tear (tear propagation to involve both supraspinatus and infraspinatus tendons), *LR* likelihood ratio

finding may help identify patients with a postero-superior cuff tear (i.e., involving the supraspina-tus and infraspinatus) since most studies report good sensitivity and specificity values (Table 4.5). The test is less useful for isolated supraspinatus tears due to conflicting clinical data [111, 115].

4.6.2.3 Subscapularis

Suspicion of internal rotation weakness involv-ing the subscapularis muscle is typically gener-ated during the initial strength survey via resisted internal rotation stress tests at both 0° and 90° of glenohumeral abduction. In addition, patients may also exhibit increased external rotation capacity due to the decreased resting tension of the subscapularis muscle (Fig. 4.26). The belly-press, lift-off, and bear-hug tests are provocative maneuvers designed to detect the presence of a subscapularis tear with moderate to good sensitivity and specificity (Table 4.6). According to a recent retrospective analysis in 52 shoulders with subscapularis tears, the overall sensitivity was found to be 81 % when at least one of these three tests were positive [121].

Belly-Press Test

The belly-press test is performed by placing both of the patient's hands on the lower abdomen with flat wrists, the elbows pointed laterally and without finger overlap. The patient presses poste-riorly with their hands while keeping the elbows anterior to the plane of the abdomen (Fig. 4.27). A positive test occurs when the affected elbow falls posteriorly due to the recruitment of ancil-lary muscles to compensate for the weakened subscapularis (Fig. 4.28).

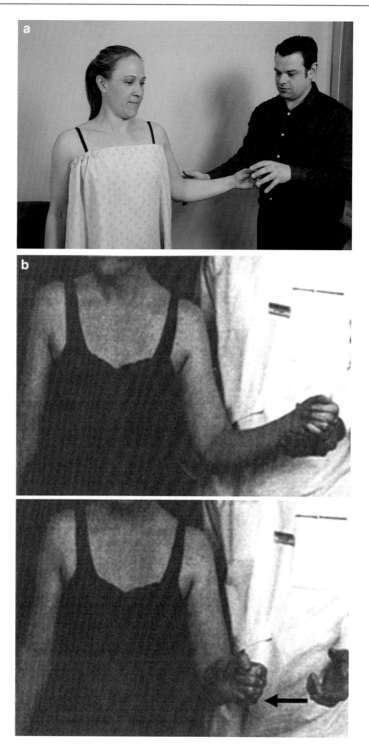

Fig. 4.25 External rotation lag sign. (**a**) With the arm at the side and the elbow flexed to 90°, the examiner passively places the humerus between 20° and 30° of external rotation. The examiner then removes their hand and asks the patient to hold this position. Inability to hold this position indicates a positive external rotation lag sign where the amount of subsequent internal rotation indicates the degrees of lag. (**b**) Clinical photographs demonstrating a positive external rotation lag sign in a patient with a massive posterosuperior cuff tear. (Part B from Hertel et al. [113]; with permission).

Table 4.5 Diagnostic efficacy of the external rotation lag sign in the detection of posterosuperior cuff tears

Diagnostic efficacy of the external rotation lag sign							
Investigators	Maneuver	Pathology	Standard	LR+	LR−	Sensitivity (%)	Specificity (%)
Bak et al. [111]	ERLS	FTT—Supraspinatus	Ultrasound	5.00	0.60	77	26
Castoldi et al. [115]	ERLS	FTT—Supraspinatus	Arthroscopy	28.0	0.45	56	98
Castoldi et al. [115]	ERLS	FTT—Supra & infra	Arthroscopy	13.9	0.03	97	93
Miller et al. [112]	ERLS	FTT—Supra/infra	Ultrasound	7.20	0.60	46	94
Castoldi et al. [115]	ERLS	FTT—Teres minor	Arthroscopy	14.3	0.00	100	93

ERLS external rotation lag sign, *FTT* full-thickness tear, *RCT* rotator cuff tear, *LR* likelihood ratio

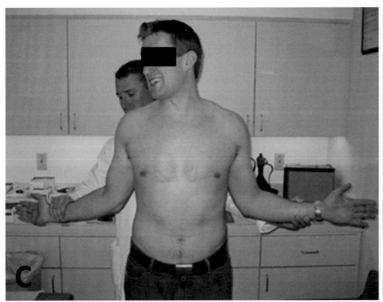 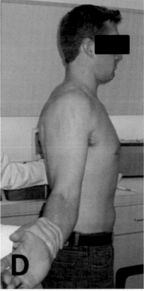

Fig. 4.26 Clinical photographs demonstrating increased passive external rotation capacity in a patient with a subscapularis tear involving the right shoulder. (**a**) Anterior view. (**b**) Sagittal view.

Table 4.6 Diagnostic efficacies of the belly-press, lift-off and bear-hug tests for the detection of subscapularis tears

Diagnostic efficacy of the subscapularis strength tests							
Investigators	Maneuver	Pathology	Standard	LR+	LR−	Sensitivity (%)	Specificity (%)
Bartsch et al. [116]	Belly press	Subscap tear	Arthroscopy	9.67	0.14	86	91
Yoon et al. [117]	Belly press	Subscap tear	Arthroscopy	28.0	0.73	28	99
Bartsch et al. [116]	Lift-off	Subscap tendinopathy	Arthroscopy	1.90	0.76	40	79
Naredo et al. [118]	Lift-off	Subscap tendinopathy	Ultrasound	7.20	0.67	50	84
Kim et al. [119]	Lift-off	Subscap tendinopathy	Ultrasound	1.30	0.70	69	48
Salaffi et al. [77]	Lift-off	Subscap tendinopathy	Ultrasound	1.45	0.85	35	75
Itoi et al. [109]	Lift-off	Subscap tear	Arthroscopy	1.90	0.4	46	69
Yoon et al. [117]	Lift-off	Subscap tear	Arthroscopy	–	0.88	12	100
Bartsch et al. [116]	Lift-off	Subscap tendinopathy	Arthroscopy	1.30	0.64	71	60
Millar et al. [68]	Lift-off	Subscap tear	Ultrasound	6.20	0.00	100	84
Yoon et al. [117]	Lift-off	Subscap tear	Arthroscopy	6.70	0.82	20	97
Barth et al. [120]	Bear-hug	Subscap tear	Arthroscopy	7.50	0.43	60	92

LR likelihood ratio

Fig. 4.27 Belly-press test. With the hand of the affected extremity placed over the abdomen with the elbow pointed laterally, the patient attempts to press posteriorly against the abdomen. A positive test occurs when the patient is unable to hold the elbows within the plane of the body during the application of the posteriorly directed force. In this image, the test is performed comparing both arms to detect subtle weakness.

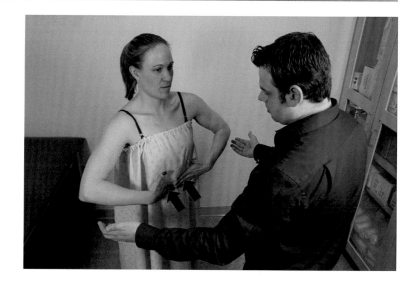

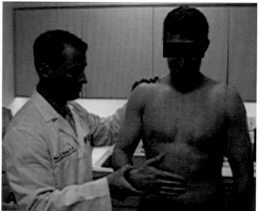
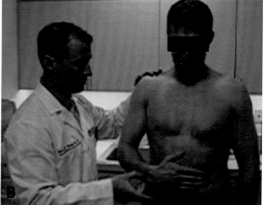

Fig. 4.28 Clinical photographs demonstrating a positive belly-press test in a patient with a subscapularis tear involving the right shoulder. In both images (**a** and **b**), the patient is attempting to pull his right hand towards the abdomen. Notice that the elbow falls posteriorly in both images when compared to the patient in Fig. 4.27.

Lift-Off Test

The lift-off test [56] is also designed to demonstrate weakness of the subscapularis muscle. The test is begun by having the patient place the dorsal aspect of the hand on the lumbar spine. The examiner then passively lifts the hand away from the lumbar spine and asks the patient to hold this position (Fig. 4.29). Inability to hold the position (the hand falls back to the spine) indicates subscapularis weakness (Fig. 4.30). The term "internal rotation lag sign" has been used on occasion to describe this test in accordance with the original terminology coined by its developer [113]; however, in contrast to the external rotation lag sign (described above for the evaluation of infraspinatus integrity), it is not often feasible to precisely measure the amount of external rotation

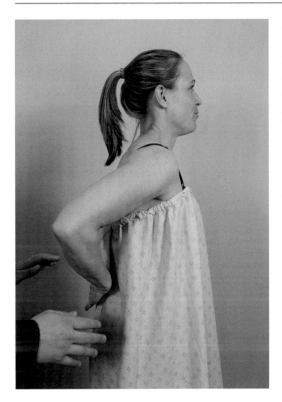

Fig. 4.29 The lift-off test. In this test, the dorsum of the patient's hand is placed over the lumbar spine. The examiner lifts the hand away from the spine and asks the patient to hold this position. A positive test occurs when the arm falls back towards the spine.

suggest less involvement whereas a stronger applied force would suggest greater involvement. Although the modified lift-off test is a clinically useful examination technique, we caution the reader that a few select patients who have subscapularis tears may actually be capable of achieving a "negative" test result since the latissimus dorsi is also highly active during this maneuver [123]. In other words, the strength of the latissimus dorsi (which primarily functions to extend and internally rotate the humerus) may overpower that of a torn subscapularis, possibly allowing some patients to demonstrate adequate strength with this test.

Bear-Hug Test

The bear-hug test is thought to cause near maximal activation of the subscapularis muscle; however, it has not been extensively studied with regard to sensitivity or specificity. We have found this test to be useful on some occasions when other subscapularis tests are inconclusive. In the most common version of the test, the patient first places the palm of the ipsilateral hand over the contralateral AC joint. With the tip of the elbow pointed directly forward, the patient is then instructed to push down onto the top of the shoulder without allowing the elbow to fall inferiorly (Fig. 4.31). A positive test occurs when the patient is unable to maintain the elbow in a horizontal plane [120, 124]. Alternatively, the examiner may also attempt to pull the arm away from the shoulder while simultaneously applying an external rotation force—a positive test occurs when the patient is unable to keep their hand on top of the shoulder. To obtain the most reliable results, it is important to confirm that the patient's fingers are extended (i.e., not wrapped over the top of the shoulder) to prevent them from generating increased resistance by grabbing the shoulder [120]. Using this method, Barth et al. [120] calculated a sensitivity of 60 % and a sensitivity of 91.7 % in a series of 68 patients who underwent subsequent diagnostic arthroscopy to confirm (or reject) the presence (or absence) of a subscapularis tear.

lag (defined as the number of degrees of involuntary external rotation that occurs following release of the patient's hand) using this test given the awkward patient-clinician positioning that is required. Using the same testing position, a positive *modified* lift-off test refers to a patient's inability to actively lift the hand away from the lumbar spine against resistance (without extending the elbow via the triceps muscle). Based on our interpretation of the results presented by Hertel et al. [113], it may be possible for an experienced examiner to estimate the extent of subscapularis involvement by judging the amount of applied force necessary to cause the humerus to externally rotate. Theoretically, a smaller applied force would

Fig. 4.30 Two sequential clinical photographs demonstrating a positive lift-off test. (**a**) The patient's hand is placed posterior to the lumbar spine and the examiner asks the patient to hold this position. The examiner may also stabilize the elbow when a massive tear is suspected. (**b**) After the examiner removed their hand, the patient's hand fell back towards the spine as the shoulder spontaneously externally rotated due to the unopposed resting tension of the infraspinatus. This patient had a massive subscapularis tear as evidenced by subsequent imaging studies. (From Costouros et al. [122]).

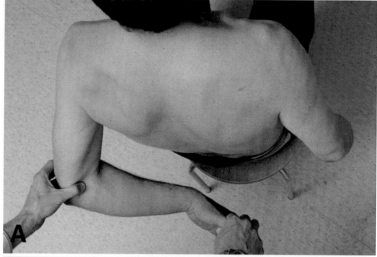

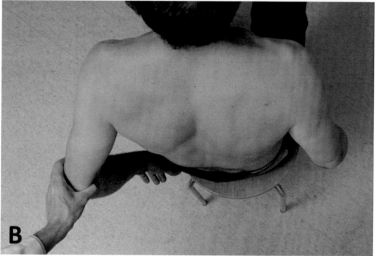

Several studies report that the upper and lower portions of the subscapularis are differentially activated with the belly-press and lift-off tests, potentially providing ancillary diagnostic utility for these tests [75, 124–127]. Although Pennock et al. [128] showed that the subscapularis muscle was electromyographically activated disproportionately more than any other rotator cuff muscle during the belly-press and lift-off tests, their results indicated that the upper and lower portions of the subscapularis were not activated at different magnitudes depending on the clinical test. Chao et al. [124] arrived at similar results regardless of whether the test was performed at

0°, 45°, or 90° of shoulder flexion. Therefore, tests for subscapularis strength should currently be viewed as an evaluation of the entire muscle-tendon unit rather than individual regions of the muscle.

4.6.2.4 Teres Minor
Hornblower's Sign

Weakness of the teres minor muscle is rarely isolated and is usually caused by inferior extension of a posterosuperior rotator cuff tear. Hornblower's sign (or "drop sign" [113]) is another type of lag sign which is primarily used to detect posterosuperior tears with inferior

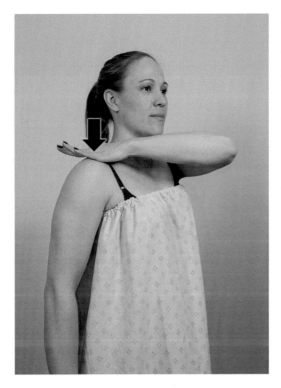

Fig. 4.31 Bear-hug test. In this test, the hand of the patient's affected extremity is placed over the contralateral shoulder with the fingers extended. The patient is instructed to use their hand to push downward onto their contralateral shoulder. A positive test occurs when the elbow of the affected extremity falls inferiorly below the horizontal plane as they attempt to apply a downward pressure onto the contralateral shoulder.

extension. In this test, the humerus is passively abducted to 90° in the scapular plane and maximally externally rotated with the elbow flexed 90°. The patient is then instructed to hold this position of maximal external rotation. A positive test occurs when the humerus involuntarily falls back to internal rotation due to teres minor weakness, thus assuming a position of "horn blowing" (Fig. 4.32).

As mentioned, the vast majority of patients with tears involving the teres minor tendon had pre-existing full-thickness posterosuperior tears that propagated inferiorly as a result of acute trauma (e.g., an acute-on-chronic injury) or chronic tendon degeneration. As a result, many of these patients will have demonstrated concomitant posterosuperior cuff weakness during both the initial strength survey (see Chap. 3 for details regarding strength testing) and subsequent provocative testing. In these cases, the hornblower's sign is performed as described above except that the examiner must help the patient maintain an abduction angle of approximately 90° by providing support beneath the elbow. This additional support is required to optimize the strength and direction of teres minor contraction in patients who would not otherwise be capable of maintaining this level humeral abduction.

Walch et al. [129] found that the sensitivity and specificity of hornblower's sign in its ability to detect teres minor tears were 100 % and 93 %, respectively. In addition, Castoldi et al. [115] found that the external rotation lag sign (described above for infraspinatus tears) was also highly sensitive and specific for the detection of teres minor tears (see Table 4.5). However, this finding should be expected since patients with massive posterior cuff tears are likely to demonstrate weakness of both the infraspinatus and teres minor muscles.

4.7 Summary

Knowledge of the pathogenesis of rotator cuff disease is critical to the interpretation of various physical examination maneuvers that test rotator cuff function. This information can be used to generate solid differential diagnoses based on the details obtained from the history and initial survey which guides the use of appropriate tests. Although having knowledge of each provocative test is useful for the clinician, performing every test on every patient is not fruitful since sensitivity and specificity data for each maneuver are widely variable. Therefore, the purpose of provocative testing is to rule in or out specific diagnoses within the focused differential that was obtained from the history and general survey rather than completing the full gamut of provocative maneuvers on every patient.

Fig. 4.32 Hornblower's sign. (**a**) The examiner passively elevates the humerus to 90° of abduction with the humerus externally rotated and the elbow flexed to 90°. The patient is asked to hold this position as the examiner releases their hand. A positive test occurs when the humerus internally rotates after the examiner releases their hand. (**b**) Clinical photograph demonstrating a positive hornblower's sign. Note that the humerus internally rotates as the arm assumes a position of "hornblowing" in this patient with a massive posterosuperior cuff tear. (From Costouros et al. [122]).

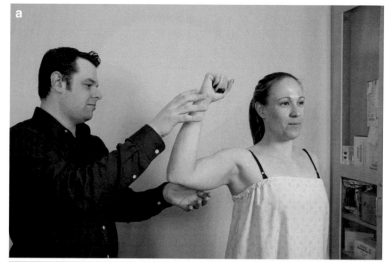

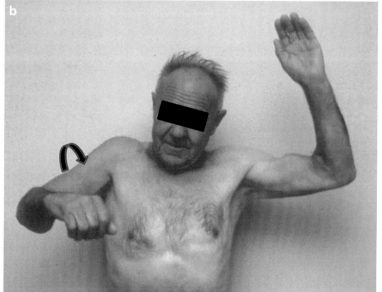

References

1. Dugas JR, Campbell DA, Warren RF, Robie BH, Millett PJ. Anatomy and dimensions of the rotator cuff insertions. J Shoulder Elbow Surg. 2002;11(5):498–503.
2. Burkhart SS. Shoulder arthroscopy. New concepts. Clin Sports Med. 1996;15(4):635–53.
3. Burkhart SS. Arthroscopic debridement and decompression for selected rotator cuff tears. Clinical results, pathomechanics, and patient selection based on biomechanical parameters. Orthop Clin North Am. 1993;24(1):111–23.
4. Burkhart SS. Arthroscopic treatment of massive rotator cuff tears: clinical results and biomechanical rationale. Clin Orthop Relat Res. 1991;267:45–56.
5. Lippitt S, Matsen F. Mechanisms of glenohumeral joint stability. Clin Orthop Relat Res. 1993;291:20–8.
6. Sano H, Hatta T, Yamamoto N, Itoi E. Stress distribution within rotator cuff tendons with a crescent-shaped and an L-shaped tear. Am J Sports Med. 2014;41(10):2262–9.
7. Sano H, Wakabayashi I, Itoi E. Stress distribution in the supraspinatus tendon with partial-thickness tears: an analysis using two-dimensional finite element model. J Shoulder Elbow Surg. 2006;15(1):100–5.

8. Hughes RE, An KN. Force analysis of rotator cuff muscles. Clin Orthop Relat Res. 1996;330: 75–83.
9. Bigliani LU, Levine WN. Subacromial impingement syndrome. J Bone Joint Surg Am. 1997;79(12): 1854–68.
10. Neer II CS. Impingement lesions. Clin Orthop Relat Res. 1983;173:70–7.
11. Vaz S, Soyer J, Pries P, Clarac JP. Subacromial impingement: influence of coracoacromial arch geometry on shoulder function. J Bone Spine. 2000; 67(4):305–9.
12. Lohr JF, Uhthoff HK. The microvascular pattern of the supraspinatus tendon. Clin Orthop. 1990;254: 35–8.
13. Flatow E, Coleman W, Kelkar R. The effect of anterior acromioplasty on rotator cuff contact: an experimental computer simulation. J Shoulder Elbow Surg. 1995;4(1):S53–4.
14. Gill T, McIrvin E, Kocher MS, Horna K, Mair S, Hawkins RJ. The relative importance of acromial morphology and age with respect to rotator cuff pathology. J Shoulder Elbow Surg. 2002;11(4): 327–30.
15. Petersilge CA, Witte DH, Sewell BO, Bosch E, Resnick D. Normal regional anatomy of the shoulder. Magn Reson Imaging Clin N Am. 1997;5(4): 667–81.
16. Pieper HG, Radas CB, Krahl H, Blank M. Anatomic variation of the coracoacromial ligament: a macroscopic and microscopic cadaveric study. J Shoulder Elbow Surg. 1997;6(3):291–6.
17. Matsen FA, Kirby RM. Office evaluation and management of shoulder pain. Orthop Clin North Am. 1982;13(3):45.
18. Lee HJ, Kim YS, Ok JH, Song HJ. Apoptosis occurs throughout the diseased rotator cuff. Am J Sports Med. 2013;41(10):2249–55.
19. Jobe FW, Moynes DR. Delineation of diagnostic criteria and a rehabilitation program for rotator cuff injuries. Am J Sports Med. 1982;10(6):336–9.
20. Fremerey R, Bastian L, Siebert WE. The coracoacromial ligament: anatomical and biomechanical properties with respect to age and rotator cuff disease. Knee Surg Sports Traumatol Arthrosc. 2000;8(5):309–13.
21. Fealy S, April EW, Khazzam M, Armengol-Barallat J, Bigliani LU. The coracoacromial ligament: morphology and study of acromial enthesopathy. J Shoulder Elbow Surg. 2005;14(5):542–8.
22. Chambler AF, Bull AM, Reilly P, Amis AA, Emery RJ. Coracoacromial ligament tension in vivo. J Shoulder Elbow Surg. 2003;12(4):365–7.
23. Yamamoto N, Muraki T, Sperling JW, Steinmann SP, Itoi E, Cofield RH, An KN. Contact between the coracoacromial arch and the rotator cuff tendons in nonpathologic situations: a cadaveric study. J Shoulder Elbow Surg. 2010;19(5):681–7.
24. Sammarco V. Os acromiale: frequency, anatomy and clinical implications. J Bone Joint Surg Am. 2000; 82(3):394–400.
25. Barbier O, Block D, Dezaly C, Sirveaux F, Mole D. Os acromiale, a cause of shoulder pain, not to be overlooked. Orthop Traumatol Surg Res. 2013;99(4): 465–72.
26. Boehm T, Matzer M, Brazda D, Gholke F. Os acromiale associated with tear of the rotator cuff treated operatively. J Bone Joint Surg Br. 2003;85(4): 545–9.
27. Boehm T, Rolf O, Martetschlaeger F, Kenn W, Gohlke F. Rotator cuff tears associated with os acromiale. Acta Orthop. 2005;76(2):241–4.
28. Mudge MK, Wood VE, Frykman GK. Rotator cuff tears associated with os acromiale. J Bone Joint Surg Am. 1984;66(3):427–9.
29. Park JG, Lee JK, Phelps CT. Os acromiale associated with rotator cuff impingement: MR imaging of the shoulder. Radiology. 1994;193(a):255–7.
30. Bigliani L, Ticker J, Flatow E. The relationship of acromial architecture to rotator cuff disease. Clin Sports Med. 1991;10(4):823–38.
31. Wang JC, Horner G, Brown ED, Shapiro MS. The relationship between acromial morphology and conservative treatment of patients with impingement syndrome. Orthopedics. 2000;23(6):557–9.
32. Natsis K, Tsikaras P, Totlis T, Gigis I, Skanalakis P, Appell HJ, Koebke J. Correlation between the four types of acromion and the existence of enthesophytes: a study on 423 dried scapulas and review of the literature. Clin Anat. 2007;20(3):267–72.
33. Hamid N, Omid R, Yamaguchi K, Steger-May K, Stobbs G, Keener JD. Relationship of radiographic acromial characteristics and rotator cuff disease: a prospective investigation of clinical, radiographic and sonographic findings. J Shoulder Elbow Surg. 2012;21(10):1289–98.
34. Balke M, Schmidt C, Dedy N, Banerjee M, Bouillon B, Liem D. Correlation of acromial morphology with impingement syndrome and rotator cuff tears. Acta Orthop. 2013;84(2):178–83.
35. Brooks CH, Revell WJ, Heatley FW. A quantitative histological study of the vascularity of the rotator cuff tendon. J Bone Joint Surg Br. 1992;74(1):151–3.
36. Chang E, Moses D, Babb J, Schweitzer M. Shoulder impingement: objective 3D shape analysis of acromial morphologic features. Radiology. 2006;239(2): 497–505.
37. Hyvönen P, Lohi S, Javovaara P. Open acromioplasty does not prevent the progression of an impingement syndrome to a tear. Nine year follow-up of 96 cases. J Bone Joint Surg Br. 1998;80(5):813–6.
38. Weber S. Arthroscopic debridement and acromioplasty versus mini-open repair in the treatment of significant partial-thickness rotator cuff tears. Arthroscopy. 1999;15(2):126–31.
39. Vanarthos WJ, Monu JU. Type 4 acromion: a new classification. Contemp Orthop. 1995;30(3):227–9.
40. Sanders TG, Miller MD. A systematic approach to magnetic resonance imaging interpretation of sports medicine injuries of the shoulder. Am J Sports Med. 2005;33(7):1088–105.

41. Tucker TJ, Snyder SJ. The keeled acromion: an aggressive acromial variant – a series of 20 patients with associated rotator cuff tears. Arthroscopy. 2004;20(7):744–53.
42. Aoki M, Ishii S, Usui M. The slope of the acromion and rotator cuff impingement. Orthop Trans. 1986;10:228.
43. Banas MP, Miller RJ, Totterman S. Relationship between the lateral acromion angle and rotator cuff disease. J Shoulder Elbow Surg. 1995;4(6):454–61.
44. McGinley JC, Agrawal S, Biswal S. Rotator cuff tears: association with acromion angulation on MRI. Clin Imaging. 2012;36(6):791–6.
45. Baechler M, Kim D. "Uncoverage" of the humeral head by anterolateral acromion and its relationship to full-thickness rotator cuff tears. Mil Med. 2006;171:1035–8.
46. Torrens C, López JM, Puente I, Cáceres E. The influence of the acromial coverage index in rotator cuff tears. J Shoulder Elbow Surg. 2007;16(3):347–51.
47. Nyffeler R, Werner C, Sukthankar A, Schmid M, Gerber C. Association of large lateral extension of the acromion with rotator cuff tears. J Bone Joint Surg Am. 2006;88(4):800–5.
48. Ames JB, Horan MP, Van der Meijden OA, Leake MJ, Millett PJ. Association between acromial index and outcomes following arthroscopic repair of full-thickness rotator cuff tears. J Bone Joint Surg Am. 2012;94(20):1862–9.
49. Kim JR, Ryu KJ, Hong IT, Kim BK, Kim JH. Can a high acromion index predict rotator cuff tears? Int Orthop. 2012;36(5):1019–24.
50. Musil D, Sadovský P, Rost M, Stehlík J, Filip L. [Relationship of acromial morphology and rotator cuff tears]. Acta Chir Orthop Traumatol Cech. 2012;79(3):238–42.
51. Hughes RE, Bryant CR, Hall JM, Wening J, Huston LJ, Kuhn JE, Carpenter JE, Blasier RB. Glenoid inclination is associated with full-thickness rotator cuff tears. Clin Orthop Relat Res. 2003;407:86–91.
52. Tétreault P, Krueger A, Zurakowski D, Gerber C. Glenoid version and rotator cuff tears. J Orthop Res. 2004;22(1):202–7.
53. Dogan M, Cay N, Tosun O, Karaglanoglu M, Bozkurt M. Glenoid axis is not related with rotator cuff tears–a magnetic resonance imaging comparative study. Int Orthop. 2012;36(3):595–8.
54. Tokgoz N, Kanatli U, Voyvoda NK, Gultekin S, Bolukbasi S, Tali ET. The relationship of glenoid and humeral version with supraspinatus tendon tears. Skeletal Radiol. 2007;36(5):509–14.
55. Wong AS, Gallo L, Kuhn JE, Carpenter JE, Hughes RE. The effect of glenoid inclination on superior humeral head migration. J Shoulder Elbow Surg. 2003;12(4):360–4.
56. Gerber C, Snedeker JG, Baumgartner D, Viehöfer AF. Supraspinatus tendon load during abduction is dependent on the size of the critical shoulder angle. A biomechanical analysis. J Orthop Res. 2014; 32(7):952–7.
57. Moor BK, Bouaicha S, Rothenfluh DA, Sukthankar A, Gerber C. Is there an association between the individual anatomy of the scapula and the development of rotator cuff tears or osteoarthritis of the glenohumeral joint? A radiological study of the critical shoulder angle. Bone Joint J. 2013;95-B(7):935–41.
58. Moor BK, Wieser K, Slankamenac K, Gerber C, Bouaicha S. Relationship of individual scapular anatomy and degenerative rotator cuff tears. J Shoulder Elbow Surg. 2014;23(4):536–41.
59. Ogata S, Uhthoff HK. Acromial enthesopathy and rotator cuff tear: a radiologic and histologic postmortem investigation of the coracoacromial arch. Clin Orthop Relat Res. 1990;254:39–48.
60. Burkhart SS, Morgan CD, Kibler WB. The disabled throwing shoulder: spectrum of pathology. Part I, pathoanatomy and biomechanics. Arthroscopy. 2003;19:404–20.
61. Chansky HA, Iannotti JP. The vascularity of the rotator cuff. Clin Sports Med. 1991;10(4):807–22.
62. Lindblom K. On pathogenesis of ruptures of the tendon aponeurosis of the shoulder joint. Acta Radiol. 1939;20:563–77.
63. Ling SC, Chen CF, Wan RX. A study on the vascular supply of the supraspinatus tendon. Surg Radiol Anat. 1990;12(3):161–5.
64. Moseley HF, Goldie I. The arterial pattern of the rotator cuff of the shoulder. J Bone Joint Surg Br. 1963;48:780–9.
65. Rathbun JB, Macnab I. The microvascular pattern of the rotator cuff. J Bone Joint Surg Br. 1970;52(3):540–53.
66. Benson RT, McDonnell SM, Knowles HJ, Rees JL, Carr AJ, Hulley PA. Tendinopathy and tears of the rotator cuff are associated with hypoxia and apoptosis. J Bone Joint Surg Br. 2010;92(3):448–53.
67. Lundgreen K, Lian Ø, Scott A, Engebretsen L. Increased levels of apoptosis and p53 in partial-thickness supraspinatus tendon tears. Knee Surg Sports Traumatol Arthrosc. 2013;21(7):1636–41.
68. Millar NL, Reilly JH, Kerr SC, Campbell AL, Little KJ, Leach WJ, Rooney BP, Murrell GA, McInnes IB. Hypoxia: a critical regulator of early human tendinopathy. Ann Rheum Dis. 2012;71(2):302–10.
69. Clark JM, Harryman II DT. Tendons, ligaments, and capsule of the rotator cuff: gross and microscopic anatomy. J Bone Joint Surg Am. 1992;74(5):713–25.
70. Hawkins RJ, Kennedy JC. Impingement syndrome in athletes. Am J Sports Med. 1980;8(3):151–7.
71. Park HB, Yokota A, Gill HS, El Rassi G, McFarland EG. Diagnostic accuracy of clinical tests for the different degrees of subacromial impingement syndrome. J Bone Joint Surg Am. 2005;87(7):1446–55.
72. Chew K, Pua YH, Chin J, Clarke M, Wong YS. Clinical predictors for the diagnosis of supraspinatus pathology. Physiother Singap. 2010;13(2):12–8.
73. Fodor D, Poanta L, Felea I, et al. Shoulder impingement syndrome: correlations between clinical tests and ultrasonographic findings. Orthop Traumatol Rehabil. 2009;11(2):120–6.

74. Fowler EM, Horsley IG, Rolf CG. Clinical and arthroscopic findings in recreationally active patients. Sports Med Arthrosc Rehabil Ther Technol. 2010;2:2.

75. Kadaba MP, Cole A, Wootten ME, McCann P, Reid M, Mulford G, April E, Bigliani L. Intramuscular wire electromyography of the subscapularis. J Orthop Res. 1992;10(3):394–7.

76. Michener LA, Walsworth MK, Doukas WC, Murphy KP. Reliability and diagnostic accuracy of 5 physical examination tests and combination of tests for subacromial impingement. Arch Phys Med Rehabil. 2009;90(11):1898–903.

77. Salaffi F, Ciapetti A, Carotti M, Gasparini S, Filippucci E, Grassi W. Clinical value of single versus composite provocative clinical tests in the assessment of painful shoulder. J Clin Rheumatol. 2010;16(3):105–8.

78. Silva L, Andréu JL, Muñoz P, Pastrana M, Millán I, Sanz J, Barbadillo C, Fernández-Castro M. Accuracy of physical examination in subacromial impingement syndrome. Rheumatology (Oxford). 2008;47(5):679–83.

79. Kelly SM, Brittle N, Allen GM. The value of physical tests for subacromial impingement syndrome: a study of diagnostic accuracy. Clin Rehabil. 2010;24(2):149–58.

80. Toprak U, Ustuner E, Ozer D, Uyanık S, Baltacı G, Sakızlıoglu SS, Karademir MA, Atay AO. Palpation tests versus impingement tests in Neer stage I and II subacromial impingement syndrome. Knee Surg Sports Traumatol Arthrosc. 2013;21(2):424–9.

81. Hegedus EJ, Goode AP, Cook CE, Michener L, Myer CA, Myer DM, Wright AA. Which physical examination tests provide clinicians with the most value when examining the shoulder? Update of a systematic review with meta-analysis of individual tests. Br J Sports Med. 2012;46(14):964–78.

82. Poppen NK, Walker PS. Forces at the glenohumeral joint in abduction. Clin Orthop Relat Res. 1978;135:165–70.

83. Dumontier C, Sautet A, Gagey O, Apoil A. Rotator interval lesions and their relation to coracoid impingement syndrome. J Shoulder Elbow Surg. 1999;8(2):130–5.

84. Ferrick MR. Coracoid impingement: a case report and review of the literature. Am J Sports Med. 2000;28(1):117–9.

85. Gerber C, Terrier F, Ganz R. The role of the coracoid process in the chronic impingement syndrome. J Bone Joint Surg Br. 1985;67(5):703–8.

86. Martetschläger F, Rios D, Boykin RE, Giphart JE, de Waha A, Millett PJ. Coracoid impingement: current concepts. Knee Surg Sports Traumatol Arthrosc. 2012;20(11):2148–55.

87. Lo IK, Burkhart SS. The etiology and assessment of subscapularis tendon tears: a case for subcoracoid impingement, the roller-wringer effect, and TUFF lesions of the subscapularis. Arthroscopy. 2003;19(10):1142–50.

88. Richards DP, Burkhart SS, Campbell SE. Relation between narrowed coracohumeral distance and subscapularis tears. Arthroscopy. 2005;21(10):1223–8.

89. Goldthwait JE. An anatomic and mechanical study of the shoulder joint, explaining many of the cases of painful shoulder, many of the recurrent dislocations and many cases of brachial neuralgias or neuritis. Am J Orthop Surg. 1909;6:579–606.

90. Bhatia D, de Beer J, Du Toit D. Coracoid process anatomy: implications in radiographic imaging and surgery. Clin Anat. 2007;20:774–84.

91. Dines D, Warrant R, Inglis A, Pavlov H. The coracoid impingement syndrome. J Bone Joint Surg Br. 1990;72(2):314–6.

92. Gumina S, Postacchini F, Orsina L, Cinotti G. The morphometry of the coracoid process – its aetiologic role in subcoracoid impingement syndrome. Int Orthop. 1999;23(4):198–201.

93. Mallon WJ, Brown HR, Vogler 3rd JB, Martinez S. Radiographic and geometric anatomy of the scapula. Clin Orthop Relat Res. 1992;277:142–5.

94. Tracy MR, Trella TA, Mazarian LN, Tuohy CJ, Williams GR. Sonography of the coracohumeral interval: a potential technique for diagnosing coracoid impingement. J Ultrasound Med. 2010;29(3):337–41.

95. Ferreira Neto A, Almeida A, Maiorino R, Zoppi Filho A, Benegas E. An anatomical study of the subcoracoid space. Clinics (Sao Paulo). 2006;61(5):467–72.

96. Jobe CM. Posterior superior glenoid impingement: expanded spectrum. Arthroscopy. 1995;11(5):530–6.

97. Jobe CM. Superior glenoid impingement: current concepts. Clin Orthop Relat Res. 1996;330:98–107.

98. McFarland EG, Hsu CY, Neira C, O'Neil O. Internal impingement of the shoulder: a clinical and arthroscopic analysis. J Shoulder Elbow Surg. 1999;8(5):458–60.

99. Walch G, Boileau P, Noel E, Donell ST. Impingement of the deep surface of the supraspinatus tendon on the posterosuperior glenoid rim: an arthroscopic study. J Shoulder Elbow Surg. 1992;1(5):238–45.

100. Walch G, Liotard JP, Boileau P, Noël E. Postero-superior glenoid impingement. Another impingement of the shoulder. J Radiol. 1993;74(1):47–50.

101. Wolf EM, Agrawal V. Transdeltoid palpation (the rent test) in the diagnosis of rotator cuff tears. J Shoulder Elbow Surg. 2001;10(5):470–3.

102. Kim HM, Teefey SA, Zelig A, Galatz LM, Keender JD, Yamaguchi K. Shoulder strength in asymptomatic individuals with intact compared with torn rotator cuffs. J Bone Joint Surg Am. 2009;91(2):289–96.

103. Yamaguchi K, Sher JS, Andersen WK, Garretson R, Uribe JW, Hechtman K, Neviaser RJ. Glenohumeral motion in patients with rotator cuff tears: a comparison of asymptomatic and symptomatic shoulders. J Shoulder Elbow Surg. 2000;9(1):6–11.

104. Yamaguchi K, Tetro AM, Blam O, Evanoff BA, Teefey SA, Middleton WD. Natural history of asymptomatic rotator cuff tears: a longitudinal analysis of asymptomatic tears detected sonographically. J Shoulder Elbow Surg. 2001;10(3):199–203.

105. Codman EA. The shoulder: rupture of the supraspinatus tendon and other lesions in or about the subacromial bursa. Chap. 5. Boston: Thomas Todd; 1934. p. 123–77.

106. Ponce BA, Kundukulam JA, Sheppard ED, Determann JR, McGwin G, Narducci CA, Crowther MJ. Rotator cuff crepitus: could Codman really feel a cuff tear? J Shoulder Elbow Surg. 2014;23(7): 1017–22.

107. Lyons AR, Tomlinson JE. Clinical diagnosis of tears of the rotator cuff. J Bone Joint Surg Br. 1992;74(3):414–5.

108. Kelly BT, Kadrmas WR, Speer KP. The manual muscle examination for rotator cuff strength. An electromyographic investigation. Am J Sports Med. 1996;24(5):581–8.

109. Itoi E, Minagawa H, Yamamoto N, Seki N, Abe H. Are pain location and physical examinations useful in locating a tear site of the rotator cuff? Am J Sports Med. 2006;34(2):256–64.

110. Kim E, Jeong HJ, Lee KW, Song JS. Interpreting positive signs of the supraspinatus test in screening for torn rotator cuff. Acta Med Okayama. 2006; 60(4):223–38.

111. Bak K, Sørensen AK, Jørgensen U, Nygaard M, Krarup AL, Thune C, Sloth C, Pedersen ST. The value of clinical tests in acute full-thickness tears of the supraspinatus tendon: does a subacromial lidocaine injection help the clinical diagnosis? A prospective study. Arthroscopy. 2010;26(6): 734–42.

112. Miller CA, Forrester GA, Lewis JS. The validity of the lag signs in diagnosing full-thickness tears of the rotator cuff: a preliminary investigation. Arch Phys Med Rehabil. 2008;89(6):1162–8.

113. Hertel R, Ballmer FT, Lombert SM, Gerber C. Lag signs in the diagnosis of rotator cuff rupture. J Shoulder Elbow Surg. 1996;5(4):307–13.

114. Blonna D, Cecchetti S, Tellini A, Bonasia DE, Rossi R, Southgate R, Castoldi F. Contribution of the supraspinatus to the external rotator lag sign: kinematic and electromyographic pattern in an in vivo model. J Shoulder Elbow Surg. 2010;19(3): 392–8.

115. Castoldi F, Blonna D, Hertel R. External rotation lag sign revisited: accuracy for diagnosis of full thickness supraspinatus tear. J Shoulder Elbow Surg. 2009;18(4):529–34.

116. Bartsch M, Greiner S, Haas NP, Scheibel M. Diagnostic values of clinical tests for subscapularis lesions. Knee Surg Sports Traumatol Arthrosc. 2010;18(12):1712–77.

117. Yoon JP, Chung SW, Kim SH, Oh JH. Diagnostic value of four clinical tests for the evaluation of subscapularis integrity. J Shoulder Elbow Surg. 2013;22(9):1186–92.

118. Naredo E, Aguado P, De Miguel E, Uson J, Mayordomo L, Gijon-Baños J, Martin-Mola E. Painful shoulder: comparison of physical examination and ultrasonographic findings. Ann Rheum Dis. 2002;61(2):132–6.

119. Kim HA, Kim SH, Seo YI. Ultrasonographic findings of painful shoulders and correlation between physical examination and ultrasonographic rotator cuff tear. Mod Rheumatol. 2007;17(3):213–9.

120. Barth JR, Burkhart SS, DeBeer JF. The bear-hug test: a new and sensitive test for diagnosing a subscapularis tear. Arthroscopy. 2006;22(10):1076–84.

121. Furuqui S, Wijdicks C, Foad A. Sensitivity of physical examination versus arthroscopy in diagnosis subscapularis tendon injury. Orthopedics. 2014;37(1): e29–33.

122. Costouros JG, Gerber C, Warner JJP. Latissimus dorsi tendon transfer. In: ElAttrache NS, Mirzayan R, Harnder CD, Sekiya JK, editors. Surgical techniques in sports medicine. 1st ed., Chap. 8. Philadelphia: Lippincott Williams & Wilkins; 2007.

123. Stefko JM, Jobe FW, VanderWilde RS, Carden E, Pink M. Electromyographic and nerve block analysis of the subscapularis liftoff test. J Shoulder Elbow Surg. 1997;6(4):347–55.

124. Chao S, Thomas S, Yucha D, Kelly 4th JD, Driban J, Swanik K. An electromyographic assessment of the "bear hug": an examination for the evaluation of the subscapularis muscle. Arthroscopy. 2008;24(11): 1265–70.

125. Greis PE, Kuhn JE, Schultheis J, Hintermeister R, Hawkins R. Validation of the lift-off tests and analysis of subscapualris activity during maximal internal rotation. Am J Sports Med. 1996;24(5):589–93.

126. Nemeth G, Kronberg M, Brostrom LA. Electromyogram (EMG) recordings from the subscapularis muscle: description of a technique. J Orthop Res. 1990;8(1):151–3.

127. Tokish JM, Decker MJ, Ellis HB, Torry MR, Hawkins RJ. The belly-press test for the physical examination of the subscapularis muscle: electromyographic validation and comparison to the lift-off test. J Shoulder Elbow Surg. 2003;12(5):427–30.

128. Pennock AT, Pennington WW, Torry MR, Decker MJ, Vaishnav SB, Provencher MT, Millett PJ, Hackett TR. The influence of arm and shoulder position on the bear-hug, belly-press and lift-off tests: an electromyographic study. Am J Sports Med. 2011;39(11):2338–46.

129. Walch G, Boulahia A, Calderone S, Robinson AH. The 'dropping' and 'hornblower's' signs in evaluation of rotator-cuff tears. J Bone Joint Surg Br. 1998;80(4):624–8.

Disorders of the Long Head of the Biceps Tendon

5

5.1 Introduction

Although its precise function remains relatively unknown, the long head of the biceps (LHB) tendon is likely a significant pain generator in a variety of shoulder conditions. Therefore, pathology related to the LHB tendon should be assessed in any patient with a condition related to the glenohumeral joint. Unfortunately, physical examination is often difficult due to confounding results and the lack of definitive research. However, an in-depth knowledge of relevant anatomy, biomechanics, and pathoanatomy can typically overcome these confounders and is instrumental in making any diagnosis or formulating a treatment plan related to the LHB tendon.

5.2 Anatomy and Biomechanics

5.2.1 Anatomy

The biceps brachii, innervated by the musculocutaneous nerve, has two heads that originate from different points on the scapula. The short head arises from the coracoid process as a single tendon combined with the coracobrachialis muscle (the conjoined tendon) and the long head arises from within the glenohumeral joint from both the supraglenoid tubercle and the adjacent glenoid labrum (Fig. 5.1). The tendon travels anterolaterally in the rotator interval and exits the joint through the bicipital groove which lies between the greater and lesser tuberosities of the proximal humerus. Travelling distally, the muscle bellies of each head coalesce, cross the cubital fossa and spiral towards their primary insertion on the bicipital tuberosity on the proximal radius (Fig. 5.2). This chapter will focus on the intra-articular portion of the LHB tendon since it is often implicated in the development of acute and chronic shoulder pain.

The supraglenoid tubercle of the scapula has historically been described as the origin of the LHB tendon. However, several cadaveric studies have found that the superior labrum contributes significantly to the LHB origin [1–5]. In a series of 105 cadaveric shoulders, Vangsness Jr et al. [5] found that 40–60 % of the LHB tendon originated from the supraglenoid tubercle while the remaining fibers originated from the superior labrum (Fig. 5.3). Tuoheti et al. [4] dissected 101 cadaveric shoulders and found that the LHB tendon originated from both the supraglenoid tubercle and the glenoid in every case. In addition, Gigis et al. [2] noted that the LHB not only arises from both the supraglenoid tubercle and the labrum, but it also forms a portion of the posterosuperior labrum itself. An anatomic study of 16 cadaveric shoulders by Arai et al. [1] found that the fibers of the labrum became stiffer and stronger as the LHB tendon origin was approached. These studies support other claims that the torsional strain placed upon the superior labrum by the LHB tendon in positions of hyperabduction and external rotation is at least one factor

R.J. Warth and P.J. Millett, *Physical Examination of the Shoulder: An Evidence-Based Approach*, DOI 10.1007/978-1-4939-2593-3_5, © Springer Science+Business Media New York 2015

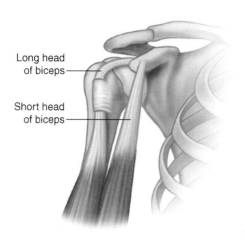

Fig. 5.1 Illustration depicting the basic anatomy of the long and short heads of the proximal biceps muscle.

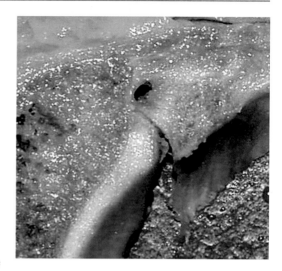

Fig. 5.3 Cadaveric photograph showing the insertion of the proximal biceps tendon on both the superior glenoid labrum and the supraglenoid tubercle.

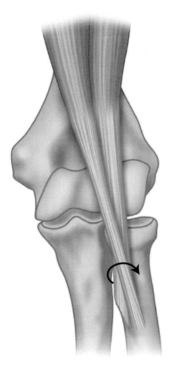

Fig. 5.2 Illustration demonstrating the rotation of the distal biceps tendon just before its insertion on the bicipital tuberosity.

involved in the development of superior labral anterior to posterior (SLAP) tears in throwing athletes (discussed later in this chapter) [6].

One of the difficulties inherent to the diagnosis of SLAP tears, especially with regard to imag-

ing studies, is the significant anatomic variability of the biceps anchor-superior labrum complex. According to Rao et al. [7], there are three predominant variations in superior labral anatomy that may be present in up to 10 % of the general population: the sublabral recess, the sublabral foramen, and the Buford complex (Figs. 5.4 and 5.5). The sublabral recess represents a potential space beneath the biceps anchor and the anterosuperior aspect of the glenoid labrum. The sublabral foramen is a small orifice located between the anterosuperior labrum and the articular cartilage of the anterior glenoid. The Buford complex is characterized by an absence of the anterosuperior labrum with a cord-like middle glenohumeral ligament that attaches directly to the superior labrum. It is crucial for the clinician to identify these findings as normal anatomic variants rather than pathologic lesions since inappropriate "repair" may lead to significant pain and external rotation loss as a result of stiffness [8, 9].

As the LHB tendon travels obliquely through the joint in an anterolateral direction, the tendon is encased in an outward-facing synovial membrane that is continuous with the joint capsule and renders the tendon extra-synovial [10]. As the tendon travels distally towards the bicipital groove of the proximal humerus, its position is

Fig. 5.4 Illustration depicting the normal anatomy of the glenohumeral capsuloligamentous structures.

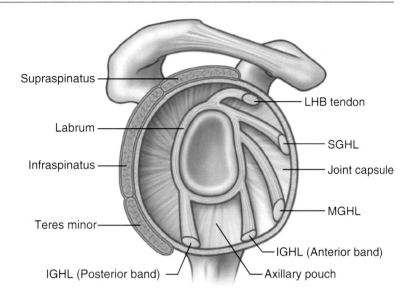

Supraspinatus

Labrum

Infraspinatus

Teres minor

LHB tendon

SGHL

Joint capsule

MGHL

IGHL (Anterior band)

IGHL (Posterior band)

Axillary pouch

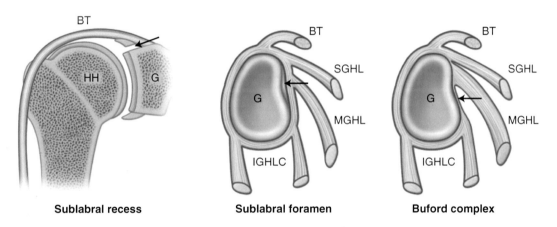

Sublabral recess   Sublabral foramen   Buford complex

Fig. 5.5 Illustrations showing the most common glenolabral anatomic variations. The sublabral recess, sublabral foramen, and Buford complex are shown.

maintained by the capsuloligamentous restraints within the rotator interval. The rotator interval is a triangular area in the anterosuperior aspect of the glenohumeral joint (Fig. 5.6). The medial base of the triangle is located at the coracoid process. The anterior margin of the supraspinatus and the superior margin of the subscapularis make up the superior and inferior borders of the rotator interval triangle, respectively. The lateral apex of the rotator interval is composed of the transverse humeral ligament which covers the

bicipital groove and contributes to the bicipital sheath (discussed below). The contents of the interval include the LHB tendon, the superior glenohumeral ligament (SGHL), the coracohumeral ligament (CHL), and the glenohumeral joint capsule [11]. A more detailed description of the structure, function, and pathologies associated with the rotator interval can be found in Chap. 6.

As the LHB tendon courses towards the bicipital groove, the SGHL and the CHL form a sling

Fig. 5.6 Illustration
highlighting the compo-
nents of the rotator interval.

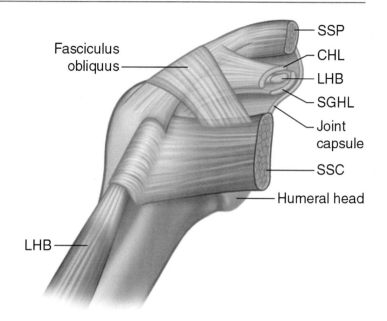

around the LHB tendon, primarily preventing its medial subluxation. This sling extends to the most anterior portion of the rotator cable and the biceps reflection pulley (BRP) at the proximal end of the bicipital groove [12]. The BRP, derived from the coalition of the SGHL, CHL, and the upper 1/3 of the subscapularis tendon, redirects the anterolateral course of the LHB tendon such that the tendon travels directly inferiorly along the anterior humeral shaft (Fig. 5.7). Habermeyer et al. [14] described a 30–40° inferior turn of the LHB tendon as it exited the joint via the BRP. Tearing of the subscapularis in this region, often known as a "pulley lesion," can allow medial subluxation of the LHB tendon producing a painful "popping" or "snapping" sensation as the arm is moved (Fig. 5.8). In addition, a biomechanical study by Braun et al. [16] found that the LHB tendon slides up to 18 mm in and out of the joint with forward flexion and internal rotation, respectively. Therefore, the LHB tendon itself is subjected to significant mechanical stresses in the area of the BRP which can lead to tendonitis, tearing or rupture of the LHB.

The bicipital sheath is another complex structure through which the LHB tendon traverses as it passes through the bicipital groove (see Fig. 5.7). The floor of this sheath is formed from the coalescence of the SGHL and the subscapularis tendons at the superior aspect of the lesser tuberosity. These fibers then travel laterally, forming the floor of the bicipital sheath. The roof of the sheath is mostly composed of fibers from both the supraspinatus and CHL ligaments. All of these fibers (the floor and the roof of the sheath) combine to form a continuous ring around the LHB tendon as it passes through the bicipital groove thus providing tendon stability (Fig. 5.9). A recent biomechanical study by Kwon et al. [17] found that the subscapularis tendon was the most important stabilizer of the LHB tendon within the bicipital groove since tears of the subscapularis in this area almost always resulted in medial subluxation of the LHB tendon.

The bony structure of the bicipital groove can also play a role in pathologies of the LHB tendon. In a radiographic study by Pfahler et al. [18], the opening angle of the groove in patients without

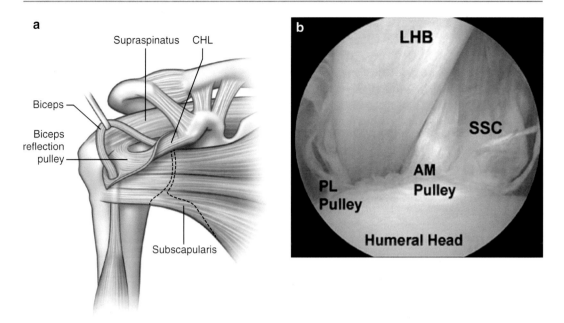

Fig. 5.7 (**a**) Illustration showing the structure of the bicipital sheath and biceps reflection pulley as the LHB tendon travels away from the glenohumeral joint. (**b**) Arthroscopic image showing anteromedial (AM) and posterolateral (PL) BRPs. (From Elser et al. [13]; with permission).

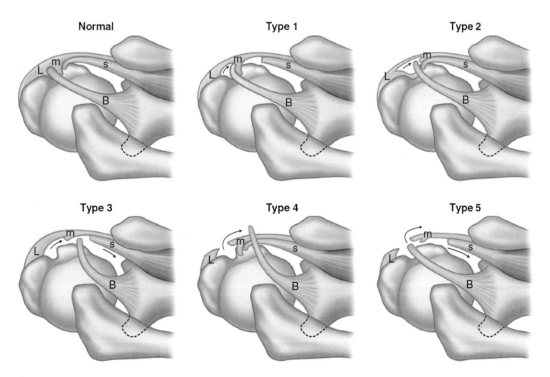

Fig. 5.8 Classification of pulley lesions as proposed by Bennett [15]. Note that medial subluxation of the LHB tendon is much more common than lateral subluxation.

LHB tendon pathology was between 101° and 120° with the medial wall having a greater height than the lateral wall. Patients with a shallow groove or a lower medial wall may also be susceptible to subluxation of the LHB tendon.

The vascular supply to the LHB tendon near the biceps-labral complex is variably derived from the suprascapular, circumflex scapular and posterior circumflex humeral arteries [10]. Vascularity of the tendon is richest near its origin and dissipates prior to entering the bicipital groove where the tendon is avascular and fibrocartilaginous. This infrastructure helps prevent tendon injury from the sliding action of the LHB within the sheath of the groove. Similarly, innervation of the LHB tendon is concentrated near its anchor and dissipates as the tendon travels distally [19]. This arrangement was described as a "net-like" pattern of sympathetic fibers by Alpantaki et al. [19] in a cadaveric study using neurofilament antibodies (Fig. 5.10). In addition, Tosounidis et al. [20] demonstrated the presence of sympathetic α_1-adrenergic receptors along the LHB tendon in cadaveric specimens with known acute and chronic shoulder conditions. These studies demonstrate that sympathetic innervation of the proximal LHB tendon may play a role in the pathogenesis of shoulder pain.

5.2.2 Biomechanics

Although the anatomy of the proximal LHB tendon has been well described, its precise function has been debated for many years. Most studies that have aimed to describe its function are based on cadaveric models that focus on glenohumeral stability.

Pagnani et al. [21] used ten cadaveric shoulders to show that decreased anterior, superior, and inferior humeral head translation occurred when a simulated load of 55 N was applied to the LHB tendon in lower angles of elevation. Rodosky et al. [22] used a dynamic cadaveric shoulder model to simulate the forces typically applied to both the rotator cuff and the LHB tendons. They found that the LHB tendon contributed to glenohumeral stability by resisting torsional forces in the abducted and externally rotated position. The authors also noted a significantly increased strain applied to the anterior band of the inferior glenohumeral ligament (IGHL) when the biceps-labral complex was detached from its anchor at the superior aspect of the glenoid. This study provides some evidence that SLAP tears may contribute to increased anterior humeral head translation that is often found during physical examination (see Chap. 6 for more details regarding glenohumeral laxity and instability). More recently, Youm et al. [23] showed that the LHB tendon contributed significantly to anterior, posterior, superior, and inferior translation of the humeral head when a 22 N load was applied.

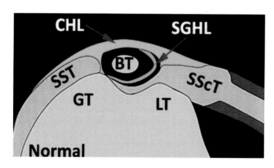

Fig. 5.9 Illustration highlighting the structures involved with a normal bicipital sheath [101].

Fig. 5.10 Photomicrograph showing the attachment of neurofilament antibodies to the proximal LHB tendon in a "net-like" pattern (from Alpantaki et al. [19]; with permission).

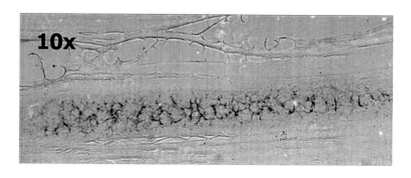

Rotational range of motion and scapulohumeral kinematics were also affected when a load was applied to the LHB tendon. Alexander et al. [102] also noted a decrease in humeral head translation in all directions when a 20 N load was applied to the LHB tendon. Su et al. [24] studied the effects of the LHB tendon in cadaveric shoulders with variably sized rotator cuff tears. In their study, a significant decrease in anterosuperior and superior humeral head translation occurred when a 55 N load was applied to the LHB tendon.

Itoi et al. [25] contested that both the LHB and the short head of the biceps contribute significantly to glenohumeral joint stability, particularly in positions of abduction and external rotation when a simulated load of 1.5 and 3.0 kg were applied. This contribution to stability was particularly robust after attenuation of anterior stabilizing structures had occurred. In another biomechanical study, Kumar et al. [26] showed that loading of the short head of the biceps alone caused superior migration of the humeral head whereas tensioning of both the short head and the LHB simultaneously did not result in humeral head translation in any direction.

Although these studies suggest the role of the LHB tendon may be associated with glenohumeral stability, interpretation of dynamic shoulder models is difficult since replication of the in vivo environment, including complex force couples and resting tension, is quite difficult to achieve. In addition, the variability of simulated loads (11–55 N) makes their results difficult to compare, especially when the precise physiologic loads applied to the LHB tendon in different angles of abduction and rotation are currently unknown. Thus, it is possible that some studies may have obtained statistically significant results due to the application of non-physiologically high loads, making the results of these studies difficult to interpret.

To help answer these questions, electromyographic (EMG) studies have been performed to evaluate the effect of the LHB tendon on glenohumeral kinematics. However, their findings have been inconsistent to date. Levy et al. [27] found that the LHB tendon aided in glenohumeral stability both passively and in association with forearm supination or flexion. In contrast, Sakurai et al. [28] determined that the LHB tendon dynamically stabilized the humeral head, regardless of elbow activity. Other studies on pitching biomechanics found that the biceps may primarily function as a stabilizer of the elbow during flexion and supination with little effect on shoulder stability [29, 30]. Thus, the effect of the LHB tendon on glenohumeral kinematics remains controversial with respect to the most current EMG literature.

Both cadaveric and EMG studies have produced an incomplete picture of how the LHB tendon actually functions with regard to glenohumeral kinematics. Therefore, in vivo studies have also been conducted to help solve the mystery. Warner and MacMahon [31] studied a group of seven patients with rupture of the proximal LHB tendon and compared humeral head translation to their unaffected shoulders by true anteroposterior radiographs. In their study, radiographs were obtained in 0°, 45°, 90°, and 120° of abduction in the scapular plane. They found that superior migration of the humeral head was significantly increased in the shoulders with a ruptured LHB tendon compared to their contralateral, unaffected shoulders at all angles of abduction. Another radiographic study by Kido et al. [32] found similar results, noting that the humeral head was depressed as the LHB tendon was stimulated. However, the accuracy of radiographic studies has been called into question. Therefore, three-dimensional biplane fluoroscopy, a modality which has sub-millimeter accuracy, has been used to study in vivo kinematics with improved accuracy during full muscle activation. A study by Giphart et al. [33] found that, in five patients who underwent unilateral open subpectoral biceps tenodesis, humeral head translations of approximately 3 mm occurred in both the affected and unaffected shoulders during active elevation. The authors also studied various loading conditions such as forward flexion with maximal biceps activity on EMG, abduction to assess superior translation and a simulated throw (hyperabduction and external rotation) to evaluate anterior translation. Despite these loading conditions, the differences in translation between tenodesed and normal shoulders was always less than 1.0 mm, suggesting that the proximal LHB tendon may actually play a minimal role in

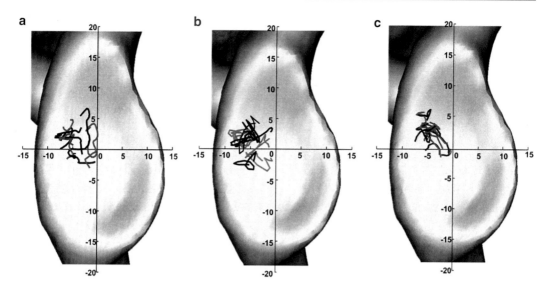

Fig. 5.11 Depiction of humeral head translation with (**a**) foward flexion, (**b**) abduction and (**c**) a simulated throwing motion. For each testing condition, biceps tenodesis resulted in minimal differences in humeral head translation when compared to the contralateral shoulder with various loading conditions.

glenohumeral kinematics in a shoulder that otherwise has an intact rotator cuff (Fig. 5.11).

The inconsistent and often contradictory findings of cadaveric, EMG, and in vivo studies have made it difficult to define the precise function of the proximal LHB tendon. While most of these studies have found that the LHB tendon may be involved with glenohumeral stability, further in vivo kinematic studies are necessary to completely elucidate the biomechanical role of the LHB tendon in shoulder motion and stability.

5.3   LHB Tendonitis, Tearing and Rupture

LHB tendonitis can occur as a result of impingement under the coracoacromial arch, subluxation out of the bicipital groove, or attrition as a result of degeneration [34]. Due to the many concurrent pathologies that are typically present in patients with LHB tendonitis, physical diagnosis is often difficult. However, a precise knowledge of the pathogenesis of LHB tendonitis will help the clinician synthesize a complete and accurate differential diagnosis with an understanding that overlapping conditions are often present.

5.3.1   Pathogenesis

Inflammation of the LHB tendon most often occurs secondarily as a result of surrounding pathologies such as impingement syndrome, pulley lesions, and/or degenerative rotator cuff tears (Fig. 5.12). Primary LHB tendonitis, in which there is isolated inflammation with no apparent cause, is not uncommon in clinical practice. Although isolated inflammation of the proximal LHB tendon can occur in overhead athletes, this may be the result of repetitive microtrauma as the tendon glides back and forth in a "sawing" motion within the bicipital groove and across the BRP. It is important to remember that because the LHB tendon is encased with synovium, inflammation within the shoulder may track proximally into the biceps-labral complex or distally into the bicipital groove.

Subacromial impingement is the most common mechanism by which LHB tendonitis occurs, especially in older patients. Subcoracoid impingement can also lead to injury involving the LHB tendon and the BRP [35]. Weak rotator cuff and periscapular musculature potentially allow increased translation of the humeral head, narrowing the space available for the subacromial or subcoracoid contents to pass thus allowing

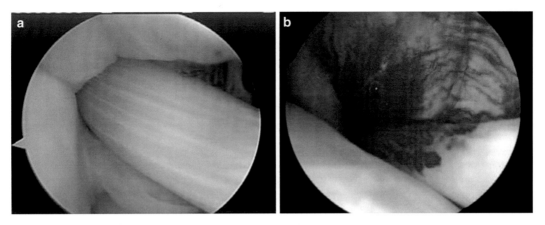

Fig. 5.12 Arthroscopic images demonstrating (**a**) a healthy LHB tendon and (**b**) an inflamed LHB tendon.

impingement of these structures between the greater tuberosity and the undersurface of the acromion or between the lesser tuberosity and the coracoid (further details on subacromial impingement and subcoracoid impingement are provided in Chap. 4). In patients with subacromial impingement, LHB tendonitis almost always occurs simultaneously since the LHB is subject to the same mechanical wear from the coracoacromial arch. In addition, because the LHB tendon is encased in an outward-facing synovial membrane extending from the glenohumeral joint, any inflammatory process within the joint can thus involve the LHB tendon, producing painful inflammation and tenosynovitis (Fig. 5.12).

The acute stage of LHB tendonitis is characterized by significant anterior shoulder pain localized within the bicipital groove. The LHB tendon will swell and sometimes develop partial-thickness tearing at points of maximal wear. Later, the tendon further degenerates and may form adhesions with surrounding structures such as the bicipital sheath and rotator interval structures. In this stage, microscopic examination reveals fibrinoid necrosis and atrophy of collagen fibers [36]. As the tendon degenerates, it can either become hypertrophic or atrophic with a deterioration of its organization and infrastructure. If, or when, rupture occurs, symptoms will often resolve immediately with the formation of a "Popeye" deformity (discussed later). On the contrary, attritional tendon degeneration may occur asymptomatically and painless rupture may occur.

5.3.2   Physical Examination

Evaluation of patients with bicipital tendonitis is often difficult due to vague symptoms and inconsistent physical examination findings. It is therefore critically important to obtain a detailed history to help guide the use of appropriate provocative testing. Some patients may describe a "popping" or "snapping" sensation, especially when internally and externally rotating the humerus in 90° of abduction. Although the most common finding in patients with bicipital tendonitis is bicipital groove tenderness, this type of pain is difficult to differentiate from pain related to the anterosuperior cuff which inserts in the area of the bicipital sheath. Patients who describe a history of anterior shoulder pain that suddenly resolved after a specific incident likely had spontaneous rupture of their LHB tendon.

Both upper extremities of every patient should be inspected for any evidence of asymmetry. Spontaneous rupture of the proximal LHB tendon can result in the classic "Popeye" deformity in which the muscle belly is distally retracted, appearing as distinct bulge in the distal aspect of the humerus just above the elbow (Fig. 5.13). Strength and range of motion should also be recorded for each extremity, particularly noting any discrepancies. Range of motion loss in patients with bicipital groove tenderness is most often associated with concomitant rotator cuff disease (see Chap. 4 for information regarding physical examination of the rotator cuff). Because

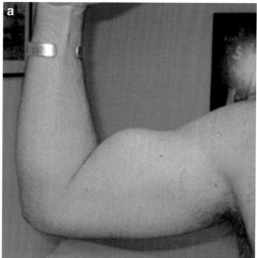
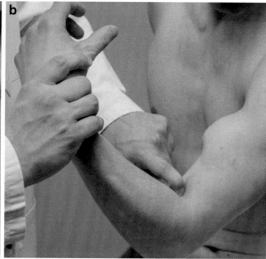

Fig. 5.13 Clinical photograph of Popeye deformity in (**a**) proximal LHB tendon rupture and (**b**) distal biceps tendon rupture. Note that proximal LHB tendon rupture

results in distal retraction of the muscle belly whereas distal biceps tendon rupture results in proximal retraction of the muscle belly.

some biomechanical data suggests that the LHB tendon functions to promote glenohumeral stability, it may also important to perform stability testing in these patients (see Chap. 6). The most important provocative tests traditionally used for the detection of bicipital tendonitis and tearing are presented below.

5.3.2.1 Palpation
There are several physical examination tests that involve palpation of the LHB tendon on the anterior aspect of the shoulder to detect peri-tendonitis or tearing. However, rather than delving into each individual palpation technique, it is most important to realize that the bicipital groove faces directly anteriorly when the humerus is slightly internally rotated and tenderness with palpation of the groove will typically move laterally as the humerus is externally rotated (Fig. 5.14). Although testing for bicipital tenderness is nonspecific and examiner dependent, when present, it is sometimes helpful to rule out other pathologies within the differential diagnosis. A recent study by Chen et al. [37] found that bicipital tenderness was 57 % sensitive and 74 % specific for the presence of biceps tendonitis after confirmation with ultrasonographic evaluation. Gill et al. [38] reported the diagnostic accuracy of bicipital

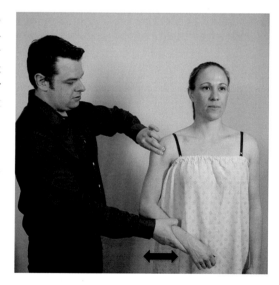

Fig. 5.14 Bicipital groove palpation. The LHB tendon is most easily palpated when the humerus is slightly internally rotated. The examiner can also simultaneously internally and externally rotate the humerus to detect any evidence of subluxation.

groove tenderness to detect partial-thickness tears of the LHB tendon; the authors calculated a sensitivity of only 53 % and a specificity of only 54 % using this diagnostic test. Thus, palpation of the bicipital groove should only be used to document the presence or absence of bicipital

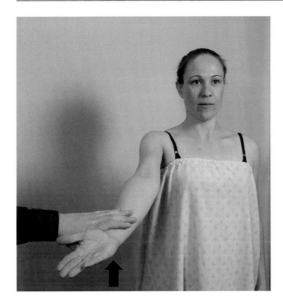

Fig. 5.15 Speed test. The patient is asked to forward flex the humerus to approximately 90° of elevation with the elbow extended and the forearm supinated (*palm upward*). The examiner then applies a downward pressure to the distal arm as the patient provides resistance.

groove tenderness since the test is not sensitive or specific for the detection of partial-thickness tears.

5.3.2.2 Speed Test

In the Speed test, the affected arm is placed in a position of 90° forward flexion with the elbow extended and the palm supinated. From this position, the examiner applies a downward force to the forearm while the patient resists (Fig. 5.15). Pain localized to the area of the bicipital groove is a positive test and may indicate the presence of bicipital tendonitis or partial tearing. The specificity for this test is much higher than its sensitivity, thus requiring a combination of historical and other physical findings to make the correct diagnosis (Table 5.1).

5.3.2.3 Yergason Test

In the Yergason test, the affected arm is placed at the side with the elbow flexed 90°. In patients with bicipital tendonitis or partial tearing, resisted supination of the forearm should produce pain over the anterior aspect of the shoulder localized to the bicipital groove (Fig. 5.16). Similar to the Speed test, the

specificity for the Yergason test is higher than its sensitivity thus requiring further information in order to make the correct diagnosis (see Table 5.1).

5.3.2.4 Lift-Off Test

Testing for rotator cuff function, especially that of the subscapularis, can also provide clues regarding the status of the proximal LHB tendon as it passes through the bicipital groove. Tearing of the subscapularis may also involve tearing of the bicipital sheath and the LHB tendon itself. Gill et al. [38] noted that the lift-off test, which tests the strength of the subscapularis, had a sensitivity of 28 % and a specificity of 89 % for the detection of partial-thickness tears of the LHB tendon. The bear-hug test can also be used to detect biceps tendinopathy with a reported sensitivity of 79 % and a specificity of 60 % [40]. See Chap. 4 for details regarding physical examination for the detection of subscapularis pathology.

5.3.2.5 Biceps Entrapment Sign

The hourglass biceps, first described by Boileau et al. [54] in 2004, occurs when the LHB tendon in the proximity of the bicipital sheath becomes inflamed and swells to a diameter that exceed that of the bicipital groove, thus preventing the LHB tendon from gliding within the sheath as shoulder motion is initiated (Fig. 5.17). Arthroscopically, the defect resembles an hourglass-shape that becomes entrapped proximal to the bicipital sheath which typically limits forward flexion capacity.

Boileau et al. [54] originally reported this entity in a series of 21 patients with a "hypertrophic intra-articular portion of the LHB tendon," all of which were associated with rotator cuff tearing. The authors noted that a 10–20° loss of passive forward flexion in the presence of bicipital groove tenderness were the most common physical findings in this group of patients. Others have suggested that both active and passive motion should be restricted where an attempt to increase the forward flexion angle results in increased shoulder pain [55]. Because this examination finding has not been formally validated, imaging studies such as those including ultrasonic evaluation [56], remain important for identification of these lesions in the clinical setting.

Table 5.1 Reported diagnostic efficacies of clinical tests used for the detection of LHB tendonitis

Maneuver	Author(s)	Year	Pathology	Diagnostic standard	Sensitivity (%)	Specificity (%)	LR+	LR−
Palpation	Chen et al. [37]	2011	Tendonitis	Ultrasound	57	74	2.2	0.58
	Gill et al. [38]	2007	Partial tear	Arthroscopy	53	54	1.15	0.87
Lift-off test	Gill et al. [38]	2007	Partial tear	Arthroscopy	28	89	2.5	0.81
	Jia et al. [39]	2009	Tendonitis	Arthroscopy	28	89	2.5	0.81
Speed test	Gill et al. [38]	2007	Partial tear	Arthroscopy	50	67	1.51	0.75
	Kibler et al. [40]	2009	Tendonitis	Arthroscopy	54	81	2.77	0.58
	Jia et al. [39]	2009	Tendonitis	Arthroscopy	50	67	1.52	0.75
	Goyal et al. [41]	2010	Tendonitis	Ultrasound	71	85	4.6	0.34
	Salaffi et al. [42]	2010	Tendonitis	Ultrasound	49	76	2.1	0.66
	Chen et al. [37]	2011	Tendonitis	Ultrasound	63	60	1.55	0.63
Yergason test	Oh et al. [43]	2007	Tendonitis	Ultrasound	75	81	4.03	0.31
	Kibler et al. [40]	2009	Tendonitis	Arthroscopy	41	79	1.94	0.74
	Chen et al. [37]	2011	Tendonitis	Ultrasound	32	78	1.47	0.87

LR likelihood ratio

Fig. 5.16 Yergason test. With the arm at the side and the elbow flexed to 90°, the patient attempts to supinate the forearm against resistance provided by the examiner.

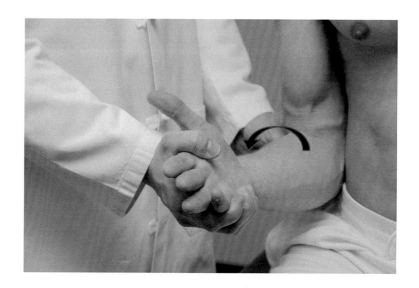

5.4 LHB Tendon Instability

Instability of the LHB tendon is most often associated with tearing of the subscapularis tendon, coracohumeral ligament, and the SGHL, all of which are components of the BRP (Fig. 5.18) [15, 57, 58]. Although several authors have proposed different classification systems to describe LHB instability [14, 57, 59], most clinicians still categorize this pathology into one of two types primarily based on the system developed by Walch et al. [59] in 1998:

(1) subluxation out of the groove, (2) dislocation out of the groove, and (3) intra-articular dislocation. In general, most episodes of instability occur with the LHB translating medially over the lesser tuberosity. Lateral instability of the LHB tendon is rare.

5.4.1 Pathogenesis

The pathogenesis of pulley lesions that lead to medial subluxation or dislocation of the LHB tendon has not been completely elucidated.

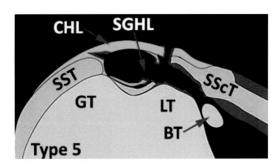

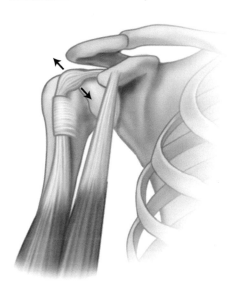

Fig. 5.18 Illustration showing medial biceps subluxation as a result of tearing of the subscapularis tendon and the SGHL. Tearing of the coracohumeral ligament can also be seen. *Source*: Stadnick ME. Pathology of the long head of the biceps tendon. Radsource Web Clinics. February 2014. http://radsource.us/pathology-of-the-long-head-of-the-biceps-tendon/.

Fig. 5.17 Illustration depicting an hourglass biceps which cannot slide efficiently into and out of the bicipital sheath with arm elevation.

Some have suggested that asymmetric loading of the LHB in positions of abduction and external rotation may be responsible for lesions of the BRP. However, in a biplane fluoroscopic study in cadavers performed by Braun et al. [16], the investigators demonstrated high shear-force vectors across the BRP in both the neutral and in internal rotation positions with or without forward flexion. Currently, there is insufficient data to suggest a specific pathomechanism responsible for the development of pulley lesions.

5.4.2 Physical Examination

While there are some physical examination maneuvers that can be used to evaluate instability of the LHB tendon [25, 60, 61], none of these methods have been formally validated. Typically, the clinician will palpate the bicipital groove while simultaneously internally and externally rotating the humerus (see Fig. 5.14). Painful "clicking" or "popping" occurs as the LHB tendon translates over the lesser tuberosity. Complete dislocation of the LHB tendon out of the bicipital groove indicates a high probability of concomitant full- or partial-thickness tearing of the upper 1/3 of the subscapularis tendon and/or the anterior aspect of the supraspinatus tendon [59, 61]. Therefore, full examination of the anterosuperior rotator cuff is necessary in cases where instability of the LHB is suspected (see Chap. 4).

5.4.2.1 Arm Wrestle Test

Recently, we have begun using an arm wrestle test to detect medial or lateral subluxation of the LHB tendon. In this test, the clinician first grasps the patient's hand in a standard "arm wrestle grip." With the elbow flexed approximately 90° and the shoulder in neutral rotation, the patient is asked to flex the elbow and supinate the forearm against resistance with perturbations (Fig. 5.19). A positive test occurs when pain or other mechanical symptoms are reproduced as the LHB tendon subluxates out of the bicipital groove. Although we are unaware of any other previous studies that utilize this test, we have anecdotally found it quite useful for the detection of medial or lateral biceps subluxation.

5.5 SLAP Tears

In 1985, Andrews et al. [62] were the first investigators to describe lesions to the proximal biceps tendon with involvement of the superior aspect of the glenoid labrum. Later, Snyder et al. [63] coined

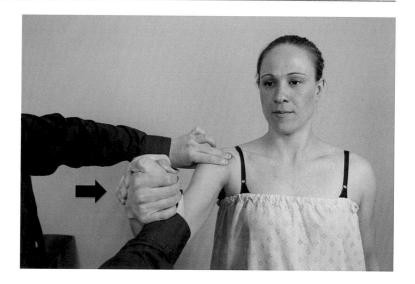

Fig. 5.19 Arm wrestle test. With the elbow flexed to 90° in neutral rotation, the examiner grasps the hand of the patient in an "arm wrestle grip." The patient then attempts to flex and supinate the forearm against resistance (perturbations) provided by the examiner.

the term "SLAP" tear due to the anterior to posterior direction of labral tearing (*Superior Labral Anterior to Posterior*; Fig. 5.20). Snyder et al. [63] also classified SLAP tears into four groups which were later supplemented by three additional groups (types I–VII) (Fig. 5.21). The incidence of non-type I SLAP (non-degenerative) tears ranges from 3.4 to 26 % in patients who present with shoulder pain [47, 63–68]; however, these figures may be increased in high-level throwing athletes. SLAP tears can occur in isolation or in conjunction with other shoulder pathologies such as rotator cuff tears, biceps tendon pathology, and/or glenohumeral instability [64, 67, 69].

5.5.1 Pathogenesis

The precise pathomechanism behind the development of SLAP tears has been debated since its first description in 1985. Investigators most commonly cite forceful traction loads, forceful compression loads, and overhead sporting activities as the most common causes of SLAP tears. A forceful traction load to the biceps tendon may create a defect at the superior labrum resulting in pain and dysfunction [10, 70]. Clavert et al. [70] and Bey et al. [71] found that forward flexion and inferior traction, respectively, facilitated the development of SLAP lesions in separate cadaveric models. A forceful compression load may trap the biceps-

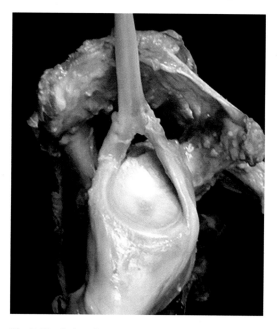

Fig. 5.20 Cadaveric photograph depicting a SLAP tear. Note that the biceps-labral complex is elevated away from the glenoid both anteriorly and posteriorly.

labrum complex between the humeral head and the superior glenoid rim which may produce a mechanical shearing effect (or "grinding," as suggested by Snyder et al. [63, 67]) resulting in a tear of the superior labrum. Repetitive traction from participation in overhead throwing sports such as baseball and softball also commonly result in tearing of the superior labrum.

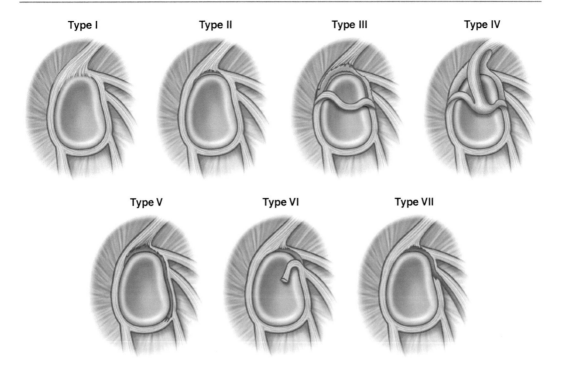

Fig. 5.21 SLAP tear classification system developed by Snyder et al. [63] and later modified by Maffett et al. [64] *Type I* = degenerative fraying; *Type II* = extension into biceps tendon; *Type III* = bucket-handle tear with intact biceps; *Type IV* = bucket-handle tear with biceps extension; *Type V* = SLAP tear combined with Bankart lesion; *Type VI* = unstable flap tear *Type VII* = extension into middle glenohumeral ligament (MGHL).

5.5.2   Physical Examination

The physical diagnosis of SLAP tears is one of the most challenging aspects of the shoulder examination for several reasons. First, there is little evidence to support any single function of the biceps anchor-superior labrum complex. Some clinicians have suggested that the glenoid labrum may have a similar function to that of the meniscus in the knee. They extrapolate that injuries to the labrum may produce similar symptoms to that of injuries to the meniscus such as clicking and/or locking with range of motion testing. While this is a convenient analogy, several studies have shown that these mechanical symptoms are not sensitive or specific for superior labral pathology, especially for type I SLAP lesions [45, 66, 72, 73]. Second, there are no proven historical features that are associated with the presence of a SLAP tear given the numerous potential mechanisms of injury. However, it is now well

recognized that sudden compression (e.g., a fall onto an outstretched arm) or traction loads (e.g., shoulder dislocation or sudden inferiorly directed traction) are probably the most common etiologies of SLAP tears in the general population [63]. Third, SLAP tears are rarely isolated and typically occur concomitantly with other painful shoulder conditions. Thus, the pain from a concomitant pathologic lesion, such as a partial-thickness rotator cuff tear, could mask, enhance, or mimic the pain produced by a possible SLAP tear, potentially confusing the clinical picture. Fourth, the location, quality, and intensity of pain related to a SLAP tear may differ across a population. In addition to making the clinical diagnosis of a SLAP tear difficult, this factor also hinders the ability to study and interpret various physical examination maneuvers designed to elicit symptoms associated with tearing of the biceps-labrum complex. Fifth, there are numerous physical examination maneuvers that are purported to elicit symptoms related to SLAP tears—deciding which techniques are most useful is one of the more daunting aspects of the shoulder examination. The most common physical examination maneuvers used to detect SLAP tears are described below. Reported sensitivity, specificity, positive and negative likelihood ratio data for the detection of types II–IV SLAP tears are presented in Table 5.2.

5.5.2.1 Anterior Slide Test

First described by Kibler [44] in 1995, the anterior slide test utilizes the rationale that a combined compression and shear force applied to the torn superior labrum will produce pain and/or mechanical symptoms such as clicking. To perform this test, the patient is asked to place each hand on the iliac crests with the thumb pointed posteriorly. The examiner stabilizes the scapula by placing one hand on the top of the affected shoulder and the other hand across the epicondyles of the affected arm. The examiner then applies an anterosuperior axial load through the humerus directed towards the anterosuperior aspect of the glenoid

(Fig. 5.22). Reproduction of the patient's symptoms is regarded as a positive test.

In Kibler's original study of five groups of athletes [44], the sensitivity and specificity of the anterior slide test was calculated to be 78.4 and 91.5 %; however, this study did not involve a diagnostic gold standard. Later, Burkhart et al. [6] calculated a sensitivity of 100 % and a specificity of 47 % for the diagnosis of type II SLAP tears using the anterior slide test. The investigators also found that the anterior slide test was more accurate in the detection of anterior lesions when compared to posterior or combined anterior–posterior SLAP lesions. A more recent study by Schlecter et al. [47] evaluated 254 patients using the anterior slide test and correlated the results with arthroscopic findings. The investigators calculated a sensitivity of 21 % and a specificity of 98 % for the detection of type II–IV SLAP tears using the anterior slide test. When the anterior slide test was performed in combination with the so-called passive distraction test described by Rubin [28] (passive forearm pronation with the humerus in 150° of abduction in the scapular plane), the sensitivity was 70 % and

Table 5.2 Reported diagnostic efficacies of clinical tests used for the detection of SLAP tears

Maneuver	Author(s)	Year	Pathology	Diagnostic standard	Sensitivity (%)	Specificity (%)	LR+	LR−
Anterior slide test	Kibler [44]	1995	SLAP tear	Arthroscopy	78	92	2.63	0.64
	McFarland et al. [45]	2002	SLAP tear	Arthroscopy	8	84	0.50	2.0
	Parentis et al. [46]	2002	SLAP tear	Arthroscopy	10	82	0.55	1.10
	Oh et al. [43]	2008	SLAP tear	Arthroscopy	21	70	0.70	1.13
	Schlecter et al. [47]	2009	SLAP tear	Arthroscopy	21	98	10.5	0.81
Crank test	Parentis et al. [46]	2002	SLAP tear	Arthroscopy	13	83	0.76	1.05
	Guanche and Jones [48]	2003	SLAP tear	Arthroscopy	39	67	1.18	0.91
Active compression test	McFarland et al. [45]	2002	SLAP tear	Arthroscopy	47	55	1.04	0.96
	Parentis et al. [46]	2002	SLAP tear	Arthroscopy	63	50	1.26	0.74
	Guanche and Jones [48]	2003	SLAP tear	Arthroscopy	54	47	1.02	0.98
	Myers et al. [49]	2005	SLAP tear	Arthroscopy	78	11	0.88	2.00
	Oh et al. [43]	2008	SLAP tear	Arthroscopy	63	53	1.34	0.70
	Ebinger et al. [50]	2008	SLAP tear	Arthroscopy	94	28	1.31	0.21
	Schlecter et al. [47]	2009	SLAP tear	Arthroscopy	59	92	7.38	0.45
	Jia et al. [39]	2009	SLAP tear	Arthroscopy	53	58	1.26	0.81
	Fowler et al. [51]	2010	SLAP tear	Arthroscopy	64	43	1.12	0.84
	Cook et al. [52]	2012	SLAP tear	Arthroscopy	91	14	1.06	0.64
Biceps load test II	Kim et al. [53]	2001	SLAP tear	Arthroscopy	90	97	30.0	0.10
	Oh et al. [43]	2008	SLAP tear	Arthroscopy	30	78	1.36	0.90
	Cook et al. [52]	2012	SLAP tear	Arthroscopy	67	51	1.4	0.66

LR likelihood ratio

the specificity was 90 % for the detection of type II–IV SLAP tears. The utility of the anterior slide test to detect type I SLAP lesions is less reliable

[45, 74]; however, the clinical relevance of the type I SLAP lesion has been questioned.

5.5.2.2 Crank Test

The crank test was first described by Liu et al. [75] in 1996 as a means to detect various types of labral tears. This test can be performed with the patient either standing or supine. The humerus is maximally elevated with the elbow in approximately 20° of flexion. The examiner uses one hand to hold the subject's wrist while the other hand is used to apply an axial force through the humerus towards the glenoid. The humerus is then rotated internally and externally against the glenoid, producing mechanical shear across the labrum (Fig. 5.23). Reproduction of the patient's symptoms is considered a positive test.

Liu et al. [75, 76] performed two studies evaluating the ability of the crank test to diagnose any labral tear. However, the investigators were unable to evaluate the difference between SLAP tears and other labral tears (such as anterior or posterior Bankart lesions) using this test. Mimori et al. [77] performed the test on 15 baseball players with shoulder pain and calculated a sensitivity of 83 % and a specificity of 100 % for the detection of SLAP tears using magnetic resonance arthrography (MRA) as the diagnostic gold standard. However, Stetson and Templin [78] calculated a sensitivity of 46 % and a specificity of 56 % for the crank test in the diagnosis of

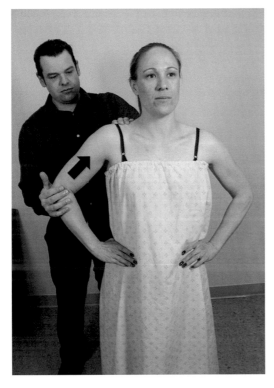

Fig. 5.22 Anterior slide test. In this test, the patient places their hands over the iliac crests with the thumbs pointed posteriorly. The examiner stabilizes the scapula with one hand and applies an anterosuperiorly directed axial load through the humerus towards the anterosuperior aspect of the glenoid.

Fig. 5.23 Crank test. With the patient standing or supine, the humerus is elevated above the horizontal plane with the elbow flexed to approximately 20°. The examiner uses one hand to hold the patient's wrist while the other hand applies an axial load through the humerus towards the glenoid. The humerus is simultaneously internally and externally rotated while an axial force is applied.

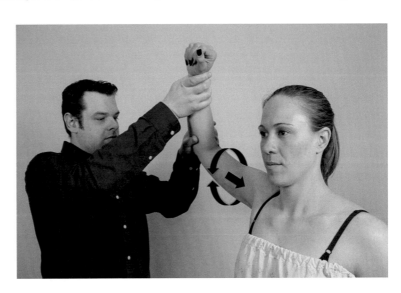

SLAP tears in a prospective series of 65 patients over 45 years of age with shoulder pain. In their study, diagnosis was made via direct arthroscopic visualization. In light of this evidence, we suggest using the crank test in combination with other more sensitive and specific tests to aid in the physical diagnosis of SLAP tears.

5.5.2.3 O'Brien Test (Active Compression Test)

The active compression test, first devised by O'Brien et al. [79] in 1998, is a two-part test that was originally designed to aid in the diagnosis of SLAP tears. With the patient standing, the humerus is placed in 90° of forward flexion and approximately 10° of horizontal adduction. From this position, the humerus is internally rotated such that the thumb points towards the floor and the palm faces laterally. The patient is then asked to resist a downward force applied to the forearm or wrist by the examiner. The arm is then positioned with the palm facing upward and an identical downward force is applied to the distal arm (Fig. 5.24). According to the original description, the presence of deep-seated pain and/or clicking with the first maneuver (thumb downward) that

was relieved by the second maneuver (palm upward) indicated a positive test. O'Brien et al. [79] calculated a sensitivity of 100 %, a specificity of 99 %, a positive predictive value (PPV) of 95 %, and a negative predictive value of 100 % for the ability of the active compression test to diagnose SLAP tears. However, these outstanding results have never been reproduced despite numerous published attempts [39, 43, 45, 47–52, 74, 80, 81].

The active compression test has several important limitations that warrant discussion. First, in the original study published by O'Brien et al. [79], the investigators noted that this maneuver also had some efficacy in the diagnosis of pathology involving the acromioclavicular (AC) joint (discussed further in Chap. 7). For these reasons, the authors recommended that clinicians determine the location and quality of the pain that was produced during the first portion of the test. Pain that occurred "deep" in the shoulder was thought to be related to superior labral pathology whereas pain that occurred at the top of the shoulder (i.e., near the AC joint) was thought to be related to pathology involving the AC joint. Second, because the perception of pain related to different shoulder pathologies can vary significantly

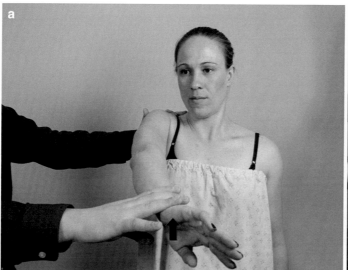
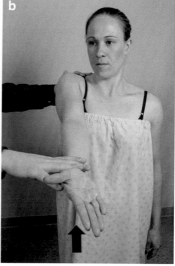

Fig. 5.24 Active compression test. (**a**) With the patient standing, the humerus is forward flexed to 90° with approximately 10° of horizontal adduction and the thumb pointed downward. The examiner then applies a down-ward force to the distal arm while the patient provides resistance. (**b**) The test is repeated with the palm facing upward. Characteristic pain with the first maneuver that is relieved by the second maneuver indicates a positive test.

between individuals [6], patients may misinterpret the location, quality, and/or intensity of the pain which may lead to an inaccurate clinical diagnosis. For example, some patients may complain of pain in areas that would not normally be indicative of a SLAP tear whereas others may complain of pain during both portions of the test. In addition, some patients who do not have pain with this test demonstrate significant superior labral pathology on subsequent imaging studies. Third, although contrary to the original description, the presence of "clicking" within the shoulder during the first portion of the test should probably not be considered a positive result since several studies have demonstrated its lack of diagnostic utility [45, 73]. It should be noted that audible clicking with this maneuver can also be caused by various pathologies involving the AC joint and, therefore, the clinician should exercise caution when interpreting this finding.

In light of these limitations and the lack of convincing clinical data, we prefer to perform this test in combination with other tests to improve the overall accuracy and reliability of the physical diagnosis.

5.5.2.4 SLAPrehension Test

This test, originally described by Berg and Ciullo [82] in 1995, is similar to O'Brien's active compression test described above. With the patient standing, the patient actively flexes the arm to 90° of forward elevation, adducts the arm by an unspecified amount (presumably 10–20°), and pronates the forearm such that the thumb points inferiorly. The clinician then applies an inferiorly directed force on the distal arm while the patient resists. The test was repeated with the forearm supinated and the palm facing upward (see Fig. 5.24). A positive test occurred when pain was reproduced in the area of the bicipital groove with the forearm supinated and subsequently relieved when the same resistance was applied with the forearm pronated. The authors hypothesized that (1) the superior labrum became entrapped between the greater tuberosity and the glenoid when the humerus was internally rotated and (2) forearm pronation increased the traction forces applied to the superior labrum through the LHB tendon

which may also generate pain in the shoulder. Therefore, it was thought both the entrapment of the superior labrum and the increased tension could be relieved by humeral external rotation and forearm supination which effectively moved the greater tuberosity away from the superior glenoid and diminished the tension applied to the biceps-labral complex, respectively.

Several years later, the same investigators published the results of a study in which 66 patients with arthroscopically confirmed SLAP tears (types I–IV according to the classification system developed by Snyder et al. [63]; see Fig. 5.21) were evaluated retrospectively to determine whether a positive SLAPrehension test was documented prior to surgical intervention. According to their results, the sensitivity of this test was found to be 87.5 % for the diagnosis of types II–IV SLAP tears and 50 % for the diagnosis of type I SLAP tears. However, we could not confirm these calculations since all patients in that study had an arthroscopically confirmed SLAP tear (i.e., there were no true negatives or false negatives for the overall prevalence of SLAP tears in their study, regardless of classification). In addition, the ability of a patient to localize pain precisely to the bicipital groove is notoriously poor and may influence the results of both this study and future studies. No other studies have evaluated the clinical utility of the SLAPrehension test in the diagnosis of SLAP tears. For these reasons, this test remains primarily of academic interest and probably should not be utilized in clinical practice.

5.5.2.5 Biceps Load Test I

The biceps load test was developed by Kim et al. [83] as a method to detect SLAP tears in the presence of anterior instability with an associated osseous or soft-tissue Bankart lesion. With the patient supine on the examination table, the affected arm was placed in neutral rotation and abducted to approximately 90°. The elbow was flexed to 90° and the forearm was supinated. From this position, the humerus was slowly externally rotated until the patient experienced pain or became apprehensive (see Chap. 6 for details regarding the apprehension sign). At this point,

Fig. 5.25 Biceps load test I. With the patient supine, the humerus is elevated to 90° of straight lateral abduction in neutral rotation. The elbow is flexed to 90° and the forearm is supinated. The examiner then passively externally rotates the humerus until pain or apprehension is felt by the patient. At this point, the patient is asked to flex the elbow against resistance provided by the examiner.

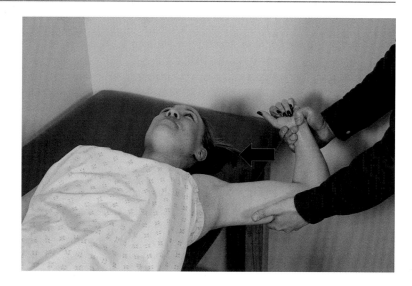

external rotation was stopped and the patient was asked to further flex the elbow while the examiner applied resistance (Fig. 5.25). When resisted elbow flexion did not relieve the patient's symptoms, the investigators suspected the presence of a Bankart lesion with a concomitant SLAP tear. When resisted elbow flexion *did* relieve the patient's symptoms, the presence of a concomitant SLAP tear was deemed less likely. Although several studies have confirmed that the LHB tendon is most active during this test [84, 85], no other studies have specifically evaluated the tension placed on the proximal biceps anchor and, therefore, the exact cause of the increased pain with this maneuver is still largely theoretical.

Kim et al. [83] also evaluated the clinical utility of the biceps load test in the diagnosis of SLAP tears with an associated Bankart lesion. According to their statistical analyses, the biceps load test had a sensitivity of 91 %, a specificity of 97 %, a PPV of 83 %, and an NPV of 98 % for the above-mentioned diagnosis. This study included only patients with recurrent anterior instability without a control group and, unfortunately, no other studies have evaluated the diagnostic efficacy of this test. For these reasons, we cannot recommend the use of this test in clinical practice.

5.5.2.6 Biceps Load Test II

A few years after their original description of the biceps load test, Kim et al. [53] devised another similar test (biceps load test II) which was thought to reproduce symptoms related to SLAP tears independent of glenohumeral stability. In this test, the arm was abducted to 120° and maximally externally rotated. With the forearm supinated and the elbow flexed to approximately 90°, the patient was asked to flex the elbow against resistance. A positive test occurred when the patient experienced an increase in shoulder pain with resisted elbow flexion (Fig. 5.26). The authors hypothesized that this maneuver increased the tension placed on the biceps anchor and, when torn, would produce an increase in shoulder pain.

Kim et al. [53] also evaluated the diagnostic utility of this test in a series of 127 patients with shoulder pain who all underwent subsequent arthroscopic evaluation. Their results indicated that the biceps load test II was 90 % sensitive and 97 % specific for the diagnosis of SLAP tears with a PPV of 92 % and an NPV of 96 %. However, no other studies have been able to confirm the diagnostic accuracy of this test (see Table 5.2) [43, 52].

5.5.2.7 Pain Provocation Test

The pain provocation test was developed by Mimori et al. [77] in 1999. Similar to the biceps load tests described above, it was hypothesized that this test would specifically activate the LHB tendon, thus generating increased tension over the

Fig. 5.26 Biceps load test II. This test is performed in the same manner as the Biceps load test I, except that the humerus is first elevated to approximately 120° of straight lateral abduction. The humerus is maximally externally rotated until pain or apprehension is felt by the patient. The patient then flexes the elbow against resistance provided by the examiner.

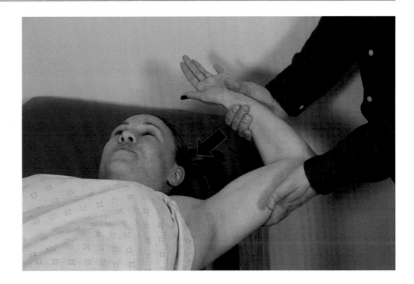

proximal biceps anchor and producing pain in a patient with a lesion involving the biceps-labral complex. With the patient sitting, the arm was abducted to 90° of elevation and the elbow was flexed to 90°. The clinician stood behind the patient, using one hand to stabilize the scapula while the other hand was placed on the distal arm/wrist to control humeral rotation along with forearm supination and pronation. The humerus was then externally rotated first with the forearm pronated and then with the forearm supinated. The patient was then asked to report which of these two positions (forearm pronated or supinated) produced the greatest amount of pain (Fig. 5.27). The test was considered positive when the intensity of pain was greatest with the forearm pronated. This description of a positive test is in contrast to the biceps load test where a positive test occurred when shoulder pain was produced by resisted elbow flexion with the forearm supinated. It is also not clear whether similar pain in both positions was considered a positive or negative test.

In the original study conducted by Mimori et al. [77], the pain provocation test was used to evaluate 32 overhead athletes with shoulder pain in the absence of instability. All patients had a negative relocation test (discussed below and in Chap. 6). Because only 15 patients underwent diagnostic arthroscopy, MRA was used to make the final diagnoses. The investigators calculated a sensitivity of 100 % and a specificity of 90 %.

Unfortunately, no other clinical studies have evaluated the efficacy of this test in the diagnosis of SLAP tears and, therefore, we cannot currently recommend its use in clinical practice.

5.5.2.8 Relocation Test

The relocation test was originally developed by Jobe et al. [29] in 1989 as a method to assess shoulder pain in overhead athletes. With the patient supine, the humerus was abducted to 90° and externally rotated into the position of apprehension that is commonly used to test for anterior instability (see Chap. 6 for more information regarding the apprehension sign). The authors hypothesized that overhead athletes, many of whom demonstrate anterior microinstability as a result of capsular laxity, would have an increased propensity for subacromial impingement as a result of anterior humeral head translation. Therefore, pain over the deltoid with the shoulder in this position was thought to represent rotator cuff impingement beneath the acromion. The shoulder was then "relocated" by applying a posteriorly directed pressure to the anterior aspect of the humeral head (Fig. 5.28). If this relocation maneuver resulted in pain relief, the patient was thought to have anterior microinstability with secondary subacromial impingement.

Several years later, both Jobe [86] and Walch et al. [87] concluded that overhead athletes were more likely to experience pain with this test as a

Fig. 5.27 Pain provocation test. With the patient sitting with the affected arm either at the side or elevated to 90° of straight lateral abduction and the elbow flexed to 90°, the examiner uses one hand to stabilize the scapula while the other hand is used to control humeral rotation. The humerus is then passively and maximally externally rotated, first with the forearm pronated (**a**) and then with the forearm supinated (**b**). When the patient reports greater pain with the forearm pronated, the test is considered positive.

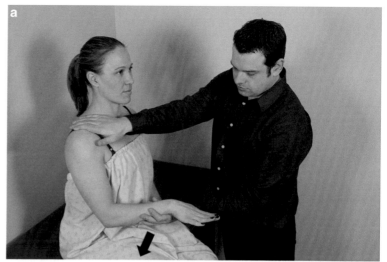
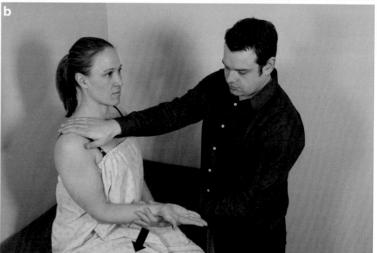

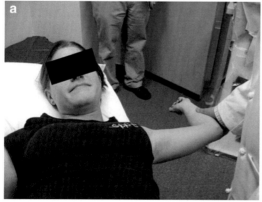
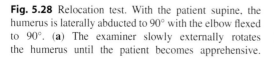
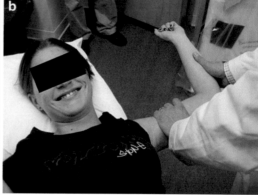

Fig. 5.28 Relocation test. With the patient supine, the humerus is laterally abducted to 90° with the elbow flexed to 90°. (**a**) The examiner slowly externally rotates the humerus until the patient becomes apprehensive. (**b**) The examiner then applies an anteriorly directed pressure on the proximal humerus to relocate the humeral head which should relieve the apprehension.

Fig. 5.29 Illustration showing the mechanism of symptomatic internal impingement. As the humerus becomes more capable of extreme amounts of external rotation, the posterosuperior cuff and posterosuperior labrum can become pinched between the greater tuberosity and the glenoid rim, producing a partial-thickness rotator cuff tear and/or a labral tear.

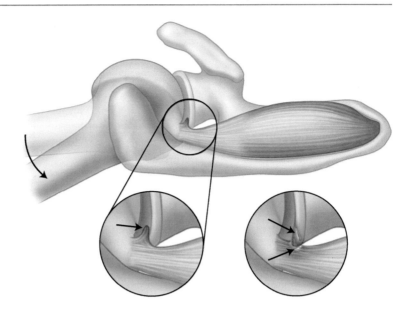

result of superior labral pathology. Under direct arthroscopic visualization, Walch et al. [87] noted that the posterosuperior labrum became pinched between the greater tuberosity and the posterosuperior glenoid rim when the arm was abducted and externally rotated (Fig. 5.29). This so-called internal impingement was subsequently relieved when the joint was relocated. While many investigators believed this condition was secondary to anterior glenohumeral laxity [86, 89–92], more recent studies have suggested a more complex mechanism involving anatomic and physiologic remodeling of the shoulder that occurs throughout the sporting careers of overhead athletes [93–96].

Burkhart et al. [80] performed a retrospective study of the relocation test in a series of patients who were all diagnosed with type II SLAP tears (anterior extension, posterior extension or combined) by direct arthroscopic visualization. According to their results, the relocation test was most sensitive for the diagnosis of SLAP tears with posterior extension (85 %). The sensitivity of the test for SLAP tears with combined anterior and posterior extension was 59 % and, for SLAP tears with anterior extension, the sensitivity was only 4 %. However, approximately one-third of the patients included in this study had concomitant rotator cuff tears which may have altered the statistical analyses. In addition, this study did not

have a control group which eliminated the ability to calculate true sensitivity and specificity data regarding the ability of the relocation test to detect either the presence or absence of a SLAP tear.

Oh et al. [43] studied the diagnostic efficacy of the relocation test in 297 patients with shoulder pain who underwent diagnostic arthroscopy. After retrospective review, 146 patients with type II SLAP lesions were identified along with an age-matched control group of 151 patients without labral pathology. Their results showed that the relocation test was 44 % sensitive and 54 % specific for the diagnosis of SLAP tears with a PPV of 52 % and an NPV of 47 %. In contrast to these results, a more recent study by van Kampen et al. [97] evaluated the relocation test in 175 patients who presented with shoulder pain. Of these, 60 patients were diagnosed with anterior instability and 109 patients were diagnosed with other conditions following MRA interpretation. The relocation test was found to be 96.7 % sensitive and 78.0 % specific for the diagnosis of SLAP tears with a PPV of 71.1 % and an NPV of 97.7 %.

Given these conflicting results and the lack of consensus regarding the actual meaning of a positive test, we conclude that the test may have some diagnostic utility in some situations; however, determining when this test is most efficacious has been challenging topic of discussion thus far.

5.5.2.9 Resisted Supination External Rotation Test

The resisted supination external rotation test, first described by Myers et al. [49] in 2005, was designed to detect SLAP lesions in overhead athletes that resulted from a "peel-back" mechanism that was previously described by Burkhart et al. (Fig. 5.30) [6]. Briefly, the peel-back mechanism for the development of SLAP tears occurs when the biceps-labral complex (particularly the posterior aspect) experiences extraphysiologic torsional strain as a result of repeated bouts of glenohumeral abduction and hyperexternal rotation as which occurs in throwing athletes. With the patient lying supine, the humerus was abducted to 90°, the elbow was flexed to 65–70° and the forearm was placed in either neutral rotation or pronation. The examiner supported the elbow and asked the patient to supinate the forearm against resistance. While resistance was being applied, the humerus was slowly and maximally externally rotated. The patient was then asked to describe their symptoms at the point of maximal external rotation (Fig. 5.31). The test was deemed positive if they experienced pain anteriorly or deep within the shoulder, clicking within the shoulder or the reproduction of similar symptoms for which they sought medical treatment. The test was considered negative when the patient experienced pain posteriorly, no pain or apprehension.

In their study, 40 overhead athletes with shoulder pain were subjected to the above-described maneuver. At diagnostic arthroscopy,

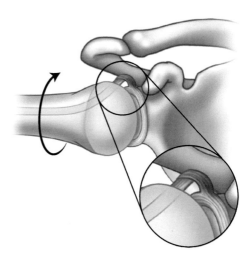

Fig. 5.30 Illustration showing the peel-back mechanism. Increasing degrees of external rotation increases the torsional strain across the biceps anchor which can lead to SLAP tears.

Fig. 5.31 Resisted supination external rotation test. With the patient supine, the humerus is laterally abducted to 90° and the elbow is flexed to 65–70° with the arm in neutral rotation. While supporting the elbow, the patient then attempts to supinate the forearm against resistance provided by the examiner. While this resistance is applied, the humerus is slowly externally rotated.

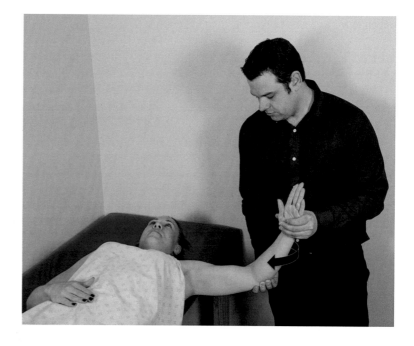

Fig. 5.32 Dynamic labral shear test. With the patient sitting or standing, the patient's arm is placed at the side and the humerus is passively abducted and externally rotated while the examiner stabilizes the scapula. The humerus is then moved upward and downward in the coronal plane between 60° and 120° of straight lateral abduction.

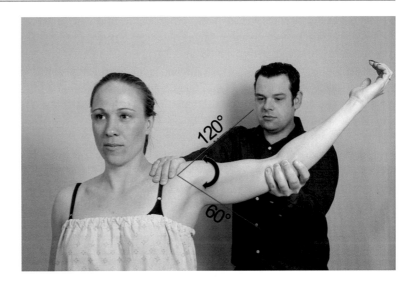

29 athletes (72.5 %) were found to have a SLAP tear. This resulted in a sensitivity of 82.8 %, a specificity of 81.8 %, a PPV of 92.3 %, and an NPV of 64.3 % for the ability of the resisted supination external rotation test to diagnose SLAP tears in overhead athletes. The authors also noted that 79 % of the shoulders with a SLAP tear also had concomitant lesions such as rotator cuff tears and chondral defects among other various injuries. Almost every patient in the control group also had other intra-articular injuries.

In at least two EMG studies [85, 98], the resisted supination external rotation test was found to selectively activate the LHB tendon which, in turn, was thought to increase the applied tension to the biceps-labral complex, especially when the humerus was maximally externally rotated. However, no study has quantified the amount of tension that this test (or any other test designed to detect SLAP tears) produces at the biceps-labral complex relative to normal physiologic loads. This information would be important to help clinicians and researchers understand the precise mechanism behind the development of SLAP tears in overhead athletes. Although this testing procedure requires further study, it appears to have some potential and may become an important diagnostic tool in the future.

5.5.2.10 Dynamic Labral Shear Test

Information regarding the dynamic labral shear test was apparently communicated to Pandya et al. [99] in late 2004 through personal communications with Dr. O'Driscoll; however, McFarland [72] suggested that the test was described as early as 2000 at various professional meetings. Because each source reported different aspects of the procedure, we combined the information obtained from both sources to describe the full procedure. Given the verbal nature of the communication and the potential for recall bias, we caution the reader that small variations in this maneuver may exist. The test can be performed with the patient sitting or standing with the clinician standing behind the affected shoulder. Beginning with the arm at the side in neutral rotation, the examiner passively externally rotates and abducts the humerus within the coronal plane using one hand while the other hand is used to stabilize the scapula. The humerus is then moved upwards and downwards between 60° and 120° of abduction (Fig. 5.32). McFarland [72] reported that an anteriorly directed force should also be applied to the posterior aspect of the humeral head in conjunction with this motion. A positive test occurred when the patient experienced posterior shoulder pain with or without a clicking sensation as the humerus was moved between abduction angles.

Pandya et al. [99] performed a study that evaluated the efficacy of the dynamic labral shear test in its ability to detect symptomatic SLAP tears. In that study, 51 consecutive patients with arthroscopically confirmed SLAP tears underwent both preoperative physical examination and magnetic resonance imaging (MRI) or MRA evaluation. Physical examination findings were compared to the findings on imaging studies and diagnostic arthroscopy for sensitivity analyses. The sensitivity of the dynamic labral shear test was found to be 80 %. The authors also calculated a sensitivity of 100 % when any one of the following three SLAP tests were positive: the active compression test, the dynamic labral shear test, or the relocation test.

Kibler et al. [40] performed a slightly modified version of this test and compared its diagnostic efficacy with other clinical tests designed to detect SLAP tears. The modified version of the test was performed as described above except that the humerus was first abducted >120° within the scapular plane and then moved directly horizontally such that the position of abduction was in the coronal plane. When the humerus was moved between 60° and 120° of elevation, a positive test occurred only when posterior shoulder pain and/or clicking was present in the interval between 90° and 120° of abduction. According to the authors, this procedural change was performed to eliminate the

high rate of false positives that were found in a pilot study when the humerus was initially abducted in the coronal plane. In their study, six clinical tests were used to make the diagnosis in 101 patients who underwent subsequent diagnostic arthroscopy. With specific regard to the modified dynamic labral shear test, the sensitivity was 72 %, the specificity was 98 %, the PPV was 97 %, and the NPV was 77 %. This test was more accurate than any of the other tests for the diagnosis of SLAP tears performed in this study. Future studies are needed to confirm these results before we can recommend its routine use in clinical practice.

5.5.2.11 SLAC Test

In 2001, Savoie et al. [100] used the term "SLAC lesion" to represent a frequently observed combination of pathologies involving the *s*uperior *l*abrum and the *a*nterior *c*uff that were thought to result in anterosuperior glenohumeral instability (i.e., labral tearing, articular-sided anterosuperior cuff tears and/or glenoid chondromalacia). The same investigators also designed a physical examination test to detect these so-called SLAC lesions. In this test, the humerus was abducted to 90° within the scapular plane with the palm facing upward. The clinician then applied a downward force to the wrist (Fig. 5.33). A positive test occurred when the humeral head "shifted" anterosuperiorly or when the patient experienced pain

Fig. 5.33 SLAC test. The humerus is abducted to approximately 90° in the scapular plane with the palm facing upward. The examiner then stabilizes the scapula and applies a downward force to the wrist while the patient provides resistance.

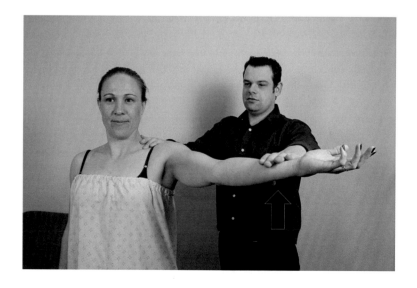

when the downward force was applied. In their study of 40 patients with arthroscopically confirmed SLAC lesions, 35 of these patients (88 %) had a positive SLAC test preoperatively. Unfortunately, no other studies have evaluated the diagnostic utility of this test and, therefore, it remains primarily of academic interest.

5.6 Conclusion

Physical examination of the LHB tendon can be complex and, at times, confusing; however, an understanding of the basic pathoanatomic features of the most common conditions can improve the accuracy of physical diagnosis by guiding the clinician through the examination process. As mentioned in previous chapters, it is not necessary to perform every test on every patient, but rather to focus the examination according to the differential diagnosis that was obtained earlier in the patient encounter.

References

1. Arai R, Kobayashi M, Harada H, Tsukiyama H, Saji T, Toda Y, Hagiwara Y, Miura T, Matsuda S. Anatomical study for SLAP lesion repair. Knee Surg Sports Traumatol Arthrosc. 2014;22(2):435–41.
2. Gigis P, Natsis C, Polyzonis M. New aspects on the topography of the tendon of the long head of the biceps brachii muscle. One more stabilizer factor of the shoulder joint. Bull Assoc Anat (Nancy). 1995;79(245):9–11.
3. Pal GP, Bhatt RH, Patel VS. Relationship between the tendon of the long head of the biceps brachii and the glenoidal labrum in humans. Anat Rec. 1991;229(2):278–80.
4. Tuoheti Y, Itoi E, Minagawa H, Yamamoto N, Saito H, Seki N, Okada K, Shimada Y, Abe H. Attachment types of the long head of the biceps tendon to the glenoid labrum and their relationships with the glenohumeral ligaments. Arthroscopy. 2005;21(10):1242–9.
5. Vangsness Jr CT, Jorgenson SS, Watson T, Johnson DL. The origin of the long head of the biceps from the scapula and glenoid labrum. An anatomical study of 100 shoulders. J Bone Joint Surg Br. 1994;76(6):951–4.
6. Burkhart SS, Morgan CD. The peel-back mechanism: its role in producing and extending posterior type II SLAP lesions and its effect on SLAP repair rehabilitation. Arthroscopy. 1998;14(6):637–40.
7. Rao AG, Kim TK, Chronopoulos E, McFarland EG. Anatomical variants in the anterosuperior aspect of the glenoid labrum: a statistical analysis of seventy-three cases. J Bone Joint Surg Am. 2003;85(4):653–9.
8. Keener JD, Brophy RH. Superior labral tears of the shoulder: pathogenesis, evaluation, and treatment. J Am Acad Orthop Surg. 2009;17(10):627–37.
9. Knesek M, Skendzel JG, Dines JS, Altchek DW, Allen AA, Bedi A. Diagnosis and management of superior labral anterior posterior tears in throwing athletes. Am J Sports Med. 2013;41(2):444–60.
10. Cooper DE, Arnoczky SP, O'Brien SJ, Warren RF, DiCarlo E, Allen AA. Anatomy, histology, and vascularity of the glenoid labrum. An anatomical study. J Bone Joint Surg Am. 1992;74(1):46–52.
11. Gaskill TR, Braun S, Millett PJ. The rotator interval: pathology and management. Arthroscopy. 2011;27(4):556–67.
12. Hulstyn MJ, Fadale PD. Arthroscopic anatomy of the shoulder. Orthop Clin North Am. 1995;26(4):597–612.
13. Elser F, Braun S, Dewing CB, Giphart JE, Millett PJ. Anatomy, function, injuries, and treatment of the long head of the biceps brachii tendon. Arthroscopy. 2011;27(4):581–92.
14. Habermeyer P, Magosch P, Pritsch M, Scheibel MT, Lichtenberg S. Anterosuperior impingement of the shoulder as a result of pulley lesions: a prospective arthroscopic study. J Shoulder Elbow Surg. 2004;13(1):5–12.
15. Bennett WF. Arthroscopic repair of anterosuperior (supraspinatus/subscapularis) rotator cuff tears: a prospective cohort with 2- to 4-year follow-up. Classification of biceps subluxation/instability. Arthroscopy. 2003;19(1):21–33.
16. Braun S, Millett PJ, Yongpravat C, Pault JD, Anstett T, Torry MR, Giphart JE. Biomechanical evaluation of shear force vectors leading to injury of the biceps reflection pulley: a biplane fluoroscopy study on cadaveric shoulders. Am J Sports Med. 2010;38(5):1015–24.
17. Kwon YW, Hurd J, Yeager K, Ishak C, Walker PS, Khan S, Bosco 3rd JA, Jazrawi LM. Proximal biceps tendon—a biomechanical analysis of the stability at the bicipital groove. Bull NYU Hosp Jt Dis. 2009;67(4):337–40.
18. Pfahler M, Branner S, Refior HJ. The role of the bicipital groove in tendopathy of the long biceps tendon. J Shoulder Elbow Surg. 1999;8(5):419–24.
19. Alpantaki K, McLaughlin D, Karagogeos D, Hadjipavlou A, Kontakis G. Sympathetic and sensory neural elements in the tendon of the long head of the biceps. J Bone Joint Surg Am. 2005;87(7):1580–3.
20. Tosounidis T, Hadjileontis C, Triantafyllou C, Sidiropoulou V, Kafanas A, Kontakis G. Evidence of sympathetic innervation and α1-adrenergic receptors of the long head of the biceps brachii tendon. J Orthop Sci. 2013;18(2):238–44.

21. Pagnani MJ, Deng XH, Warren RF, Torzilli PA, O'Brien SJ. Role of the long head of the biceps brachii in glenohumeral stability: a biomechanical study in cadaver. J Shoulder Elbow Surg. 1996;5(4):255–62.

22. Rodosky MW, Harner CD, Fu FH. The role of the long head of the biceps muscle and superior glenoid labrum in anterior stability of the shoulder. Am J Sports Med. 1994;22(1):121–30.

23. Youm T, ElAttrache NS, Tibone JE, McGarry MH, Lee TQ. The effect of the long head of the biceps on glenohumeral kinematics. J Shoulder Elbow Surg. 2009;18(1):122–9.

24. Su WR, Budoff JE, Luo ZP. The effect of posterosuperior rotator cuff tears and biceps loading on glenohumeral translation. Arthroscopy. 2010;26(5):578–86.

25. Itoi E, Kuechle DK, Newman SR, Morrey BF, An KN. Stabilising function of the biceps in stable and unstable shoulders. J Bone Joint Surg Br. 1993; 75(4):546–50.

26. Kumar VP, Satku K, Balasumbramaniam P. The role of the long head of the biceps brachii in the stabilization of the head of the humerus. Clin Orthop Relat Res. 1989;244:172–5.

27. Levy AS, Kelly BT, Lintner SA, Osbahr DC, Speer KP. Function of the long head of the biceps at the shoulder: electromyographic analysis. J Shoulder Elbow Surg. 2001;10(3):250–5.

28. Sakurai G, Ozaki J, Tomita Y, Nishimoto K, Tamai S. Electromyographic analysis of shoulder joint function of the biceps brachii muscle during isometric contraction. Clin Orthop Relat Res 1998;(354): 123–131.

29. Jobe FW, Kvitne RS, Giangarra CE. Shoulder pain in the overhead or throwing athletes. The relationship of anterior instability and rotator cuff impingement. Orthop Rev. 1989;18(9):963–75.

30. Rojas IL, Provencher MT, Bhatia S, Foucher KC, Bach Jr BR, Romeo AA, Wimmer MA, Verma NN. Biceps activity during windmill softball pitching: injury implications and comparison with overhand throwing. Am J Sports Med. 2009;37(3): 558–65.

31. Warner JJ, McMahon PJ. The role of the long head of the biceps brachii in superior stability of the glenohumeral joint. J Bone Joint Surg Am. 1995; 77(3):366–72.

32. Kido T, Itoi E, Konno N, Sano A, Urayama M, Sato K. The depressor function of the biceps on the head of the humerus in shoulders with tears of the rotator cuff. J Bone Joint Surg Br. 2000;82(3):416–9.

33. Giphart JE, Elser F, Dewing CB, Torry MR, Millett PJ. The long head of the biceps tendon has minimal effect on in vivo glenohumeral kinematics: a biplane fluoroscopy study. Am J Sports Med. 2012;40(1): 202–12.

34. Slätis P, Aalto K. Medial dislocation of the tendon of the long head of the biceps brachii. Acta Orthop Scand. 1979;50(1):73–7.

35. Millett PJ, Braun S, Horan MP, Tello TL. Coracoid impingement: a prospective cohort study on the association between coracohumeral interval narrowing and anterior shoulder pathologies. Arthroscopy. 2009;25(6):e5.

36. Claessens H, Snoeck H. Tendinitis of the long head of the biceps brachii. Acta Orthop Belg. 1972;58(1): 124–8.

37. Chen HS, Lin SH, Hsu YH, Chen SC, Kang JH. A comparison of physical examinations with musculoskeletal ultrasound in the diagnosis of biceps long head tendinitis. Ultrasound Med Biol. 2011;37(9):1392–8.

38. Gill HS, El Rassi G, Bahk MS, Castillo RCX, McFarland EG. Physical examination for partial tears of the biceps tendon. Am J Sports Med. 2007;35(8):1334–40.

39. Jia X, Petersen SA, Khosravi AH, Almareddi V, Pannirselvam V, McFarland EG. Examination of the shoulder: the past, the present, and the future. J Bone Joint Surg Am. 2009;91 Suppl 6:10–8.

40. Kibler WB, Sciascia AD, Hester P, Dome D, Jacobs C. Clinical utility of traditional and new tests in the diagnosis of biceps tendon injuries and superior labrum anterior and posterior lesions in the shoulder. Am J Sports Med. 2009;37(9):1840–7.

41. Goyal P, Hemal U, Kumar R. High resolution sonographic evaluation of painful shoulder. Internet J Radiol. 2009;12(1):22.

42. Salaffi F, Ciapetti A, Carotti M, Gasparini S, Filippucci E, Grassi W. Clinical value of single versus composite provocative clinical tests in the assessment of painful shoulder. J Clin Rheumatol. 2010;16(3):105–8.

43. Oh JH, Kim JY, Kim WS, Gong HS, Lee JH. The evaluation of various physical examinations for the diagnosis of type II superior labrum anterior and posterior lesion. Am J Sports Med. 2008;36(2):353–9.

44. Kibler WB. Specificity and sensitivity of the anterior slide test in throwing athletes with superior labral tears. Arthroscopy. 1995;11(3):296–300.

45. McFarland EG, Kim TK, Savino RM. Clinical assessment of three common tests for superior labral anterior-posterior lesions. Am J Sports Med. 2002;30(6):810–5.

46. Parentis MA, Mohr KJ, ElAttrache NS. Disorders of the superior labrum: review and treatment guidelines. Clin Orthop Relat Res. 2002;400:77–87.

47. Schlecter JA, Summa S, Rubin BD. The passive distraction test: a new diagnostic aid for clinically significant superior labral pathology. Arthroscopy. 2009;25(12):1374–9.

48. Guanche CA, Jones DC. Clinical testing for tears of the glenoid labrum. Arthroscopy. 2003;19(5):517–23.

49. Myers TH, Zemanovic JR, Andrews JR. The resisted supination external rotation test: a new test for the diagnosis of superior labral anterior posterior lesions. Am J Sports Med. 2005;33(9):1315–20.

50. Ebinger N, Magosch P, Lichtenberg S, Habermeyer P. A new SLAP test: the supine flexion resistance test. Arthroscopy. 2008;24(5):500–5.

51. Fowler EM, Horsley IG, Rolf CG. Clinical and arthroscopic findings in recreationally active patients. Sports Med Arthrosc Rehabil Ther Technol. 2010;2:2.

52. Cook C, Beaty S, Kissenberth MJ, Siffri P, Pill SG, Hawkins RJ. Diagnostic accuracy of five orthopedic clinical tests for diagnosis of superior labrum anterior posterior (SLAP) lesions. J Shoulder Elbow Surg. 2012;21(1):13–22.

53. Kim SH, Ha KI, Ahn JH, Kim SH, Choi HJ. Biceps load test II: a clinical test for SLAP lesions of the shoulder. Arthroscopy. 2001;17(2):160–4.

54. Boileau P, Ahrens PM, Hatzidakis AM. Entrapment of the long head of the biceps tendon: the hourglass biceps—a cause of pain and locking of the shoulder. J Shoulder Elbow Surg. 2004;13(3):249–57.

55. Werner A, Mueller T, Boehm D, Gohlke F. The stabilization sling for the long head of the biceps tendon in the rotator cuff interval. A histoanatomic study. Am J Sports Med. 2000;28(1):28–31.

56. Pujol N, Hargunani R, Gadikoppula S, Holloway B, Ahrens PM. Dynamic ultrasound assessment in the diagnosis of intra-articular entrapment of the biceps tendon (hourglass biceps): a preliminary investigation. Int J Shoulder Surg. 2009;3(4):80–4.

57. Bennett WF. Correlation of the SLAP lesion with lesions of the medial sheath of the biceps tendon and intra-articular subscapularis tendon. Indian J Orthop. 2009;43(4):342–6.

58. Resnick D, Kang HS, Pretterklieber M. Shoulder. In: Internal derangement of joints. 2nd ed. Philadelphia: Saunders Elsevier; 2007. p. 713–1122.

59. Walch G, Nove-Josserand L, Boileau P, Levigne C. Subluxations and dislocations of the tendon of the long head of the biceps. J Shoulder Elbow Surg. 1998;7(2):100–8.

60. Gilchrist EL. Dislocation and elongation of the long head of the biceps brachii. Ann Surg. 1936;104(1):118–38.

61. O'Donoghue DH. Subluxing biceps tendon in the athlete. Clin Orthop Relat Res. 1982;164:26–9.

62. Andrews JR, Carson Jr WG, McLeod WD. Glenoid labrum tears related to the long head of the biceps. Am J Sports Med. 1985;13(5):337–41.

63. Snyder SJ, Karzel RP, Del Pizzo W, Ferkel RD, Friedman MJ. SLAP lesions of the shoulder. Arthroscopy. 1990;6(4):274–9.

64. Maffet MW, Gartsman GM, Moseley B. Superior labrum-biceps tendon complex lesions of the shoulder. Am J Sports Med. 1995;23(1):93–8.

65. Handelberg F, Willems S, Shahabpour M, Huskin JP, Kuta J. SLAP lesions: a retrospective multicenter study. Arthroscopy. 1998;14(8):856–62.

66. Kim TK, Queale WS, Cosgarea AJ, McFarland EG. Clinical features of the different types of SLAP lesions: an analysis of one hundred and thirty-nine cases. Superior labrum anterior posterior. J Bone Joint Surg Am. 2003;85-A(1):66–71.

67. Snyder SJ, Banas MP, Karzel RP. An analysis of 140 injuries to the superior glenoid labrum. J Shoulder Elbow Surg. 1995;4(4):243–8.

68. Tomonobu H, Masaaki K, Kihumi S, Kenji O, Sunao F, Akihiko K, Mituhiro A, Masamichi U, Seiichi I. The incidence of glenohumeral joint abnormalities concomitant to rotator cuff tears. J Shoulder Elbow Surg. 1999;8(4):383.

69. Grauer JD, Paulos LE, Smutz WP. Biceps tendon and superior labral injuries. Arthroscopy. 1992;8(4):488–97.

70. Clavert P, Bonnomet F, Kempf JF, Boutemy P, Braun M, Kahn L. Contribution to the study of the pathogenesis of type II superior labrum anterior-posterior lesions: a cadaveric model of a fall on the outstretched hand. J Shoulder Elbow Surg. 2004;13(1):45–50.

71. Bey MJ, Elders GJ, Huston LJ, Kuhn JE, Blasier RB, Soslowsky LJ. The mechanism of creation of superior labrum, anterior, and posterior lesions in a dynamic biomechanical model of the shoulder: the role of inferior subluxation. J Shoulder Elbow Surg. 1998;7(4):397–401.

72. McFarland EG. Examination of the biceps tendon and superior labrum anterior and posterior (SLAP) lesions. In: McFarland EG, editor. Examination of the shoulder: the complete guide. New York: Thieme Medical Publishers, Inc; 2006.

73. Michener LA, Doukas WC, Murphy KP, Walsworth MK. Diagnostic accuracy of history and physical examination of superior labrum anterior-posterior lesions. J Athl Train. 2011;46(4):343–8.

74. Morgan CD, Burkhart SS, Palmeri M, Gillespie M. Type II SLAP lesions: three subtypes and their relationships to superior instability and rotator cuff tears. Arthroscopy. 1998;14(6):553–65.

75. Liu SH, Henry MH, Nuccion SL. A prospective evaluation of a new physical examination in predicting glenoid labral tears. Am J Sports Med. 1996;24(6):721–5.

76. Liu SH, Henry MH, Nuccion S, Shapiro MS, Dorey F. Diagnosis of glenoid labral tears. A comparison between magnetic resonance imaging and clinical examinations. Am J Sports Med. 1996;24(2):149–54.

77. Mimori K, Muneta T, Nakagawa T, Shinomiya K. A new pain provocation test for superior labral tears of the shoulder. Am J Sports Med. 1999;27(2):137–42.

78. Stetson WB, Templin K. The crank test, the O'Brien test, and routine magnetic resonance imaging scans in the diagnosis of labral tears. Am J Sports Med. 2002;30(6):806–9.

79. O'Brien SJ, Pagnani MJ, Fealy S, McGlynn SR, Wilson JB. The active compression test: a new and effective test for diagnosing labral tears and acromioclavicular joint abnormalities. Am J Sports Med. 1998;26(5):610–3.

80. Burkhart SS, Morgan CD, Kibler WB. Shoulder injures in overhead athletes. The "dead arm" revisited. Clin Sports Med. 2000;19(1):125–58.

81. Chronopoulos E, Kim TK, Park HB, Ashenbrenner D, McFarland EG. Diagnostic value of physical tests for isolated chronic acromioclavicular lesions. Am J Sports Med. 2004;32(3):655–61.

82. Berg EE, Ciullo JV. The SLAP prehension test. J South Orthop Assoc. 1995;4(3):237–8.

83. Kim SH, Ha KI, Han KY. Biceps load test: a clinical test for superior labrum anterior and posterior lesions in shoulders with recurrent anterior dislocations. Am J Sports Med. 1999;27(3):300–3.

84. Swaringen JC, Mell AG, Langenderfer J, LaScalza S, Hughes RE, Kuhn JE. Electromyographic analysis of physical examination tests for type II superior labrum anterior-posterior lesions. J Shoulder Elbow Surg. 2006;15(5):576–9.

85. Wood VJ, Sabick MB, Pfeiffer RP, Kuhlman SM, Christensen JH, Curtin MJ. Glenohumeral muscle activation during provocative tests designed to diagnose superior labrum anterior-posterior lesions. Am J Sports Med. 2011;39(12):2670–8.

86. Jobe CM. Posterior superior glenoid impingement: expanded spectrum. Arthroscopy. 1995;11(5):530–6.

87. Walch G, Boileau P, Noel E, Donnel ST. Impingement of the deep surface of the supraspinatus tendon on the posterosuperior glenoid rim: an arthroscopic study. J Shoulder Elbow Surg. 1992;1(5):238–45.

88. Spiegl UJ, Warth RJ, Millett PJ. Symptomatic internal impingement of the shoulder in overhead athletes. Sports Med Arthrosc. 2014;22(2):120–9.

89. Andrews JR, Broussard TS, Carson WG. Arthroscopy of the shoulder in the management of partial tears of the rotator cuff: a preliminary report. Arthroscopy. 1985;1(2):117–22.

90. Bigliani LU, Codd TP, Connor PM, Levine WN, Littlefield MA, Hershon SJ. Shoulder motion and laxity in the professional baseball player. Am J Sports Med. 1997;25(5):609–13.

91. Conway JE. Arthroscopic repair of partial-thickness rotator cuff tears and SLAP lesions in professional baseball players. Orthop Clin North Am. 2001;32(3):443–56.

92. Paley KJ, Jobe FW, Pink MM, Kvitne RS, ElAttrache NS. Arthroscopic findings in the overhand throwing athlete: evidence for posterior internal impingement of the rotator cuff. Arthroscopy. 2000;16(1):35–40.

93. Burkhart SS, Morgan CD, Kibler WB. The disabled throwing shoulder: spectrum of pathology. Part I: pathoanatomy and biomechanics. Arthroscopy. 2003;19(4):404–20.

94. Burkhart SS, Morgan CD, Kibler WB. The disabled throwing shoulder: spectrum of pathology. Part II, evaluation and treatment of SLAP lesions in throwers. Arthroscopy. 2003;19(5):531–9.

95. Kuhn JE, Lindholm SR, Huston LJ, Soslowsky LJ, Blasier RB. Failure of the biceps superior labral complex: a cadaveric biomechanical investigation comparing the late cocking and early deceleration positions of throwing. Arthroscopy. 2003;19(4):373–9.

96. Pradhan RL, Itoi E, Hatakeyama Y, Urayama M, Sato K. Superior labral strain during the throwing motion. A cadaveric study. Am J Sports Med. 2001;29(4):488–92.

97. van Kampen DA, van den Berg T, van der Woude HJ, Castelein RM, Terwee CB, Willems WJ. Diagnostic value of patient characteristics, history, and six clinical tests for traumatic anterior shoulder instability. J Shoulder Elbow Surg. 2013;22(10):1310–9.

98. McCaughey R, Green RA, Taylor NF. The anatomical basis of the resisted supination external rotation test for superior labral anterior to posterior lesions. Clin Anat. 2009;22(6):665–70.

99. Pandya NK, Colton A, Webner D, Sennett B, Huffman GR. Physical examination and magnetic resonance imaging in the diagnosis of superior labrum anterior-posterior lesions of the shoulder: a sensitivity analysis. Arthroscopy. 2008;24(3):311–7.

100. Savoie 3rd FH, Field LD, Atchinson S. Anterior superior instability with rotator cuff tearing: SLAC lesion. Orthop Clin North Am. 2001;32(3):457–61. 3.

101. Stadnick ME. Pathology of the long head of the biceps tendon. Radsource Web Clinics. February 2014 http://radsource.us/pathology-of-the-long-head-of-the-biceps-tendon/

102. Alexander S, Southgate DF, Bull AM, Wallace AL. The role of negative intraarticular pressure and the long head of biceps tendon on passive stability of the glenohumeral joint. J Shoulder Elbow Surg 2013;22(1):94–101.

Glenohumeral Instability

6

6.1 Introduction

The structure of the glenohumeral joint allows for a large arc of shoulder motion. Since approximately one-fourth of the humeral head articular surface remains in contact with the glenoid throughout the range of shoulder motion [1], instability can result when static and/or dynamic stabilizers are disrupted. Static stabilizers include bony articular congruency, the glenohumeral ligaments, the glenoid labrum, the rotator interval, and the negative intra-articular pressure whereas dynamic stabilizers include the rotator cuff and periscapular musculature. The long head of the biceps (LHB) tendon is probably not significantly involved with glenohumeral stability since Walch et al. [2], Boileau et al. [3], and Giphart et al. [4] all demonstrated that neither proximal humeral head migration nor glenohumeral instability occurred after biceps tenodesis.

As a result of the numerous structures involved with the maintenance of glenohumeral stability, physical examination of the patient with instability can be particularly challenging. However, an effective examination most often reveals a characteristic pattern of signs and symptoms that typically lead the clinician towards the correct diagnosis.

6.2 Anatomy and Biomechanics

6.2.1 Basic Structure and Function

The balance between mobility and stability of the glenohumeral joint is achieved through the coordinated, complex interactions between multiple static and dynamic stabilizers that function to center the humeral head within the glenoid fossa throughout the full range of shoulder motion. Static constraints include articular congruency, glenoid version, the coracoacromial arch, the glenoid labrum, capsuloligamentous structures, the rotator interval, and the inherent negative intra-articular pressure. Dynamic constraints include the rotator cuff and periscapular musculature which both contribute to the well-described concavity compression mechanism. The LHB tendon should not be considered a dynamic constraint since a recent biplane fluoroscopic study found no difference in humeral head translation in any plane after biceps tenodesis when compared to the contralateral, unoperated shoulder [4]. These findings have also been noted by others [2, 3].

R.J. Warth and P.J. Millett, *Physical Examination of the Shoulder: An Evidence-Based Approach*, DOI 10.1007/978-1-4939-2593-3_6, © Springer Science+Business Media New York 2015

Fig. 6.1 Illustrations of
(**a**) a normal glenoid, (**b**)
a fractured anteroinferior
glenoid (bony Bankart
lesion), and (**c**) an
"inverted pear" glenoid.

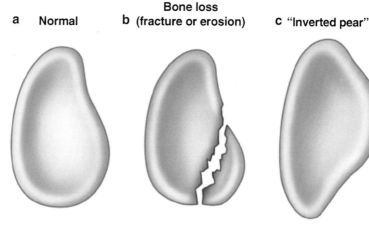

6.2.1.1 Static Constraints
Articular Congruency

The glenoid takes the shape of a teardrop or a pear—that is, the diameter of the superior aspect of the glenoid is approximately 20 % less than that of the inferior glenoid [5, 6]. The inferior aspect of the glenoid is more circular and its symmetry is often used to measure the amount of acute or attritional bone loss in cases of recurrent instability (e.g., "inverted pear glenoid") via pre-operative imaging or direct visualization at arthroscopy (Fig. 6.1) [7, 8]. Approximately one-fourth of the humeral head makes contact with the glenoid at any point throughout the entire range of shoulder motion, thus highlighting the importance of strong soft-tissue stabilizers that serve to maintain the constant balance between motion and stability (Fig. 6.2) [9]. Geometrically, the glenohumeral ratio (maximum glenoid diameter divided by the maximum diameter of the humeral head) is approximately 0.75 in the sagittal plane and 0.60 in the transverse plane [10]. Biomechanically, glenohumeral stability is determined by the balance stability angle (maximum angle of the axial force vector applied by the humeral head to the glenoid center line) and the effective glenoid arc (radius of curvature of the glenoid able to support the joint reaction force produced by the humeral head), a parameter which includes the increased depth produced by an intact labrum (Fig. 6.3) [11]. Both the balance stability angle and the effective glenoid arc

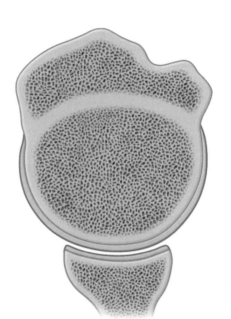

Fig. 6.2 Illustration showing the articular congruency of the glenohumeral joint. Note that only approximately 25 % of the humeral head articular cartilage makes contact with the glenoid throughout the entire arc of motion.

are affected by the morphology of the articular cartilage, labrum, and osseous anatomy of both the humeral head and the glenoid (Fig. 6.4).

Glenoid Version

Churchill et al. [12] reported that the normal glenoid is retroverted a mean of 1.2°. Their study reported a range between 9.5° of anteversion to

Fig. 6.3 Illustrations demonstrating (**a**) the effective glenoid arc and (**b**) the balance stability angle. The effective glenoid arc refers to the radius of curvature of the glenoid able to support joint reaction forces across the joint that would otherwise lead to humeral head translation. The balance stability angle is the maximum scapulo-humeral angle at which humeral head translation can be prevented by the effective glenoid arc when an axial load is applied through the humerus.

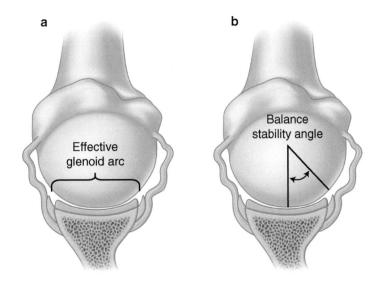

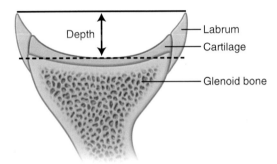

Fig. 6.4 Axial cut-away view showing the structure of the glenoid, articular cartilage, and labrum.

10.5° of retroversion in 344 human scapulae with a mean age of 25.6 years, indicating that a high degree of anatomic variability exists across the general population. Although it is unknown whether these shoulders were afflicted with recurrent instability, most evidence suggests that excessive glenoid version (anterior, posterior, superior, or inferior) or humeral torsion may be associated with decreased glenohumeral stability [12–17] and rotator cuff tears (Fig. 6.5) [18].

Coracoacromial Arch

The coracoacromial arch is situated anterosuperi-orly above the humeral head and is composed of the anterior acromion and the coracoid with the coracoacromial ligament spanning between these structures. This arch is known to prevent excessive anterosuperior migration of the humeral head (Fig. 6.6). However, contact of the humeral head with the undersurface of the acromion can be both a cause and effect of significant rotator cuff disease (see Chap. 4). In general, clinical instability as a result of superior humeral head migration in the absence of a large rotator cuff tear is an extremely rare entity.

Glenoid Labrum

The glenoid labrum is a triangular, fibrocartilagi-nous structure that adheres to the circumference of the glenoid rim (see Fig. 6.1). Its primary function is to provide an extension of the bony glenoid by increasing both its depth and surface area (Fig. 6.7)—factors that have been shown to contribute to approximately 10 % of glenohumeral stability [19, 20]. Recently, Park et al. [21] studied the effect of labral height on subjective outcomes in 40 patients who underwent arthroscopic repair of soft-tissue lesions of the anteroinferior glenoid (i.e., Bankart lesions). Patients with decreased labral height after repair demonstrated inferior clinical outcomes 1 year postoperatively (via Rowe scores) when compared to those with higher labral height. In addition to improving glenoid depth and contact surface area, the glenoid labrum also serves as an attachment site for the joint capsule and the glenohumeral ligaments.

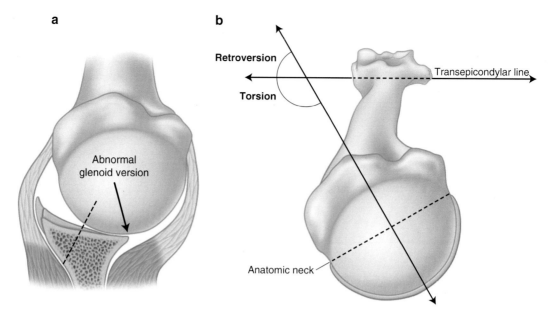

Fig. 6.5 (**a**) Increased glenoid retroversion can lead to recurrent instability due to absence of the effective glenoid arc. Severe anterior instability may cause tearing of the subscapularis tendon. (**b**) Increased humeral retrotorsion can lead to recurrent instability by overcoming the native balance stability angle of the glenohumeral joint.

Fig. 6.6 (**a**) Normal coracoacromial arch. (**b**) Surgical release of the coracoacromial ligament and removal of the anterior acromion can result in anterosuperior instability. This is extremely uncommon when the rotator cuff is intact.

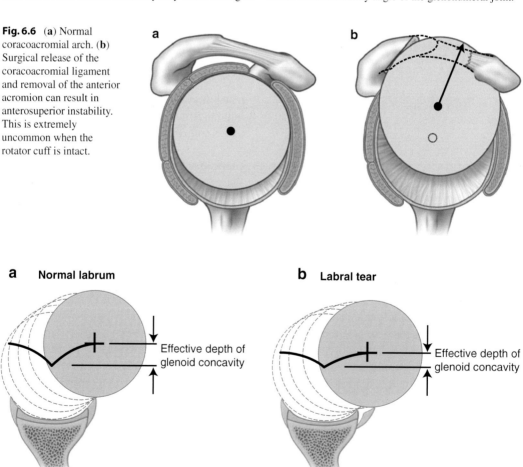

Fig. 6.7 (**a**) Effective glenoid depth with an intact labrum. (**b**) Effective glenoid depth with a labral tear.

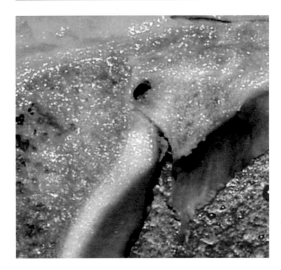

Fig. 6.8 Cadaveric photograph showing the origin of the LHB tendon from both the superior labrum and the supraglenoid tubercle.

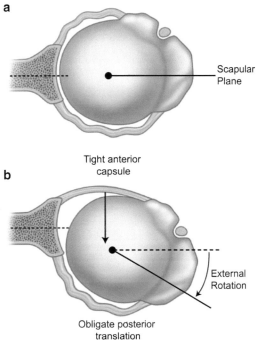

Fig. 6.9 (**a**) Loose pack position. Note that in the scapular plane, the humerus and glenoid are in neutral alignment and the anterior and posterior capsule are in a normal resting position. (**b**) Increased tension of anterior structures occurs when the humerus is externally rotated. The posterior structures become taut when the humerus is internally rotated.

Approximately 40–60 % of the LHB substance originates from the superior labrum (the remaining percentage originates from the supraglenoid tubercle) (Fig. 6.8) [22].

Capsuloligamentous Structures

With the humerus in a neutral position (such as the "loose pack position" described in Chap. 2), stability is achieved through dynamic muscle contraction since the glenohumeral joint capsule and associated ligamentous structures are somewhat lax in this position [23]. However, these structures become variably taught with both active and passive shoulder motion which both maximizes articular surface contact and prevents abnormal humeral head translation (Fig. 6.9). The joint capsule itself, the coracohumeral ligament (CHL) and the superior, middle, and inferior glenohumeral ligaments (SGHL, MGHL, and IGHL, respectively) make up this important capsuloligamentous complex (Fig. 6.10).

The glenohumeral joint capsule is one of the primary static restraints involved in maintaining shoulder stability. It is primarily composed of collagen fiber bundles with varying degrees of thickness and fiber orientation [24, 25]. The CHL, SGHL, MGHL and IGHL make up distinct bands or areas of capsular thickening that are important for the maintenance of glenohumeral stability in any plane of shoulder motion. These structures become variably taught with both active and passive motion, thus maximizing articular surface contact and preventing abnormal humeral head translation. The shape and function of each individual ligament is determined by the position of the humerus in space.

The CHL has two distinct bands (anterior and posterior) that originate from the lateral base of the coracoid and travel between the supraspinatus and subscapularis tendons. The anterior band merges with the insertional fibers of the subscapularis tendon and the joint capsule near the lesser tuberosity whereas the posterior band inserts over the anterior aspect of the greater tuberosity. With the arm at the side, the anterior band primarily resists excessive external rotation and the posterior band

Fig. 6.10 Illustration showing the major labroligamentous structures surrounding the glenoid. The rotator cuff musculature is also shown.

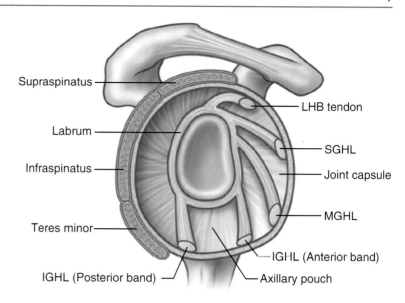

primarily functions to prevent excessive internal rotation. Both the anterior and posterior bands of the CHL also provide resistance to inferior humeral head translation with the arm at the side and posterior humeral head translation when the arm is horizontally adducted [26–29].

The SGHL originates from the superior rim of the glenoid near the biceps-labral complex, travels parallel to the much larger CHL, and inserts on the lesser tuberosity, blending with the fibers of the subscapularis tendon. Its usual functions are similar to that of the CHL, preventing excessive external rotation [30] and inferior translation [31] when the arm is at the side and preventing posterior translation when the arm is horizontally adducted. However, its diameter, strength, and relative contribution to shoulder stability are highly variable across the population.

The anatomy of the MGHL is also highly variable. It can originate from the scapular neck, the anterosuperior glenoid rim or the supraglenoid tubercle with the biceps-labral complex. Similar to the CHL and the SGHL, the distal insertion of the MGHL blends with the fibers of the subscapularis tendon. The morphologic phenotype of the MGHL can also range in appearance from a round, cord-like ligament to a flat, sheet-like structure that blends with the IGHL inferiorly.

Biomechanical ligament sectioning studies have shown that the MGHL primarily functions as a restraint to anterior translation when the humerus is between 0° and 45° of abduction and externally rotated [23]. In addition, the MGHL may also be important in limiting external rotation when the humerus is abducted greater than 60°.

The IGHL complex circumferentially attaches to the inferior aspect of the glenoid labrum anteriorly, inferiorly, and posteriorly and runs laterally to widely insert over an area extending between the lesser tuberosity anteriorly and the triceps tendon posteriorly. The IGHL is composed of thick anterior and posterior bands with an interposed "hammock-like" pouch that loosely cradles the inferior aspect of the humeral head (see Fig. 6.10). Its function is to resist both anterior and posterior humeral head translation when the humerus is abducted more than 60° [30]. Specifically, as the humerus is abducted and externally rotated, the anterior band of the IGHL complex along with the anteroinferior capsule becomes taut and prevents anterior humeral head translation. When the humerus is flexed, adducted, and internally rotated, the posterior band of the IGHL complex and the posterior capsule become taut and prevent posterior humeral head translation (see Fig. 6.9).

Fig. 6.11 Illustration highlighting the components of the rotator interval.

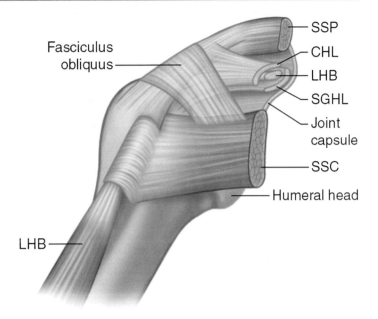

Rotator Interval

The rotator interval is a triangular space over the anterosuperior aspect of the joint capsule. The supraspinatus forms the superior border, the subscapularis forms the inferior border, and the coracoid process forms the medial base (Fig. 6.11). The CHL, the SGHL, the MGHL, the LHB tendon and the anterosuperior joint capsule all reside within this triangular space. Jost et al. [32] performed one of the more detailed cadaveric studies in which the rotator interval was described as being composed of several layers. However, the precise anatomy of the rotator interval is still under investigation and is beyond the scope of this chapter.

The exact function of the rotator interval is also the subject of numerous biomechanical studies [26, 32–39]. However, many of their reported results have been conflicting. Harryman et al. [36] performed one of the first comprehensive and descriptive studies that examined the function of the structures within the rotator interval. After dividing the capsule and ligamentous structures within the rotator interval in a series of 80 cadaveric shoulders, the investigators noted an increase in passive glenohumeral flexion, extension, external rotation, and adduction capacity.

Medial–lateral imbrication of the same structures resulted in the opposite effect, thus decreasing these motions. The authors concluded that the rotator interval provided resistance against excessive motion while also functioning to limit posteroinferior glenohumeral translation. Nobuhara and Ikeda [39] also showed that tightening of the rotator interval decreased the propensity for humeral head translation in the posteroinferior direction. As a result of these studies, most surgeons believe that the rotator interval does provide some degree of stability, especially inferiorly when the humerus is externally rotated.

As mentioned in Chap. 5, the rotator interval also contributes to stability of the LHB tendon as it travels through the bicipital groove towards the superior labrum and supraglenoid tubercle. Specifically, the SGHL, CHL, and subscapularis tendon together form a structure known as the biceps reflection pulley which supports the tendon as it enters the glenohumeral joint (Fig. 6.12) [2, 26, 27, 40].

Negative Intra-Articular Pressure

Within the closed joint, a negative intra-articular pressure is produced by either a "piston-in-valve"

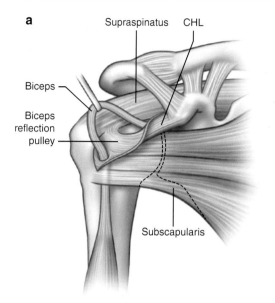

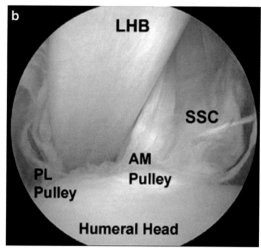

Fig. 6.12 (**a**) Illustration showing the structure of the bicipital sheath and biceps reflection pulley (BRP) as the LHB
tendon travels into the glenohumeral joint. (**b**) Arthroscopic
image showing anteromedial (AM) and posterolateral (PL)
BRPs. (Part B from Elser F, Braun S, Dewing CB, Giphart
JE, Millett PJ. Anatomy, function, injuries, and treatment of
the long head of the biceps brachii tendon. Arthroscopy.
2011;27(4):581–92; with permission).

mechanism, an adhesion-cohesion effect of the
viscous synovial fluid, or both, which exist to
provide some degree of stability to the glenohumeral joint [41]. Any perforation of the joint
capsule can "vent" the joint, eliminating this
nascent pressure gradient (Table 6.1) [41–43].
However, although this mechanism may provide
some joint stability, capsular venting alone is not
an apparent cause of clinical instability.

6.2.1.2 Dynamic Constraints
Rotator Cuff
The rotator cuff contributes to glenohumeral stability through several different mechanisms.
First, contraction of the rotator cuff muscles
serves to compress the humeral head within the
glenoid concavity, thus maximizing contact
between the articular surfaces during active
motion (the "concavity compression" mechanism is discussed below). Second, the physical
presence of the rotator cuff musculature prevents
humeral head migration. Specifically, the supraspinatus (along with the coracoacromial arch)
helps prevent superior translation, the infraspinatus and teres minor resist posterior translation

Table 6.1 Mean intra-articular pressures with the neutral
and abduction/axial traction positions[a]

	Neutral position (mm Hg)	Abduction/axial traction (mm Hg)
Cadaveric shoulders (n = 18)	−34	−111
Stable shoulders (n = 15)	−32	−133
Unstable shoulders (n = 17)	0	−2

Table adapted from Habermeyer et al. [41]; with
permission
[a]The values given are the mean intra-articular pressures
with each position in each population sample

and the subscapularis helps to stabilize the joint
anteriorly. Third, the rotator cuff forms direct
attachments with the joint capsule and contributes to stability by increasing capsular tension
during active motion. Finally, the glenohumeral
joint capsule has proprioceptors that are activated
by capsular stretching [44]. Afferent nerve
impulses travel through the dorsal root ganglia
and return via efferent fibers to produce contraction of the rotator cuff and deltoid muscles which

Posterior view

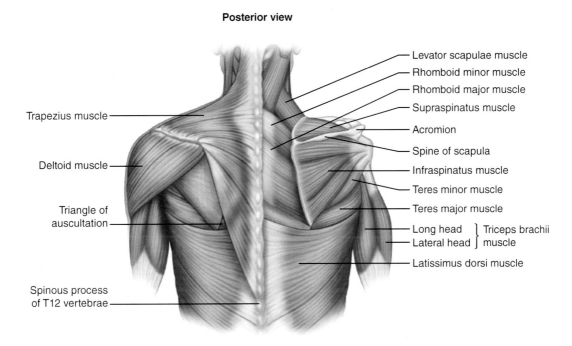

Fig. 6.13   Illustration highlighting the anatomy of the periscapular musculature.

effectively counteracts the initial stimulus (i.e., capsular stretching).

Periscapular Musculature

The periscapular muscles, including the trapezius, rhomboids, levator scapulae, serratus anterior, latissimus dorsi, and pectoralis minor, function in synchrony to optimize the position of the scapula during rotation, elevation, and horizontal adduction of the humerus, thus maintaining the humeral head in a centered position within the glenoid fossa in any motion plane (Fig. 6.13). See Chaps. 2, 3 and 9 for more information regarding basic scapulohumeral kinematics and related physical examination techniques.

Concavity Compression

Contraction of the rotator cuff and deltoid muscles compresses the humeral head against the glenoid fossa during active motion (also known as "concavity compression"; Fig. 6.14). As discussed in Chap. 4, the rotator cuff and deltoid muscles produce parallel force vectors that act against the glenoid surface. Simultaneous contraction of

parallel muscles on opposite sides of the joint (e.g., the subscapularis anteriorly and the infraspinatus posteriorly) compresses the humeral head into the glenoid while contraction of muscles on the same side of the joint (e.g., the supraspinatus and the deltoid superiorly) produces humeral head rotation (e.g., abduction). In addition, the relative strength of contraction of each muscle determines the plane of elevation or rotation. For example, if the concentric contraction strength of the subscapularis was 1.0 units and the eccentric contraction strength of the infraspinatus was 0.5 units, the net rotational moment would favor subscapularis and, thus, internal rotation with simultaneous glenohumeral compression would result. This dynamic mechanism favors both motion and stability and can be applied to other muscles and joints throughout the body.

6.2.2   Anatomic Variations

Many of the structures described above have several anatomic variations that are important

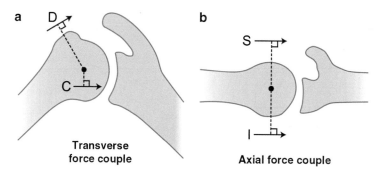

Fig. 6.14 Illustration highlighting the important force couples that help maintain concavity compression and overall glenohumeral stability. (**a**) The combined actions of the deltoid muscle (D) and the rotator cuff (C) make up the transverse plane force couple and pull the humeral head medially towards the glenoid fossa. (**b**) The combined actions of the subscapularis (S) and the infraspinatus (I) make up the axial plane force couple and also work to drive the humeral head medially towards the glenoid fossa.

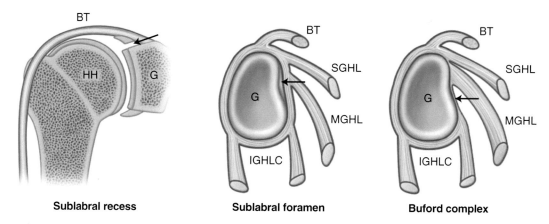

Fig. 6.15 Illustrations showing the most common glenolabral anatomic variations. The sublabral recess, sublabral foramen, and Buford complex are shown.

to recognize from a management perspective (Fig. 6.15). However, because these variations are not discernible by physical examination, an in-depth discussion of each variation would not be helpful in the context of this chapter. Rather, we have provided a summary of this information with their corresponding references in Table 6.2 in an effort to direct the reader towards the most relevant published evidence related to these anatomic variations. In addition, we recommend reviewing the article published by Tischer et al. [53] which provides a detailed discussion of the relevance of each anatomic variation as they relate to the arthroscopic management of instability.

6.3 Classification of Instability

Instability is typically described according to severity (microinstability, subluxation, or dislocation), direction (anterior, posterior, inferior, or multidirectional), and chronicity (acute, chronic, or acute on chronic). In other cases, instability can also be described as being voluntary or involuntary [54] and hereditary or acquired [55]. Although several classification systems have been proposed, none of these have been comprehensive nor have they been proven to adequately facilitate communication between physicians,

Table 6.2 Anatomic variations of the glenoid and glenoid labrum

Structure	Anatomic variation	Prevalence	References
Glenoid	Teardrop glenoid with notch	59 %	Anetzberger and Putz [5]
	Teardrop glenoid without notch	29 %	Anetzberger and Putz [5]
	Oval glenoid	12 %	Anetzberger and Putz [5]
Glenoid labrum	Any anterosuperior variation	13.4–25 %	Cooper and Brems [45] and Kanatli et al. [46]
	Sublabral recess	Highly variable	Kanatli et al. [46] and Smith et al. [47]
	Sublabral foramen	12–18.5 %	Ilahi et al. [48], Pfahler et al. [49], and Williams et al. [50]
	Buford complex	1–6.5 %	Williams et al. [50], Ilahi et al. [48], and Ide et al. [51]

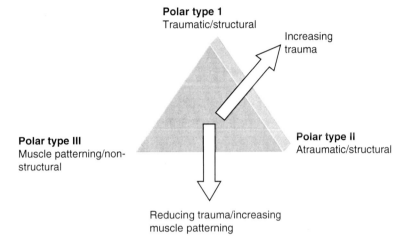

Fig. 6.16 Stanmore classification [58]. See text for explanation and interpretation. (From Lewis et al. [58]; with permission).

guide treatment decisions or predict outcomes. In 1989, Thomas and Matsen [56] categorically divided those with instability into two distinct groups according to the distinctive characteristics of their condition. In one group, the acronym TUBS was used to describe individuals with *T*raumatic, *U*nilateral instability with a *B*ankart lesion that generally requires *S*urgical repair. The other group was described using the acronym AMBRI which included patients with *A*traumatic, *M*ultidirectional instability which was typically *B*ilateral, *R*esponded to physical therapy and sometimes required *I*nferior capsular plication to prevent recurrence. In this group, many individuals are afflicted with underlying multiligamentous laxity who gradually develop instability as they age. However, although this classification system has some academic merit, its usefulness in clinical practice is very limited since most patients present with pathologic traits that overlap

between the TUBS and AMBRI groups. For example, many patients with generalized hyperlaxity present with uni- or bi-directional instability [57] whereas up to one-fourth of patients with traumatic instability display evidence of contralateral involvement and increased capsular elastin content which suggests the possibility of familial inheritance [55]. This overlap indicates that the term "instability" most likely encompasses a continuous spectrum of pathologic features where the TUBS and AMBRI groups represent the terminal ends.

As a result, other classification systems were proposed to account for this continuum of pathologies associated with glenohumeral instability. Particularly noteworthy is the Stanmore classification developed by Lewis et al. [58] in 2004 in which the three points of a triangle represent the polar pathologic characteristics associated with instability (Fig. 6.16). Type I represented traumatic instability, type II represented atraumatic instability, and type III represented neurologic dysfunction and muscle patterning (i.e., voluntary instability). The line between types I and II corresponded with the spectrum of disease between traumatic (TUBS) and atraumatic (AMBRI) etiologies. The line connecting types II and III corresponded with the spectrum of disease in those with atraumatic instability and neurologic dysfunction. As one moves towards the apex of the triangle (i.e., towards the polar type I pathology), the involved pathology increasingly resembles the clinical picture of traumatic instability. The opposite is true when one moves towards the base of the triangle. While this system adequately represents the variability in clinical presentation, it fails to guide the clinician towards a specific treatment option for individual clinical scenarios.

In 2008, Kuhn et al. [59] systematically reviewed the literature to determine the frequency of various criteria that have been used to classify glenohumeral instability. The authors observed that four of these criteria were used in more than 50 % of the proposed classification systems. They also noted that a survey conducted by the American Shoulder and Elbow Surgeons (ASES) echoed these same results. As a result, a classification system that accounts for *F*requency, *E*tiology, *D*irection and *S*everity of instability (FEDS system) was developed since these features were found to be the most important factors involved in treatment decision-making. Subsequent analysis revealed that the FEDS classification had high inter- and intra-rater agreement [60]. However, the major drawback of the FEDS system is its inability to categorize all patients who present with instability. Therefore, further studies that correlate this classification system with treatment outcomes are needed. With this information, clinical results could be predicted at the time of initial clinical evaluation.

Due to the lack of a single validated classification system for glenohumeral instability, the clinician must utilize the concepts derived from several different classification schemes and published literature to make individual treatment decisions based on the etiology and underlying pathologic lesions associated with the injury.

6.4   Pathoanatomic Features of Traumatic Instability

6.4.1   Soft-Tissue Defects

6.4.1.1 Capsular Distention

As mentioned above, the IGHL complex is the most important static restraint that prevents abnormal anterior–posterior humeral head translations. In the normal shoulder, anterior (or posterior) dislocation occurs when a force is applied to the humeral head that exceeds the peak load required to displace the humeral head from the glenoid fossa, to stretch and deform the anterior (or posterior) band of the IGHL complex and, in most cases of acute dislocation, detachment of the glenoid labrum (i.e., Bankart Lesions—discussed below). Once the microstructure of the ligament has been damaged via plastic deformation, a return to its previous shape and function is unlikely in most cases [61]. This is particularly true for the mid-substance of the ligament where strain to failure has been found to be less than that of the other portions of the ligament substance (e.g., the bony insertion sites) [62]. Bigliani et al. [62] noted that failure of the anterior band occurred either at its glenoid insertion (40 %), in its mid-substance (35 %) or at its humeral insertion (25 %). However, significant elongation of the ligament occurred regardless of the mode of failure in this study. After reduction of the joint, the anterior (or posterior) band of the IGHL complex remains irrecoverably elongated and patulous, thus substantially increasing the risk for future dislocations (Fig. 6.17). Rowe et al. [63] found that up to 28 % of patients with recurrent instability had some degree of capsular redundancy. Furthermore, recurrent episodes of instability increase the severity of capsular distention which can lead to significant disability through a variety of other mechanisms [13, 64].

6.4.1.2 Bankart Lesions

Detachment of the anteroinferior glenoid labrum (also known as a Bankart lesion) is thought to occur in up to 90 % of cases of traumatic anterior instability and has traditionally been referred to

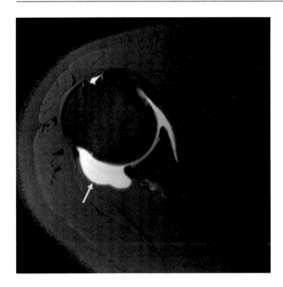

Fig. 6.17 Magnetic resonance arthrogram (MRA) of the right shoulder following an acute posterior glenohumeral dislocation. Note the significant distention of the posterior capsule (*arrow*).

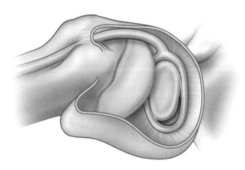

Fig. 6.18 Illustration depicting an anteroinferior labral tear (Bankart lesion).

as the "essential lesion" of traumatic shoulder dislocation (Figs. 6.18 and 6.19b). When the soft-tissue defect is associated with periosteal stripping of the glenoid neck without medial displacement of the labral tissue, it is typically referred to as a "Perthes lesion" (Fig. 6.19c) [65]. Despite its near-universal presence in cases of traumatic instability [66, 67], soft-tissue Bankart lesions alone are not a frequent cause recurrent instability. Rather, the underlying cause is most often multifactorial with particular focus on redundancy and plastic deformation of the IGHL complex [68].

6.4.1.3 ALPSA Lesions

The anterior labral periosteal sleeve avulsion (ALPSA) lesion is an entity similar to that of the Bankart lesion; however, in this case, the periosteum along the anterior glenoid neck elevates from the underlying bone in a "sleeve-like" pattern along with the IGHL-labrum complex which typically appears in a medialized position (Fig. 6.19d) [69].

6.4.1.4 SLAP Tears

Superior labral anterior to posterior (SLAP) tears (discussed in Chap. 5) are more common in overhead athletes probably as a result of the peel-back mechanism as described by Burkhart and Morgan [70] (Fig. 6.20). The deceleration phase of the throwing motion may also produce extraphysio-

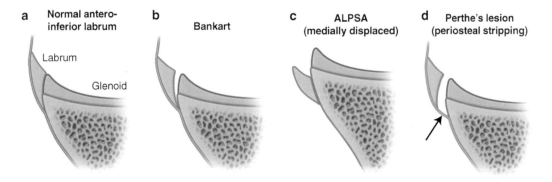

Fig. 6.19 Axial cut-away view showing (**a**) a normal glenoid labrum, (**b**) a Bankart lesion, (**c**) a Perthes lesion, and (**d**) an ALPSA lesion.

logic eccentric loads on the biceps anchor that can result in tearing or rupture. Complete tears of the biceps anchor increased superior–inferior and anterior–posterior humeral head translation in a cadaveric study [71]. However, more recent evidence suggests that posterosuperior migration of the humeral head in overhead athletes as a result of posterior capsular contracture may produce a greater degree of anterior translation that can easily be perceived as clinical laxity (i.e., "pseudolaxity"). This perceived laxity is more likely to be the result of posterior capsule contracture rather than the presence of a SLAP lesion in these patients; however, it should be noted that SLAP tears that extend into the MGHL can also produce increased anterior humeral head translation. Chapter 5 provides further details regarding SLAP tears.

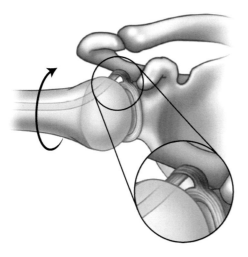

Fig. 6.20 Illustration showing the peel-back mechanism described by Burkhart and Morgan [70]. Increasing degrees of external rotation increases the torsional strain across the biceps anchor which can lead to SLAP tears.

6.4.1.5 HAGL Lesions

The humeral avulsion of the glenohumeral ligament (HAGL) lesion occurs when the insertion of the IGHL complex avulses or otherwise separates from the humeral neck (Fig. 6.21a). Although its incidence is relatively low, this injury most commonly occurs after a first-time anterior shoulder dislocation. When combined with a Bankart lesion, the anterior band of the IGHL complex is referred to as a "floating segment." The same combination of injuries can also occur posteriorly thus involving the posterior band of the IGHL complex (Fig. 6.21b) [72, 73].

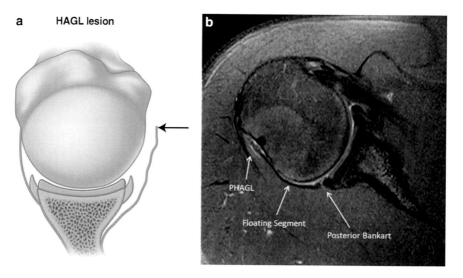

Fig. 6.21 (a) Axial image of HAGL lesion. (b) Axial MRI demonstrating a floating posterior HAGL lesion. (From Martetschläger et al. [72]; with permission).

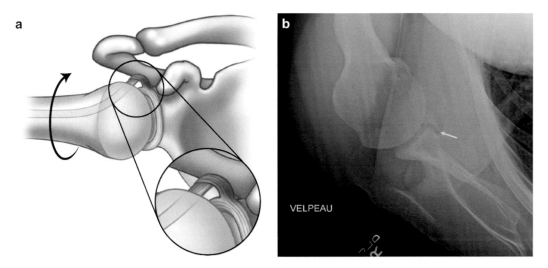

Fig. 6.22 (**a**) Illustration of an anteroinferior glenoid fracture (bony Bankart lesion). (**b**) Velpeau axillary radiograph of a right shoulder showing a fracture of the anterior glenoid.

6.4.1.6 Rotator Interval Lesions

Due to the significant anatomic variability inherent to the rotator interval, it is sometimes difficult to determine whether a physical finding is normal or abnormal. However, in our experience, laxity of the rotator interval can be detected on physical examination by inducing a sulcus sign of >2 cm when the humerus is externally rotated (discussed below).

6.4.2   Osseous Defects

6.4.2.1 Bony Bankart Lesions

Anterior shoulder dislocations can also create fractures of the anteroinferior glenoid rim (i.e., bony Bankart lesions; Fig. 6.22). These fractures can range in morphology and size depending on the direction of load transmission. Loss of bone from the anterior glenoid from any cause decreases glenoid concavity and increases the potential for recurrent dislocations. In general, as the size of the lesion increases, glenohumeral stability decreases [74]. Several biomechanical studies have shown that defects measuring more than one half of the glenoid length decrease joint stability by up to 30 % [75, 76]. Others have

shown that soft-tissue Bankart repair is not adequate for defects involving at least 20–25 % of the inferior glenoid diameter [7]. Although there are numerous methods for measuring anteroinferior glenoid bone loss, discussion of their significance is beyond the scope of this chapter.

6.4.2.2 Attritional Glenoid Bone Loss

Erosion of the anteroinferior glenoid rim as a result of repeated dislocations is another cause for glenoid bone loss (Fig. 6.23). These patients must rely on soft-tissue constraints to maintain anterior stability; however, these restraints are insufficient due to the capsuloligamentous stretching from previous anterior dislocations. Although these patients present similarly to those with other causes of instability, there are many fewer treatment options. For example, there is often no bony fragment that can be used for surgical fixation and, in many cases, soft-tissue repair would not be adequate to prevent recurrent instability [63]. Bony reconstruction of the anterior glenoid is typically indicated which may involve iliac crest bone grafting, the Latarjet procedure, or distal tibial osteochondral allograft (Figs. 6.24 and 6.25).

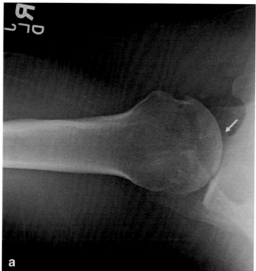

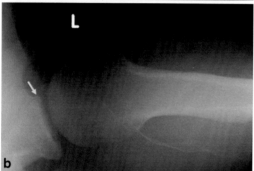

Fig. 6.23 (**a**) Axillary radiograph of a right shoulder demonstrating attritional bone loss involving the anterior glenoid. Note that the humeral head appears to be resting anterior to the axis of glenoid. (**b**) Axillary radiograph of a left shoulder demonstrating attritional bone loss involving the anterior glenoid. The humeral head appears to be positioned anterior to the glenoid axis.

6.4.2.3 Hill–Sachs Lesions

The Hill–Sachs lesion is characterized by an impression fracture of the posterosuperior aspect of the humeral head. These fractures can occur as a result of anterior dislocation when the soft bone of the posterosuperior humeral head impacts the much harder bone of the anteroinferior glenoid rim. Although most lesions are small and generally do not affect glenohumeral stability, other larger lesions can cause recurrent dislocations especially in positions of 90° of abduction and 90° of external rotation (i.e., the 90/90 position) where the humeral head defect can "engage" with the glenoid rim (Fig. 6.26) [7, 77–79].

6.4.2.4 Glenoid Version

Glenoid version, especially retroversion, has been cited as an uncommon, but potential contributory factor involved in recurrent shoulder instability due to the absence of an effective glenoid arc (see Fig. 6.5a) [12, 80]. Due to conflicting data suggesting a possible link between mild glenoid version and recurrent instability, this entity is generally considered a diagnosis of exclusion after all other causes of recurrent instability have been ruled out [14, 81, 82]. On the other hand, more severe cases of glenoid version can result in debilitating instability (Fig. 6.27); most of these cases involve significant retroversion that lead to posterior instability.

Fig. 6.24 Illustration depicting the Latarjet procedure for the treatment of recurrent anterior instability in the setting of glenoid bone loss.

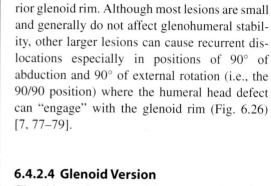

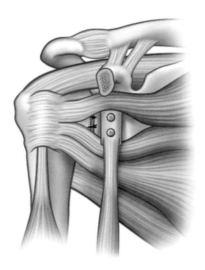

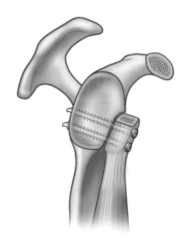

Fig. 6.25 Other bony reconstruction options for the treatment of glenoid bone loss include iliac crest bone grafting and distal tibial osteochondral allograft. (**a**) Surgical photograph demonstrating fixation of a bone graft to the anterior glenoid in a patient with recurrent anterior instability. (**b**) Example of an iliac crest bone graft. (**c**) Example of a distal tibial osteochondral allograft.

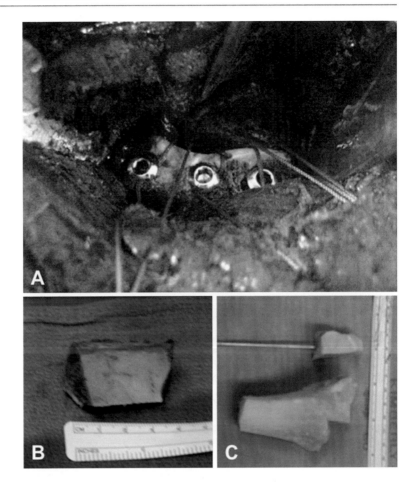

6.5   Pathoanatomic Features of Atraumatic Instability

It is often difficult for clinicians to define which patients are afflicted with atraumatic instability because the effects of activities of daily living and/or sporting activities may lead to undetectable glenohumeral joint damage. The cumulative effects of this damage may lead to unilateral or bilateral instability without an apparent cause. However, some degree of genetic predisposition is implied when patients present with atraumatic bilateral shoulder instability [83]. For example, multidirectional instability (MDI) is defined as atraumatic anterior or posterior instability with a component of increased inferior translation. Studies have demonstrated increased elastin con-

tent in both the skin and capsular tissue of many patients with MDI [84] in addition to increased capsular volume [57, 85, 86] and, in some cases, laxity of the rotator interval [87]. These findings suggest that undiagnosed Ehlers–Danlos syndrome or multiligamentous laxity may be a substantial contributing factor involved in the development of instability in many of these patients. It should be also noted that traumatic and atraumatic instability can occur simultaneously in the same patient and thus should not be considered entirely independent from one another. For example, a patient diagnosed with MDI can also present to the clinic after a traumatic dislocation, potentially resulting in any of the pathologic lesions associated with traumatic instability (i.e., bony Bankart lesion, Hill–Sachs lesion, HAGL lesion, etc.).

Fig. 6.26 (**a**) Hill–Sachs lesions can engage with the anterior glenoid when the humerus is externally rotated. Bone loss or fracture of the anterior glenoid can exacerbate the problem. Engagement of the Hill–Sachs lesion with the anterior glenoid can deepen the humeral head defect. (**b**) Axial computed tomography (CT) scan showing an engaging Hill–Sachs lesion in a patient with debilitating instability.

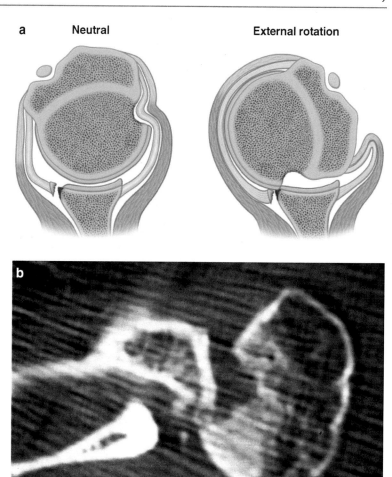

a   Neutral   External rotation

b

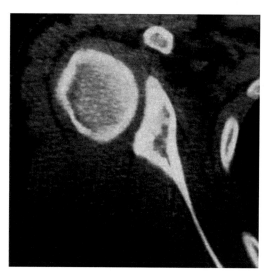

Fig. 6.27 Axial computed tomography (CT) scan demonstrating severe glenoid retroversion. This patient presented with recurrent posterior instability.

6.6 Instability or Increased Laxity?

The semantic relationship between laxity and instability should be recognized and understood by all clinicians who evaluate patients with various shoulder pathologies. The term "laxity" refers to the normal physiologic motion allowed as a result of the position and tension of the ligaments that maintains stability of a joint [88–90]. Without this physiologic laxity, joint motion would not be possible. Because the shoulder requires a large range of motion, its physiologic laxity has a greater magnitude than the other joints within the body. Therefore, laxity testing in the shoulder requires that the clinician understands the difference between "normal" and "abnormal" joint motion as they relate to the entire clinical picture. Along the same lines, the clinician should also understand that increased joint laxity does not necessarily equate pathologic instability, even if this finding occurs unilaterally. As mentioned above, these conditions lie along a spectrum of disease that is most frequently and conveniently labeled as "instability."

6.7   Quantifying Humeral Head Translation

Currently, there are three basic methods by which humeral head motion is quantified: (1) translation in millimeters, (2) translation as a percentage of the humeral head diameter, and (3) the sensations felt when the humeral head is translated. A fourth modality includes the use of instrumentation or imaging; however, these methods are currently under development.

6.7.1   Humeral Head Translation in Millimeters

There are four grades of anterior and/or posterior translation of the humeral head [91].
- Grade 0 = minimal or no translation
- Grade 1 = <10 mm of translation
- Grade 2 = 10–20 mm of translation
- Grade 3 = >20 mm of translation or subluxation

A similar system exists for the measurement of inferior translation [92–95]. The primary limitation of this method of measurement is its subjectivity—that is, each measurement is an approximation made by the examiner and extensive practice is needed before one becomes proficient and accurate. As of this writing, these methods of measurement have not been biomechanically or clinically validated; however, they are widely used in the setting of a busy clinical practice due to their convenience and, when performed by the most experienced clinicians, sufficient accuracy.

6.7.2   Humeral Head Translation as a Percentage of Humeral Head Diameter

Measurement of humeral head translation can also be estimated using the humeral head diameter as described by Cofield and Irving [96]. Specifically, the amount of translation as a percentage of the humeral head diameter is used. This method accounts for the size of the individual being tested and may theoretically provide a more accurate estimate of glenohumeral translation. However, several studies have provided conflicting results regarding the amount of translation that should be considered abnormal. Reported estimates for normal anterior and posterior translations have ranged from 0 to 50 % and from 26 to 50 %, respectively [79, 89, 93, 97–99]. In addition, humeral head diameters vary widely across the population and its estimation may be difficult without some sort of radiographic measurement. This method has not been formally validated for the measurement of humeral head translation and, in at least one case, has been reported as invalid [89].

6.7.3   Tactile Sensation of Humeral Head Translation

Another way to quantify humeral head translation is to report what is felt by the examiner when the humeral head is translated anteriorly or posteriorly. The primary advantage of the classification scheme is that the measurement does not rely upon absolute numbers to define certain pathologies. There are four grades of translation according to Hawkins and Bokor [100]:
- Grade 0: Normal physiologic motion
- Grade 1: Translation to the glenoid rim
- Grade 2: Translation over the glenoid rim
- Grade 3: Humeral head remains out of joint after examiner removes hands (i.e., "lock out")

Levy et al. [94] investigated the reliability and accuracy of the original Hawkins system to detect humeral head translations in a series of 43 athletes. Two fellows in sports medicine, a senior orthopedic resident or an attending physician in orthopedic

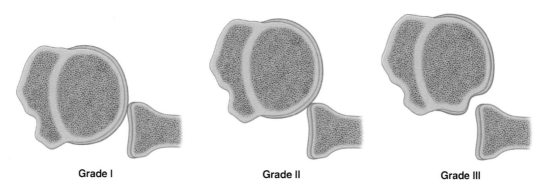

Grade I   Grade II   Grade III

Fig. 6.28 Illustration of the modified Hawkins classification of glenohumeral translation (grades 1, 2 and 3) [100].

surgery performed all of the physical examinations. These researchers found an overall inter-rater reliability of less than 50 %. However, they found that the inter-rater agreement increased to a mean of 73 % when grades 0 and 1 were considered together. The intra-rater agreement also increased from 46 to 73 % when grades 0 and 1 were consolidated. Using this modified Hawkins scale, McFarland et al. [101] demonstrated an intra-rater reliability of 100 % and 86 % for anterior and posterior humeral head translations, respectively. As a result of these studies, the original Hawkins system was modified due to the difficulty in distinguishing between patients with grade 0 and grade 1 translations. Currently, grade 1 represents humeral head translation "not over the rim," grade 2 represents "over the rim," and grade 3 represents "lock out" (Fig. 6.28). However, the clinical significance of the modified Hawkins system is still heavily debated. For example, using the anterior and posterior drawer tests (described below), several studies have demonstrated grade 2 laxity in physiologically normal shoulders without clinical instability [102–104]. In addition, these studies also found that glenohumeral joint laxity may be increased in the non-dominant shoulder, suggesting that asymmetric findings with laxity testing is most likely normal in the majority of cases. Additional research is necessary to determine the applicability of the modified Hawkins classification as it relates to the diagnosis of shoulder instability.

6.7.4 Objective Instrumentation

In the shoulder, humeral head translation in any direction is primarily measured by tactile sensation and requires a great deal of practice and experience. When a clinician becomes proficient, abnormal joint motions of <1 mm can reliably be detected, especially when the patient is under general anesthesia. Although this practice has some element of subjectivity, it is widely accepted since there are currently no validated devices that can accurately and reproducibly detect small amounts of joint motion. These types of instruments for the shoulder are currently in development and use a similar design to that of the KT-1000 [105–107] a device used to measure tibial translation relative to the femur. However, measuring humeral head translation using these new instruments is limited due to the effects of soft-tissue compliance and patient apprehension. In addition, there is no single amount of humeral head translation beyond which instability or increased laxity can be diagnosed [36, 109, 110]. Further research is necessary before these types of instruments can be recommended for clinical practice. The use of ultrasound and stress radiographs have also been proposed as methods to measure joint translation; however, these methods are unreliable and, again, further testing is needed before they can be recommended for use in the clinical setting.

6.8 Laxity Testing

Patient guarding or apprehension is one of the main challenges associated with laxity testing of the shoulder in the office setting. With these maneuvers, it is required that the patient remains relaxed to allow the humeral head to translate appropriately during testing. While many of these tests can be performed in the sitting or supine position, several authors have noted that laxity testing with the patient in the supine position may produce the best results because the patient is generally more relaxed [111, 112]. Another challenge associated with laxity testing is the interpretation of the clinical findings. Although the end feel classification system derived by Cyriax and Cyriax [113] in 1947 has been used in the past (see Chap. 2), defining the quality of the end point in shoulder laxity testing is not practical since none of these qualities can be associated with any specific pathology, treatment or outcome. However, in the clinical setting, the reproduction of symptoms is often a strong indicator of the underlying diagnosis and may also direct the use of other provocative maneuvers.

6.8.1 Drawer Signs

Drawer signs can be used to assess anterior or posterior humeral head translation as long as the patient remains in a relaxed state throughout the

maneuver. This is sometimes difficult in patients who present with overt instability where significant guarding and/or apprehension may be present. As mentioned above, it may be helpful to place the patient in the supine position to promote patient relaxation. When the patient is supine, it is also important to confirm that the humeral head is not supported by the examination table beneath as this will prevent posterior translation. On the other hand, posterior support of the scapula is advantageous since increased scapular rotation (internal or external rotation) may produce inaccurate results when attempting to manipulate the humeral head. Although the original developers of this maneuver recommended that the arm be placed between 80° and 120° of abduction, it is preferred to place the humerus in the approximate "loose pack" position [102, 114, 115] to (1) minimize the effects of proprioceptive muscle contraction (generated by increased capsular tension [16]), (2) to prevent scapular motion during testing, and (3) to more accurately assess true humeral head translation (Fig. 6.29). The glenohumeral resting position (or the "loose pack" position, discussed in Chap. 2) is debated; however, it is generally thought to occur between 55° and 70° of abduction within the scapular plane and with neutral rotation [116, 117].

The posterior drawer test is performed with the patient supine and the shoulder in the "loose pack" position as described above. The examiner holds the wrist to minimize patient-controlled contraction of the deltoid in an effort to actively hold the

Fig. 6.29 Demonstration of the approximate glenohumeral resting position with the humerus abducted to 55–70° within scapular plane and in neutral rotation.

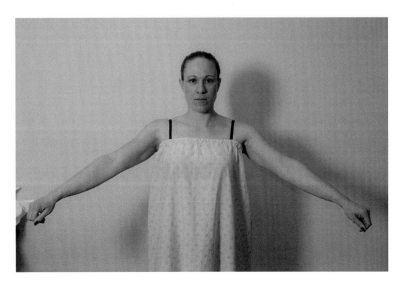

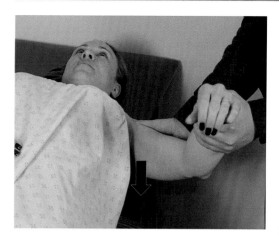

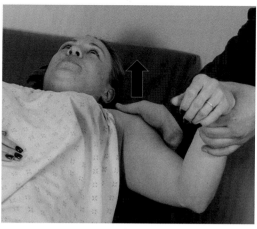

Fig. 6.30 Posterior drawer test. With the patient supine, the extremity is placed in the approximate "loose pack" position. The examiner holds the patient's wrist to prevent biceps contraction while the other hand is placed over the shoulder such that the thumb is anterior and the fingers are posterior. The examiner then applies a posteriorly directed force with the thumb and the amount of translation is estimated.

Fig. 6.31 Anterior drawer test. The patient is placed in an identical position to that which is presented in Fig. 6.33. In this case, the fingers are used to pull the humerus anteriorly. The amount of humeral head translation is then estimated. It may be helpful to apply a gentle axial load during drawer testing to aid in the detection of translation relative to the glenoid rim.

arm in position. This also allows for passive flexion of the elbow and subsequent relaxation of the biceps muscle which may have some effect on glenohumeral stability via the proximal LHB tendon. The examiner's other hand is placed over the shoulder such that the thumb lies on the anterior aspect of the humeral head and the fingers span over the top of the shoulder. From this position, the thumb is used to apply a posteriorly directed force on the humeral head to a point of subluxation which is felt by the examiner's fingers. Pressure from the thumb is then removed while the fingers continue to monitor the subluxation status of the humeral head (Fig. 6.30). At this point, the modified Hawkins classification is used to quantify the degree of glenohumeral laxity (discussed above). When the humeral head does not subluxate posteriorly, the patient has grade 1 laxity (a normal finding). If subluxation does occur, grade 2 laxity is diagnosed when the removal of thumb pressure allows the humeral head to spontaneously reduce whereas grade 3 laxity is diagnosed when the humeral head remains subluxated even after the removal of anterior thumb pressure (i.e., "lock out") (see Fig. 6.28).

The anterior drawer test has a similar biomechanical premise; however, the examiner must also control scapular motion which can affect translation measurements. One method involves placing one hand over the top of the shoulder to stabilize the scapula while the other hand is wrapped around the upper arm near the humeral head. A posterior to anterior force is then applied to the humeral head, producing anterior translation [112]. In most cases, it is preferred to hold the wrist with one hand and the proximal humerus with the other hand while simultaneously applying a medially directed force on the humeral head towards the glenoid fossa (Fig. 6.31). This method helps prevent scapular motion and also helps the examiner detect the precise moment of joint subluxation [95, 118]. The results of this maneuver are classified using the modified Hawkins criteria as described above for the posterior drawer test.

6.8.2   Load-and-Shift Test

The load-and-shift test was first described by Silliman and Hawkins [95] in 1993 as a method to assess anterior and posterior laxity. With the patient sitting, the examiner places one hand over the top of the shoulder to stabilize the scapula while the other hand is placed over the proximal humerus. The examiner then applies gentle pressure to the proximal humerus in the direction of the glenoid fossa, thus "loading" the joint as described by its original developers [79, 95]. The purpose of this initial joint loading is to ensure adequate joint reduction and to assist the examiner in detecting joint subluxation. The humeral head is then grasped with the examiner's thumb placed posteriorly and the fingers placed anteriorly. An anteriorly directed force is applied to the humeral head in an attempt to translate the humeral head over the anterior rim of the glenoid. This is followed by a similar maneuver in which a posteriorly directed force is applied to induce posterior subluxation (Fig. 6.32).

Although the original developers placed the arm in 20° of abduction and 20° of forward flexion before applying the translation force, we have not found this positioning to be helpful. This test can also be performed with the patient supine.

6.8.3   Sulcus Signs

First described by Neer and Foster [119] in 1980, sulcus signs have traditionally been utilized as a measure of inferior glenohumeral laxity. The test is typically performed with the patient sitting since this places the humerus in a relative resting position, especially when the hands and forearms are placed on the patient's lap. Each arm can be tested individually; however, we recommend first testing both extremities simultaneously in new patients since this method allows direct comparison between extremities. If asymmetry is present, then the affected shoulder can be evaluated in more detail (Fig. 6.33). With the patient seated on the examination table, the examiner grasps both arms just above the elbow and applies gentle inferior traction to the glenohumeral joint. Each shoulder should also be tested individually with the humerus in maximum external rotation to evaluate laxity of the rotator interval structures (Fig. 6.34) [31, 36, 120]. The patient should

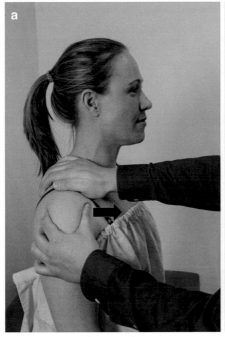
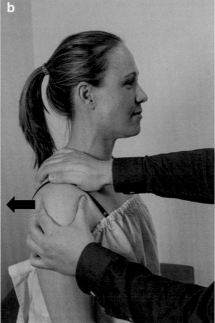

Fig. 6.32 Load-and-shift test. With the patient sitting and the arms at the side, the examiner places one hand over the top of the shoulder to stabilize the scapula and the other hand is placed over the proximal humerus. The examiner then applies a medially directed force to the proximal humerus in the direction of the glenoid fossa while simultaneously translating the humeral head (**a**) anteriorly and then (**b**) posteriorly.

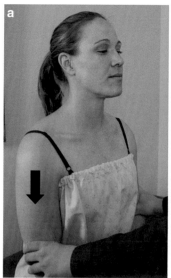
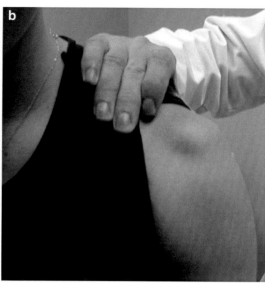

Fig. 6.33 Sulcus sign. (**a**) While the patient is seated with the hands resting on their lap, the examiner grasps each arm just above the elbow and applies a distraction force to the glenohumeral joint bilaterally to detect asymmetric joint laxity. (**b**) Clinical photograph demonstrating a positive sulcus sign (>2 cm step-off between the lateral edge of the acromion and the top of the humeral head).

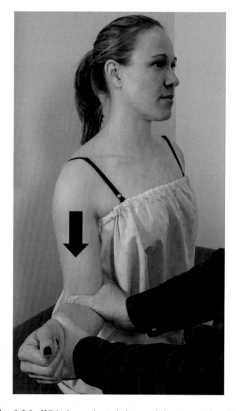

Fig. 6.34 With the patient sitting and the arm at the side, the humerus is placed at approximately 90° of external rotation. The examiner grasps the arm just above the elbow and applies an inferiorly directed distraction force to the glenohumeral joint. A positive sulcus sign with this maneuver is indicative of rotator interval pathology.

always be asked if the maneuver reproduces their symptoms. In most cases, sulcus signs are graded according to the degree of inferior translation that is produced: grade I indicates <1 cm inferior translation, grade II indicates 1–2 cm inferior translation, and grade III indicates >2 cm inferior translation [92–95]. Of course, this grading system is most useful when correlated with other findings within the history and physical examination.

6.8.4   Hyperabduction Test

The hyperabduction test was first described by Gagey and Gagey [121] in 2001 as a method to evaluate the patency of the IGHL complex. With the patient sitting, the examiner stands behind the affected shoulder. While a downward pressure is applied to the top of the shoulder to stabilize the scapula, the humerus is passively abducted until the scapula begins to rotate (Fig. 6.35). The degree of abduction at which scapular motion begins was originally termed the maximum range of passive abduction (RPA). When the RPA was exceeded 105°, the test was considered positive for increased laxity of the IGHL complex. This cut-off point is derived from the original study

Fig. 6.35 Hyperabduction test. With the patient sitting, the examiner stabilizes the scapula and passively abducts the humerus in the coronal plane until the scapula begins to rotate upward. When upward rotation of the scapula begins at >105° of humeral abduction, the test is considered positive.

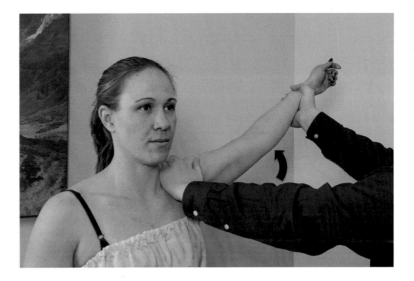

which involved performing the test on 100 cadavers (both before and after sequential sectioning of the IGHL complex; however, other soft tissues were not left intact), 100 volunteers without shoulder complaints and 90 volunteers with documented shoulder instability. In that study, 85 % of unstable shoulders demonstrated an RPA of >105° whereas stable shoulders demonstrated a mean RPA of approximately 90°. The authors concluded that laxity of the IGHL complex could be suspected in patients with an RPA >105°. The intra-class correlation coefficients (ICCs) were found to be excellent in this study (inter-observer ICC: 0.87–0.90; intra-observer ICC: 0.84–0.89). More recently, van Kampen et al. [122] studied six clinical tests for instability in 169 consecutive patients at an orthopedic outpatient clinic (apprehension, relocation, release, anterior drawer, load-and-shift and hyperabduction tests). Magnetic resonance arthrography was used as the diagnostic gold standard. Of the 169 patients, 60 patients were diagnosed with anterior instability according to imaging studies. Overall, the diagnostic accuracy of the clinical tests for increased glenohumeral laxity ranged between 80.5 and 86.4 % where the hyperabduction test was found to be 81.1 % accurate with a sensitivity of 66.7 % and a specificity of 89.0 %.

6.9 Testing for Anterior Instability

6.9.1 Drawer Signs

Although the drawer signs are typically used to assess glenohumeral laxity (discussed above), there are specific scenarios in which these signs may increase the clinical suspicion for instability (see Figs. 6.30 and 6.31). For example, some clinicians consider the maneuver to be "positive" for instability when the patient experiences apprehension. In the study by van Kampen et al. (mentioned above) [122], the anterior drawer sign was also evaluated with regard to its diagnostic efficacy for clinical instability. A "positive" test was defined as either increased anterior humeral head translation as detected by the examiner when compared to the contralateral shoulder *or* when the patient experienced feelings of apprehension during the maneuver. In this study, the sensitivity of the anterior drawer sign was calculated to be 58.3 % (high rate of false negatives) whereas the specificity was calculated to be 92.7 % (low rate of false positives). It should be remembered that asymmetric laxity measurements do not always indicate instability.

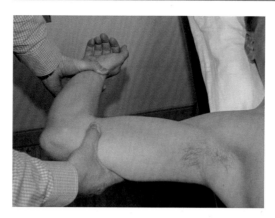

Fig. 6.36 Anterior apprehension. This test can be performed with the patient sitting or standing. The humerus is laterally abducted to 90° and externally rotated to 90°. The examiner then applies a gentle anteriorly directed force to the posterior aspect of the humeral head.

6.9.2 Anterior Apprehension Sign

The apprehension sign was initially described by Rowe and Zarins [123] in 1981 as a method to reproduce symptoms related to clinical instability. With the patient sitting or standing, the humerus is externally rotated and abducted to approximately 90° within the coronal plane. The examiner then applies a gentle anteriorly directed force to the posterior aspect of the humeral head (Fig. 6.36). A positive test occurs when the patient initiates a sudden guarding reflex to prevent dislocation, sometimes in the presence of pain. The anterior apprehension sign can also be elicited with the patient lying supine on the examination table [95, 122–124]. In this variation of the test, the patient is asked to slide to the edge of the table such that the extremity to be tested must be held against gravity using voluntary muscle contraction. The scapula must remain supported by the examination table to prevent erroneously increased external rotation estimations as a result of compensatory scapular motion. With the elbows flexed to 90°, the humerus is then externally rotated using the edge of the table as a fulcrum to generate an anteriorly directed force over the posterior aspect of the humeral head. The test is positive when the patient experiences apprehension with or without the production of pain

during the maneuver. Other variations of the anterior apprehension sign have been proposed, such as performing the test at both lower and higher levels of glenohumeral abduction [96, 125]; however, currently, there is no solid evidence to support their potential diagnostic utility.

Although the apprehension signs are relatively simple to understand from a conceptual standpoint, there are several caveats that should be noted. First, given the nature of the test, a patient who had been examined on multiple prior occasions may either become accustomed to the discomfort or they may adopt compensatory mechanisms to reduce the symptoms related to subluxation or dislocation [126]. Both of these factors may produce inaccurate results in patients who require frequent clinic visits for instability. As a potential solution, McFarland [103] suggested that the test may also be performed during range of motion testing to surprise the patient, especially during the evaluation of passive external rotation capacity. With the patient sitting or standing, each arm is abducted to approximately 90°, the elbows are flexed to 90° and each arm is slowly and passively externally rotated (similar to that which is performed during range of motion testing). The patient is then asked to indicate the point at which pain or apprehension is felt. This technique eliminates the need to perform a separate maneuver and may decrease the patient's ability to mentally prepare for the apprehension test. Second, patients who experience pain during the apprehension test may have a tendency to become apprehensive at smaller degrees of external rotation during future examinations. Third, most patients with instability will display apprehension at different levels of humeral abduction, external rotation, and/or extension. Lo et al. [124] performed a study to determine the mean degrees of external rotation required to produce apprehension in patients with anterior instability, posterior instability, or MDI. In that study, mean external rotation of 83°, 100°, and 131° was required to generate apprehension in patients with anterior instability, posterior instability, and MDI, respectively. These data suggest that external rotation beyond the common 90° landmark may be necessary to elicit anterior apprehension in some patients, especially in those who display evidence of increased glenohumeral laxity during other clinical examination maneuvers. Finally, although it has been suggested on numerous occasions, a positive apprehension test following a first-time traumatic dislocation does not necessarily correspond to an increased risk of future dislocations [1].

Several studies have evaluated the diagnostic efficacy of the anterior apprehension sign as it relates to clinical instability. In most studies, both the sensitivity and specificity of the anterior apprehension test in the diagnosis of anterior instability has ranged from 70 to 90 % with excellent intra-class correlation [110, 122, 124, 127]. However, in one study, Speer et al. [128] performed the test in a series of patients with various shoulder pathologies to specifically determine whether pain was needed to define a "positive" apprehension test. In those with anterior instability, 63 % of patients demonstrated apprehension during the test whereas 46 % experienced pain during the test. In addition, many other patients with stable shoulders also experienced pain during the maneuver. This study provides evidence that pain during the anterior apprehension test may not be a necessary criterion for the diagnosis of anterior instability. Both Lo et al. [124] and Tzannes et al. [110] came to similar conclusions when they noted precipitous decreases in their calculated specificity and ICCs, respectively, when pain alone (as opposed to apprehension alone) was used to make the diagnosis of anterior instability.

6.9.3   Relocation Sign

Although there is no clear consensus regarding who actually provided the first description of the relocation sign, Jobe et al. [129] is most often credited with its development and subsequent implementation into clinical practice. The authors suggested that stretching of the IGHL complex increased the propensity for mechanical impingement of the rotator cuff tendons on the undersurface of the acromion as a result of hyperexternal rotation. Thus, increased glenohumeral translation and/or subluxation was thought to produce a "secondary impingement" of the rotator cuff. To perform this test, the patient should be in the supine position with the affected arm over the edge of the examination table. The humerus is abducted 90° and externally rotated to approximately 90° (i.e., the 90/90 position). From this starting position, the humerus is then slowly abducted and externally rotated until the patient reports pain. Jobe et al. [129] indicated that patients most commonly reported pain over the anterior aspect of the deltoid. The examiner then applies a posteriorly directed pressure over the humeral head to reduce (or "relocate") the subluxated joint (Fig. 6.37). A positive test occurs when this posteriorly

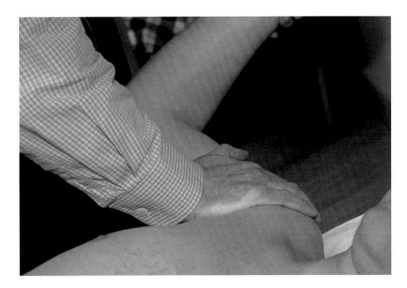

Fig. 6.37 Relocation sign. This test can also be performed with the patient sitting or standing. The anterior apprehension test is performed as described in Fig. 6.36. The examiner then applies a posteriorly directed force to the anterior aspect of the humeral head to "relocate" the joint and relieve the patient's pain and/or apprehension.

directed pressure results in symptomatic relief, potentially indicating the relief of secondary impingement beneath the acromion.

However, even Jobe et al. [129] questioned the clinical efficacy of this test to diagnose instability in overhead athletes since the starting position can produce pain in athletes with rotator cuff disease, instability or both. As a result, the authors described a basic algorithm which was thought to be useful in differentiating between athletes with and without rotator cuff disease. In this description, the test was performed using the same technique; however, when the posteriorly directed pressure failed to relieve the patient's symptoms, the pain was assumed to be the result of rotator cuff disease rather than occult instability. More recent studies have suggested that the relief of posterior pain with this maneuver may be an important clinical sign in the diagnosis of symptomatic internal impingement and posterior SLAP tears in overhead athletes [7, 70, 130–132].

The test can also be used as a method to detect clinical instability in both athletes and non-athletes alike when the posteriorly directed pressure relieves the patient's feeling of apprehension in the abducted and externally rotated position. In fact, this is the most widely utilized version of the relocation sign and has been heavily scrutinized in the literature. As a part of the study mentioned above for the apprehension sign, Speer et al. [128] calculated a sensitivity and specificity of 68 % and 100 %, respectively, when the relief of apprehension was considered a positive relocation sign. In this study, the resolution of pain with the relocation test was not a reliable method to diagnose clinical instability (sensitivity: 30 %; specificity: 58 %). Tzannes et al. [110] calculated the reliability of the relocation test in a series of 25 patients with overt instability (patients with occult instability or internal impingement were excluded). In that study, they found high inter-observer agreement when the relief of apprehension was considered a positive test (ICC: 0.71) and low inter-observer agreement when the relief of pain was considered a positive test (ICC: 0.31).

6.9.4 Release Test

The release test was originally described by Silliman and Hawkins [95] in 1993 as an extension of the relocation test. With the patient supine, the humerus is placed in 90° of abduction and 90° of external rotation. The arm is slowly externally rotated until the patient becomes apprehensive. A posteriorly directed forced is applied to the humeral head to relieve the patient's symptoms. At this point, the humerus is further externally rotated and the examiner removes their hand from the anterior shoulder (Fig. 6.38).

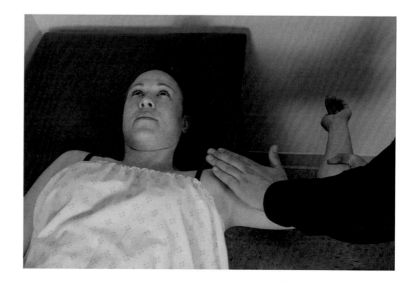

Fig. 6.38 Release test. With the patient supine, the arm is placed in the 90/90 position. The examiner applies a gentle posteriorly directed force on the anterior aspect of the humeral head. The examiner then suddenly removes, or "releases" their hand from the anterior shoulder. A sudden increase in pain or apprehension signifies a positive test.

After releasing the shoulder, the patient should experience a sudden increase in pain and apprehension. It should be noted that the primary purpose of this test is to detect subtle anterior instability and should not be used in patients with more severe patterns of instability due to the production of unnecessary discomfort and the high risk of shoulder dislocation.

Gross and Distefano [133] evaluated the diagnostic efficacy of a slightly modified version of the release test in a series of 100 patients with various pathologies who were scheduled to undergo arthroscopic shoulder surgery. According to their description, the patient was positioned supine and the humerus was abducted to 90°. A posteriorly directed forced was applied to the anterior aspect of the humeral head to maintain the humerus within the glenoid fossa while the humerus was simultaneously externally rotated. The examiner then suddenly removed their hand from the anterior shoulder. A positive test occurred when removal of the examiner's hand resulted in a sudden increase in pain intensity or the reproduction of symptoms. According to their surgical findings, the patients were divided into either an instability group or a non-instability group. After the exclusion of 18 patients with instability related to another condition, 37 patients were placed in the instability group and 45 patients were placed in the non-instability group. Following review of preoperative clinical examination findings, the investigators calculated a sensitivity of 92 % and a specificity of 89 % for the release test in its ability to accurately diagnose shoulder instability. However, these results should be interpreted with caution due to the retrospective study design, the use of pain as an indicator for a positive test and the incomplete description of the surgeons' arthroscopic findings. Nevertheless, the sensitivity and specificity values calculated by Van Kampen et al. [22] for the release test were actually quite similar: the sensitivity was calculated to be 91.7 % and the specificity was calculated to be 83.5 %. Of note, the study by van Kampen et al. [122] utilized MRA as the diagnostic gold standard and did not consider pain as an indicator of a positive release test.

6.9.5 Surprise Test

Currently, many surgeons use the terms "surprise test" and "release test" interchangeably; however, there are subtle differences that should be noted. The surprise test was actually described by Lo et al. [124] in 2004 as a slight modification to the original release test developed by Silliman and Hawkins [95] a decade earlier. In their version of the test, the investigators first performed the relocation test as described above. After stabilizing the proximal humerus by applying a posteriorly directed force, the examiner simply removed their hand from the patient's anterior shoulder without increasing the degree of external rotation. The reproduction of pain or apprehension defined a positive test. In their study, the investigators evaluated and compared the diagnostic efficacy of the apprehension sign, relocation sign and the surprise test (as described above) in a series of 46 shoulders with various diagnoses. They found that the surprise test had the highest positive predictive value (PPV) (98 %) and the highest specificity (99 %) than any of the other tests; however, the sensitivity was found to be 64 %. The authors suggested that a positive test on all three clinical exams for instability was highly predictive of traumatic anterior instability. In addition, they recommended performing the apprehension sign and the relocation test before attempting the surprise test since this maneuver can actually startle the patient and produce abnormal measurements when performing subsequent examinations.

6.10 Testing for Posterior Instability

Posterior instability most often results from an acute traumatic injury, such as a fall onto an outstretched hand or, in some cases, following a seizure or an electric shock, that forces the humeral head to subluxate or dislocate posteriorly as result of uncoordinated muscle contraction. Chronic posterior instability can then result through a series of pathoanatomic changes similar to that which occurs for anterior instability (discussed above).

Patients who present with either an acute or chronic posterior dislocation typically hold the arm internally rotated and slightly abducted since this position produces the least amount of pain. Examination under anesthesia usually reveals adequate external rotation capacity due to the elimination of pain. Inspection of the shoulder with a chronic posterior dislocation often reveals a prominence posteriorly (i.e., the humeral head), especially in thin patients with minimal overlying soft tissues. On the other hand, this prominence may not be detectable after an acute posterior dislocation due to significant swelling and/or spontaneous relocation.

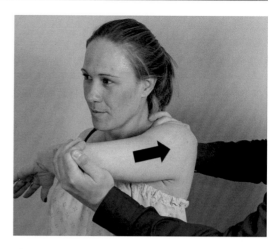

Fig. 6.39 Posterior apprehension sign. The patient's arm is placed at approximately 90° of forward flexion with slight internal rotation and adduction. An axial load is applied through the long axis of the humerus, thus forcing the humeral head to translate posteriorly.

6.10.1 Posterior Apprehension Sign

First mention of the posterior apprehension sign presumably occurred in a textbook published in 1982 by Kessel [134]. According to his original description, the posterior apprehension sign was performed by applying an axial load through the humerus via the elbow with the humerus in 90° of forward flexion, slight internal rotation, and slight adduction (Fig. 6.39). A positive test occurred when the patient initiated a guarding reflex or complained of apprehension.

Since its first description, the posterior apprehension sign has been modified on several occasions. For example, Rowe [135] performed the test by applying a posteriorly directed force through the long axis of the humerus with the arm in 90° of forward flexion and slight internal rotation (no adduction). A positive test was declared when the patient experienced apprehension or posterior shoulder pain. O'Driscoll and Evans [83] incorporated subacromial injection of local anesthetic to help differentiate between pain resulting from rotator cuff impingement and pain resulting from posterior instability. In their version of the test, the arm was flexed to 90°, internally rotated and adducted (similar to the original description by Kessel [134]). When this position produced pain in the shoulder, the examiner then injected local anesthetic into the subacromial

bursa. If the injection resulted in significant pain relief, the pain was presumably caused by rotator cuff pathology. If the injection did not result in pain relief, it was assumed that the pain was related to posterior instability.

Although the posterior apprehension sign (and its variations) is a commonly used test, its diagnostic efficacy and validity have been questioned. Hawkins et al. [93] reported the results of an electromyographic and photographic analysis to determine the position at which the humerus was most likely to subluxate or dislocate posteriorly in a series of patients with voluntary posterior instability. They found that while each patient demonstrated different patterns of instability, the position of the humerus most conducive to subluxation was actually near the glenohumeral resting position (or the "loose pack position"; see Fig. 6.29) which occurs when the humerus is between 55° and 70° of abduction, in neutral rotation and within the plane of the scapula (discussed in Chap. 2) [102, 114, 115]. Until future studies address the clinical utility of the posterior apprehension sign for the diagnosis of posterior instability, we cannot recommend its use in isolation given the potential for widely varying results and the high rates of false positive and false negative findings.

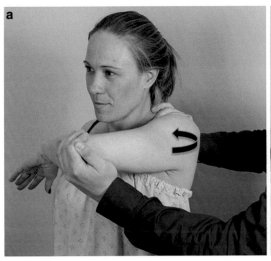
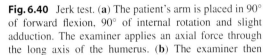
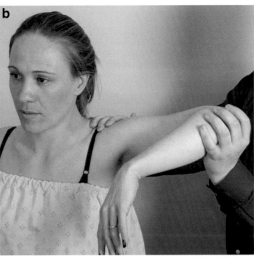

Fig. 6.40 Jerk test. (**a**) The patient's arm is placed in 90° of forward flexion, 90° of internal rotation and slight adduction. The examiner applies an axial force through the long axis of the humerus. (**b**) The examiner then rotates the shoulder towards a position of 90° of lateral abduction. A positive test occurs when a "clunk" or "jerk" is felt during this motion as the subluxated humeral head relocates back into the glenoid fossa.

6.10.2 Jerk Test

The jerk test (also known as the clunk test) was originally described by Matsen et al. [136] in 1990 as a method used to detect posterior glenohumeral instability. In this test, the examiner placed the arm in approximately 90° of forward flexion and 90° of internal rotation with the humerus slightly adducted. The examiner then applied a gentle axial force along the long axis of the humerus through the elbow to allow the humeral head to subluxate over the posterior glenoid rim. The examiner felt a so-called "jerk" as the humeral head subluxated posteriorly. At this point, the examiner then moved the shoulder towards a position of 90° of abduction (i.e., the humerus was extended from the initial position of adduction) (Fig. 6.40). During this motion, the humeral head spontaneously reduced back into the glenoid fossa, producing a second "jerk" sensation (a positive test). Although we have found this maneuver helpful in the physical diagnosis of posterior instability, few studies have formally validated its clinical efficacy despite satisfactory anecdotal reports [137]. In one study, Kim et al. [137] calculated a sensitivity of 73 %, a specificity of 98 %, a PPV of 88 %, and a negative pre-

dictive value (NPV) of 95 % for the jerk test in a series of 172 painful shoulders; however, these values are related to the diagnosis of a posteroinferior labral tear rather than clinical instability. In addition, the investigators used the incidence of posterior shoulder pain as an indicator of a positive test, regardless of whether a "jerk" occurred during extension of the humerus. Nevertheless, the authors noted that posterior instability was more common in shoulders that demonstrated a "jerk" on clinical examination whereas isolated posteroinferior labral tears (without posterior instability) were less likely to demonstrate a "jerk" on clinical examination.

6.10.3 Kim Test

The Kim test (developed by Kim et al. [138] in 2005) was initially used as a method to detect posteroinferior labral pathology. In this test, the patient was placed in a sitting position with the humerus abducted to approximately 90°. The examiner then used one hand to grasp the elbow and used the other hand to grasp the proximal arm. A strong axial load was applied through the long axis of the humerus while the arm was

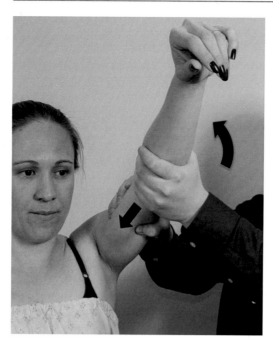

Fig. 6.41 Kim test. The humerus is first laterally abducted to 90°. The examiner then applies and axial load through the long axis of the humerus while simultaneously adducting the arm to a position of 90° of forward flexion. During the adduction maneuver, the examiner can also elevate (up to 45° of upward angulation) and lower the humerus (down to the horizontal plane) to stimulate the posteroinferior and posterior aspects of the glenoid labrum, respectively.

simultaneously adducted and forward flexed (up to 45° of upward angulation) (Fig. 6.41). The sudden onset of posterior shoulder pain, regardless of whether a "jerk" or a "clunk" occurred, defined a positive test. The developers also suggested that the test could be performed in a chair with a solid backing (or supine on the examination table, as we suggest) to help stabilize the scapula during axial loading.

The investigators performed a study in which the diagnostic efficacy of the Kim test was compared to that of the jerk test in the diagnosis of posteroinferior labral lesions in 172 painful shoulders (as mentioned above). Two clinicians performed the examinations in order to calculate inter-observer reliability. In that study, 33 shoulders had a positive Kim test, of which 24 actually had a posteroinferior labral lesion (nine false positives). Of the remaining 139 shoulders that had a

negative Kim test, 6 shoulders actually did have a posteroinferior labral lesion (six false negatives). Based on this data, the sensitivity of the Kim test was 80 %, the specificity was 94 %, the PPV was 73 %, and the NPV was 96 % with an excellent inter-observer ICC of 0.96. The results of their study indicated that the Kim test was more sensitive in the detection of predominantly inferior labral lesions whereas the jerk test was more sensitive in the detection of predominantly posterior labral lesions. The combination of tests improved the overall sensitivity to approximately 97 % for the detection of posteroinferior labral lesions.

6.10.4 Fukada Test

The first description of the Fukada test occurred in a textbook published by Neer [139] in 1990. This test is performed with the patient sitting on the examination table with the examiner standing directly behind the patient. The examiner places the thumb of each hand in-line with the scapular spine with the fingers wrapped around each humeral head. With the thumb of each hand stabilizing the scapula, the fingers of each hand are used to apply a posteriorly directed force to the anterior aspect of the humeral head (Fig. 6.42). The detected amount of translation is then compared between the affected and unaffected shoulders. Although use of this test has been documented in the literature, its clinical efficacy in the diagnosis of posterior instability has not been clearly established [45]. We believe this test is most useful in the estimation of posterior humeral head translation rather than a diagnostic tool for posterior instability.

6.10.5 Push–Pull Test

The push–pull test, described by Matsen et al. [136] in 1990, is a type of load-and-shift test designed to detect posterior shoulder instability. With the patient supine on the examination table, the clinician places the humerus in approximately 90° of abduction and 30° of forward flexion. With one hand stabilizing the distal arm at the wrist, the

Fig. 6.42 Fukada test. While standing behind the patient, the examiner places their thumbs in-line with each scapular spine bilaterally with the fingers reaching anteriorly over the humeral head. The examiner uses their fingers to apply a posteriorly directed load to the humeral head while using the scapular spine as a fulcrum. Both shoulders are tested simultaneously for comparison.

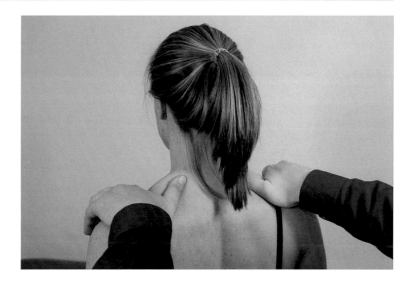

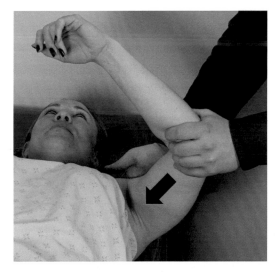

Fig. 6.43 Push–pull test. The patient is positioned supine with the humerus in 90° of abduction slightly anterior to the scapular plane. The examiner stabilizes the distal arm at the wrist or elbow with one hand while the other hand is used to apply a posteriorly directed force through the long axis of the humerus via the elbow.

other hand is used to apply a posteriorly directed force through the long axis of the humerus (Fig. 6.43). Reproduction of pain or apprehension represents a positive test. At least two cadaveric studies have been performed to evaluate the push–pull test with regard to its ability to produce posterior glenohumeral translation [89, 109]. We are unaware of any clinical studies that have assessed

the diagnostic validity of the push–pull test with regard to posterior instability or the presence of a pathologic lesion.

6.11 Testing for Inferior Instability

Fortunately, inferior dislocations of the humerus (also known as luxatio erecta humeri) are infrequently encountered in clinical practice [140–142]. In most cases, these injuries are the result of high-energy trauma such as that which occurs in a motor vehicle accident or a fall from significant height. As a result, inferior shoulder dislocations are frequently associated with concomitant injuries such as fractures (especially greater tuberosity fractures), neurovascular injuries [143–146] and, most likely, complete rupture of the IGHL complex. Patients with inferior dislocations typically present with the arm locked in an abducted, overhead position. Closed reduction maneuvers usually involve conversion of the injury to an anteroinferior dislocation followed by reduction [123, 147, 148].

Symptomatic inferior subluxation of the humeral head is also rarely seen in clinical practice despite the reportedly high prevalence of "inferior instability" diagnosed using the sulcus sign (see Fig. 6.33). Although Neer [149] clearly indicated that the reproduction of symptoms related to infe-

Fig. 6.44 Inferior apprehension. The patient's arm is laterally abducted to 90° with the forearm resting on the examiner's shoulder. The examiner then applies a gentle, downward pressure on the proximal humerus to produce inferior humeral head translation. Because of the difficulty in estimating the amount of translation, this test should be performed bilaterally for comparison.

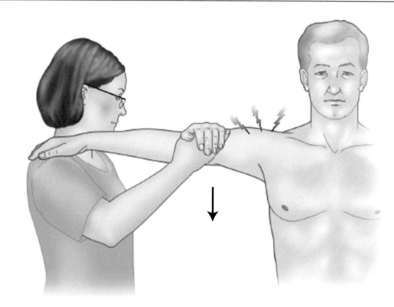

rior instability was required to produce a "positive" sulcus sign, most clinicians still adhere to the "2 cm rule" as a determinant of the test outcome and, as a result, often incorrectly diagnose patients with inferior instability (or multidirectional instability) despite the lack of symptoms.

6.11.1 Inferior Apprehension Sign

Often attributed to Dr. John Feagin, the inferior apprehension sign was first mentioned in a textbook published by Rockwood [64] in 1984 as a method to assess inferior joint laxity or to detect inferior glenohumeral instability, especially in very large patients. According to the original description, the patient's arm was abducted to 90° with the forearm resting on the examiner's shoulder. The examiner then applied a gentle, downward pressure on the proximal humerus (Fig. 6.44). The test was considered positive if the patient became apprehensive or reported the reproduction of symptoms. This maneuver could also be used to assess joint laxity by estimating the degree of inferior humeral head translation relative to the contralateral shoulder.

Itoi et al. [15, 16] referred to this test as the Abduction Inferior Stability (ABIS) test and used it to study the effects of scapular inclination on inferior glenohumeral stability in two cadaveric studies. When compared to the sulcus sign, increased superior scapular inclination (i.e., increased abduction angle), as which occurred during the ABIS test, significantly increased the translational force necessary to inferiorly dislocate the humerus in each study. These results were later confirmed by Kikuchi et al. [17] who also concluded that there was an increased resistance to inferior humeral head dislocation when the scapula was angled superiorly. Another recent clinical study reached similar conclusions [150].

Although there is no evidence to suggest that the inferior apprehension sign (or the ABIS test) has any clinical utility in the diagnosis of inferior instability, the maneuver could feasibly be used as a method to assess laxity of the IGHL complex. However, it should be noted that the inferior apprehension sign offers no advantage over the more traditional sulcus sign in the evaluation of glenohumeral laxity and/or inferior stability and may also produce extreme discomfort in those being evaluated following a traumatic dislocation. We have limited experience with this test in clinical practice and it remains primarily of academic interest.

6.12 Voluntary Instability

Some patients are capable of demonstrating their ability to subluxate and/or dislocate the glenohumeral joint at any time they wish. In the literature, many different terms have been used to describe this type of instability including voluntary, volitional, unintentional, non-structural, habitual, muscular, demonstrable, persistent, and positional. Most individuals with this type of instability have some form of multiligamentous laxity that (1) allows the arm to be placed in an awkward, unstable position through learned asymmetric muscle contraction patterns and (2) allows the humerus to subluxate or dislocate as a result of inherited capsular laxity (Figs. 6.45 and 6.46). Patients with voluntary instability very

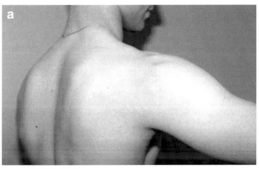
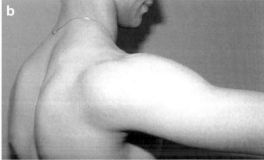

Fig. 6.45 Clinical photographs of a patient with voluntary posterior instability utilizing the "push" mechanism to dislocate the humerus (voluntary positional instability). In this case, the patient has learned the exact position of the humerus that subsequently allows the humeral head to dislocate posteriorly. (**a**) The patient elevates the humerus to the provocative position and (**b**) relaxes the posterior musculature to allow the humerus to dislocate posteriorly without experiencing pain or apprehension. (Courtesy of J.P. Warner, MD).

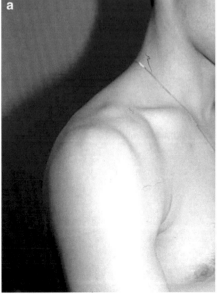
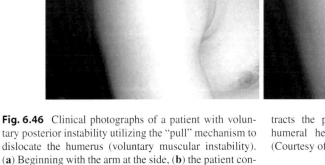

Fig. 6.46 Clinical photographs of a patient with voluntary posterior instability utilizing the "pull" mechanism to dislocate the humerus (voluntary muscular instability). (**a**) Beginning with the arm at the side, (**b**) the patient contracts the posterior musculature in order to pull the humeral head posteriorly out of the glenoid fossa. (Courtesy of J.P. Warner, MD).

rarely present with anatomic defects such as Bankart or reverse Bankart lesions. Because only a small proportion of these individuals actually seek medical attention for symptoms related to shoulder instability, the prevalence of the condition is still unknown.

Unfortunately, some patients with voluntary shoulder instability may seek medical attention for reasons involving the potential for secondary gain or other psychological issues. This is especially true in Workers' compensation cases in which the patient may claim that their shoulder instability was somehow related to an occupational hazard. The clinician should be especially weary of patients seeking narcotic medications for their condition and patients reporting early failure of surgical treatment in the absence of a traumatic injury [135]. However, it is extremely important to recognize that some patients with voluntary instability seek medical treatment because they actually *are* functionally disabled as a result of their condition. In this scenario, patients may be capable of demonstrating the instability, however, they often complain that the shoulder also occasionally subluxates or dislocates outside of the patient's control at inopportune times.

An accurate assessment of patients who present with voluntary instability is often difficult as a result of overlapping pathologies, the potential for secondary gain and, in some cases, abnormal psychology. However, despite these challenges, the clinician must still perform a thorough, objective evaluation to determine the correct course of treatment.

The clinical evaluation should adhere to the same principles that have been outlined throughout this book. A patient-centered approach to history-taking should always be performed regardless of the clinician's initial perception of the patient's reasons for seeking medical treatment. In patients with a history of voluntary instability, the clinician should especially ask about the primary direction of instability, the presence or absence of pain related to the instability and the family history to identify a possible predisposition to structural collagen disorders. Other patient-related historical factors such as

poor wound-healing, easy bruising, and visual defects should be ascertained to identify potential risk factors for multiligamentous laxity.

The physical examination should also adhere to the same principles that have been outlined throughout this book. Inspection, palpation, range of motion testing, strength testing, and neurovascular testing should all be performed to generate a solid differential diagnosis before attempting any provocative maneuvers. Testing for generalized hyperlaxity is another important component of the physical examination in this subset of patients (Fig. 6.47) [151]. Assessment of shoulder laxity (as described above) often reveals an extremely abnormal amount of humeral head translation, most commonly in the absence of anterior or posterior apprehension. In fact, some patients can be completely dislocated without showing any evidence of pain or discomfort. Patients who display some degree of apprehension with laxity testing and/or instability testing are more likely to have an involuntary component related to their instability. It is also possible for a patient to sustain a traumatic injury that converts their instability from a voluntary type to an involuntary type. Although it is more difficult to determine the precise nature of the instability in these cases, many of these patients will experience pain when the clinician forces the humeral head to translate over the injured area (e.g., Bankart and bony Bankart lesions).

6.12.1 Posterior Subluxation

Posterior subluxation or dislocation is the most common form of voluntary shoulder instability encountered in clinical practice and result from learned asymmetric muscle firing patterns that lead to posterior humeral head translation and subluxation [101, 152]. Pande et al. [152] utilized electromyography (EMG) to evaluate the timing and sequence of shoulder muscle activation during both joint subluxation and relocation in four patients with voluntary posterior instability. In that study, the investigators identified two distinct patterns of muscle firing that led to posterior humeral head subluxation: a "push" mechanism

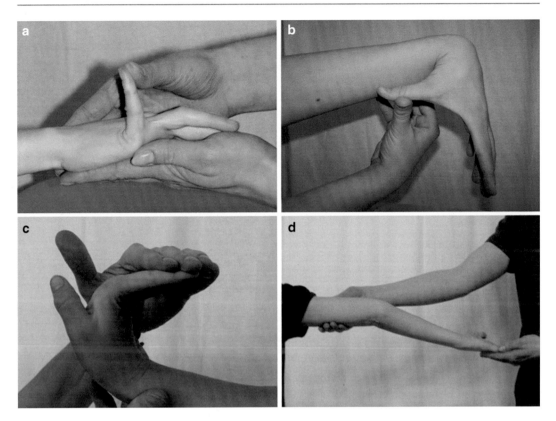

Fig. 6.47 Methods to assess generalized ligamentous laxity [151]. (**a**) Hyperextension of the metacarpophalangeal (MCP) joint. (**b**) Thumb abducted to make contact with the forearm. (**c**) Passive hyperextension of digits 2–5 until parallel with the top of the forearm. (**d**) Hyperextension of the elbow.

(with the arm flexed 20–30°) and a "pull" mechanism (with the arm at the side). In the "push" firing pattern (also known as voluntary positional instability), near-maximal activation of the anterior musculature (i.e. the anterior deltoid and biceps brachii muscles) with simultaneous relaxation of the posterior musculature (i.e., the infraspinatus and posterior deltoid muscles) was required to *push* the humeral head posteriorly (see Fig. 6.45). Conversely, in the "pull" firing pattern (also known as voluntary muscular instability), near-maximal activation of the posterior musculature with simultaneous relaxation of the anterior musculature was required to *pull* the humeral head posteriorly (see Fig. 6.46). Each patient in the study demonstrated scapular winging and characteristic EMG patterns indicating that selective inhibition of the periscapular musculature was necessary to posteriorly translate and subluxate the humeral head. In either case, joint relocation was achieved by extending the arm posteriorly (via contraction of the posterior deltoid) to lever the humeral head back into the glenoid fossa.

6.12.2 Anterior Subluxation

To produce a voluntary anterior subluxation, the patient will typically keep the arm in an adducted position (i.e., at the side). Simultaneous contraction of the anterior musculature and extensors *pulls* the humeral head anteriorly and out of the glenoid fossa [101]. In most cases, the humeral head appears to rest in an anteroinferior position relative to the glenoid as a result of the unopposed tension generated by the musculature in the anterior arm.

6.12.3 Inferior Subluxation

Voluntary inferior subluxation of the shoulder is extremely uncommon. These patients will inferiorly translate the humeral head by abducting the arm overhead and initiating an asymmetric muscle firing pattern that drives the humeral head directly downward and out of the glenoid fossa. We are not aware of any studies that have clinically or biomechanically evaluated this small subgroup of patients with voluntary inferior instability.

6.13 Summary

There are numerous static and dynamic stabilizers of the glenohumeral joint and their interactions are particularly complex. This complexity can produce confusing findings during the physical examination process. However, a working knowledge of the characteristic pathoanatomic features and patterns of glenohumeral instability will help the clinician synthesize an accurate diagnosis and an effective treatment plan.

References

1. Safran O, Milgrom C, Radeva-Petrova DR, Jaber S, Finestone A. Accuracy of the anterior apprehension test as a predictor of risk for redislocation after a first traumatic shoulder dislocation. Am J Sports Med. 2010;38(5):972–5.
2. Walch G, Edwards TB, Boulahia A, Nove-Josserand L, Neyton L, Szabo I. Arthroscopic tenotomy of the long head of the biceps in the treatment of rotator cuff tears: clinical and radiographic results of 307 cases. J Shoulder Elbow Surg. 2005;14(3):238–46.
3. Boileau P, O'Shea K, Vargas P, Pinedo M, Old J, Zumstein M. Anatomical and functional results after arthroscopic Hill–Sachs remplissage. J Bone Joint Surg Am. 2012;94(7):618–26.
4. Giphart JE, Elser F, Dewing CB, Torry MR, Millett PJ. The long head of the biceps tendon has minimal effect on in vivo glenohumeral kinematics: a biplane fluoroscopy study. Am J Sports Med. 2012;40(1):202–12.
5. Anetzberger H, Putz R. The scapula: principles of construction and stress. Acta Anat (Basel). 1996;156(1):70–80.
6. Huysmans PE, Haen PS, Kidd M, Dhert WJ, Willems JW. The shape of the inferior part of the glenoid: a cadaveric study. J Shoulder Elbow Surg. 2006;15(6):759–63.
7. Burkhart SS, De Beer JF. Traumatic glenohumeral bone defects and their relationship to failure of arthroscopic Bankart repairs: significance of the inverted-pear glenoid and the humeral engaging Hill–Sachs lesion. Arthroscopy. 2000;16(7):677–94.
8. Lo IK, Parten PM, Burkhart SS. The inverted pear glenoid: an indicator of significant glenoid bone loss. Arthroscopy. 2004;20(2):169–74.
9. Saha AK. Dynamic stability of the glenohumeral joint. Acta Orthop Scand. 1971;42(6):491–505.
10. Sauers EL, Borsa PA, Herling DE, Stanley RD. Instrumented measurement of glenohumeral joint laxity and its relationship to passive range of motion and generalized joint laxity. Am J Sports Med. 2001;29(2):143–50.
11. Lee T. Clinical anatomy and biomechanics of the glenohumeral joint (including stabilizers). In: Romeo A, Provencher MT, editors. Shoulder instability: a comprehensive approach. Philadelphia: Saunders; 2012. p. 3–19.
12. Churchill RS, Brems JJ, Kotschi H. Glenoid size, inclination, and version: an anatomic study. J Shoulder Elbow Surg. 2001;10(4):327–32.
13. Brewer BJ, Wubben RC, Carrera GF. Excessive retroversion of the glenoid cavity. A cause of nontraumatic posterior instability of the shoulder. J Bone Joint Surg Am. 1986;68(5):724–31.
14. Hurley JA, Anderson TE, Dear W, Andrish JT, Bergfeld JA, Weiker GG. Posterior shoulder instability. Surgical versus conservative results with evaluation of glenoid version. Am J Sports Med. 1992;20(4):396–400.
15. Itoi E, Motzkin NE, Morrey BF, An KN. Bulk effect of rotator cuff on inferior glenohumeral stability as a function of scapular inclination angle: a cadaver study. Tohoku J Exp Med. 1993;171(4):267–76.
16. Itoi E, Motzkin NE, Morrey BF, An KN. Scapular inclination and inferior stability of the shoulder. J Shoulder Elbow Surg. 1992;1(3):131–9.
17. Kikuchi K, Itoi E, Yamamoto N, Seki N, Abe H, Minagawa H, Shimada Y. Scapular inclination and glenohumeral joint stability: a cadaveric study. J Orthop Sci. 2008;13(1):72–7.
18. Tétreault P, Krueger A, Zurakowski D, Gerber C. Glenoid version and rotator cuff tears. J Orthop Res. 2004;22(1):202–7.
19. Halder AM, Kuhl SG, Zobitz ME, Larson D, An KN. Effects of the glenoid labrum and glenohumeral abduction on stability of the shoulder joint through concavity-compression: an in vitro study. J Bone Joint Surg Am. 2001;83-A(7):1062–9.
20. Howell SM, Galinat BJ. The glenoid-labral socket. A constrained articular surface. Clin Orthop Relat Res. 1989;243:122–5.
21. Park JY, Lee SJ, Lhee SH, Oh JH. Change in labrum height after arthroscopic Bankart repair: correlation with preoperative tissue quality and clinical outcomes. J Shoulder Elbow Surg. 2012;21(12):1712–20.
22. Vangsness Jr CT, Jorgenson SS, Watson T, Johnson DL. The origin of the long head of the biceps from the scapula and glenoid labrum. An anatomical

study of 100 shoulders. J Bone Joint Surg Br. 1994;76(6):951–4.

23. Felli L, Biglieni L, Fiore M, Coviello M, Borri R, Cutolo M. Functional study of glenohumeral ligaments. J Orthop Sci. 2012;17(5):634–7.

24. Debski RE, Moore SM, Mercer JL, Sacks MS, McMahon PJ. The collagen fibers of the anteroinferior capsulolabrum have multiaxial orientation to resist shoulder dislocation. J Shoulder Elbow Surg. 2003;12(3):247–52.

25. O'Brien SJ, Neves MC, Arnoczky SP, Rozbruck SR, Dicarlo EF, Warren RF, Schwartz R, Wickiewicz TL. The anatomy and histology of the inferior glenohumeral ligament complex of the shoulder. Am J Sports Med. 1990;18(5):449–56.

26. Arai R, Mochizuki T, Yamaguchi K, Sugaya H, Kobayashi M, Nakamura T, Akita K. Functional anatomy of the superior glenohumeral and coracohumeral ligaments and the subscapularis tendon in view of stabilization of the long head of the biceps tendon. J Shoulder Elbow Surg. 2010;19(1):58–64.

27. Arai R, Nimura A, Yamaguchi K, Yoshimura H, Sugaya H, Saji T, Matsuda S, Akita K. The anatomy of the coracohumeral ligament and its relation to the subscapularis muscle. J Shoulder Elbow Surg. 2014;23(10):1575–81.

28. Izumi T, Aoki M, Tanaka Y, Uchiyama E, Suzuki D, Miyamoto S, Fujimiya M. Stretching positions for the coracohumeral ligament: strain measurement during passive motion using fresh/frozen cadaver shoulders. Sports Med Arthrosc Rehabil Ther Technol. 2011;3(1):2.

29. Yamamoto N, Itoi E, Abe H, Minagawa H, Seki N, Shimada Y, Okada K. Contact between the glenoid and the humeral head in abduction, external rotation, and horizontal extension: a new concept of glenoid track. J Shoulder Elbow Surg. 2007;16(5):649–56.

30. Burkart AC, Debski RE. Anatomy and function of the glenohumeral ligaments in anterior shoulder instability. Clin Orthop Relat Res. 2002;400:32–9.

31. Warner JJP, Deng XH, Warren RJ, Torzilli PA. Static capsuloligamentous restraints to superior-inferior translation of the glenohumeral joint. Am J Sports Med. 1992;20(6):675–85.

32. Jost B, Koch PP, Gerber C. Anatomy and functional aspects of the rotator interval. J Shoulder Elbow Surg. 2000;9(4):336–41.

33. Bennett WF. Subscapularis, medial, and lateral head coracohumeral ligament insertion anatomy. Arthroscopic appearance and incidence of "hidden" rotator interval lesions. Arthroscopy. 2001;17(2):173–80.

34. Field LD, Warren RF, O'Brien SJ, Altchek DW, Wickiewicz TL. Isolated closure of rotator interval defects for shoulder instability. Am J Sports Med. 1995;23(5):557–63.

35. Giaroli EL, Major NM, Lemley DE, Lee J. Coracohumeral interval imaging in subcoracoid impingement syndrome on MRI. AJR Am J Roentgenol. 2006;186(1):242–6.

36. Harryman 2nd DT, Sidles JA, Harris SL, Matsen 3rd FA. The role of the rotator interval capsule in passive motion and stability of the shoulder. J Bone Joint Surg Am. 1992;74(1):53–66.

37. Itoi E, Berglund LJ, Grabowski JJ, Naggar L, Morrey BF, An KN. Superior-inferior stability of the shoulder: role of the coracohumeral ligament and the rotator interval capsule. Mayo Clin Proc. 1998;73(6):508–15.

38. Neer II CS, Satterlee CC, Dalsey RM, Flatow EL. The anatomy and potential effects of contracture of the coracohumeral ligament. Clin Orthop Relat Res. 1992;280:182–5.

39. Nobuhara K, Ikeda H. Rotator interval lesion. Clin Orthop Relat Res. 1987;223:44–50.

40. Gambill ML, Mologne TS, Provencher MT. Dislocation of the long head of the biceps tendon with intact subscapularis and supraspinatus tendons. J Shoulder Elbow Surg. 2006;15(6):e20–2.

41. Habermeyer P, Schuller U, Wiedemann E. The intra-articular pressure of the shoulder: an experimental study on the role of the glenoid labrum in stabilizing the joint. Arthroscopy. 1992;8(2):166–72.

42. Gibb TD, Sidles JA, Harryman 2nd DT, McQuade KJ, Matsen 3rd FA. The effect of capsular venting on glenohumeral laxity. Clin Orthop Relat Res. 1991;268:120–7.

43. Warner J, Deng X, Warren R, Torzilli P, O'Brien S. Superoinferior translation in the intact and vented glenohumeral joint. J Shoulder Elbow Surg. 1993;2(2):99–105.

44. Jerosch J, Steinbeck J, Schröder M, Westhues M, Reer R. Intraoperative EMG response of the musculature after stimulation of the glenohumeral joint capsule. Acta Orthop Belg. 1997;63(1):8–14.

45. Cooper RA, Brems JJ. The inferior capsular-shift procedure for multidirectional instability of the shoulder. J Bone Joint Surg Am. 1992;74(10):1516–21.

46. Kanatli U, Ozturk BY, Bolukbasi S. Anatomical variations of the anterosuperior labrum: prevalence and association with type II superior labrum anterior-posterior (SLAP) lesions. J Shoulder Elbow Surg. 2010;19(8):1199–203.

47. Smith DK, Chopp TM, Aufdemorte TB, Witkowski EG, Jones RC. Sublabral recess of the superior glenoid labrum: study of cadavers with conventional nonenhanced MR imaging, MR arthrography, anatomic dissection, and limited histologic examination. Radiology. 1996;201(1):251–6.

48. Ilahi OA, Labbe MR, Cosculluela P. Variants of the anterosuperior glenoid labrum and associated pathology. Arthroscopy. 2002;18(8):882–6.

49. Pfahler M, Haraida S, Schulz C, Anetzberger H, Refior HJ, Bauer GS, Bigliani LU. Age-related changes of the glenoid labrum in normal shoulders. J Shoulder Elbow Surg. 2003;12(1):40–52.

50. Williams MM, Snyder SJ, Buford Jr D. The Buford complex–the "cord-like" middle glenohumeral ligament and absent anterosuperior labrum complex: a normal anatomic capsulolabral variant. Arthroscopy. 1994;10(3):241–7.

51. Ide J, Maeda S, Takagi K. Normal variations of the glenohumeral ligament complex: an anatomic study for arthroscopic Bankart repair. Arthroscopy. 2004;20(2):164–8.

52. Tibone JE, Lee TQ, Csintalan RP, Dettling J, McMahon PJ. Quantitative assessment of glenohumeral translation. Clin Orthop Relat Res. 2002;400:93–7.

53. Tischer T, Vogt S, Kreuz PC, Imhoff AB. Arthroscopic anatomy, variants, and pathologic findings in shoulder instability. Arthroscopy. 2011;27(10):1434–43.

54. Gerber C, Nyffeler RW. Classification of glenohumeral joint instability. Clin Orthop Relat Res. 2002;400:65–76.

55. Dowdy PA, O'Driscoll SW. Shoulder instability. An analysis of family history. J Bone Joint Surg Br. 1993;75(5):782–4.

56. Thomas SC, Matsen 3rd FA. An approach to the repair of avulsion of the glenohumeral ligaments in the management of traumatic anterior glenohumeral instability. J Bone Joint Surg Am. 1989;71(4):506–13.

57. Johnson SM, Robinson CM. Shoulder instability in patients with joint hyperlaxity. J Bone Joint Surg Am. 2010;92(6):1545–7.

58. Lewis A, Kitamura T, Bayley JIL. Mini symposium: shoulder instability (ii). The classification of shoulder instability: new light through old windows. Curr Orthop. 2004;18(2):97–108.

59. Kuhn JE, Holmes TT, Throckmorton TW, et al. Development and reliability testing of a system for classifying glenohumeral joint instability. American Academy of Orthopaedic Surgeons 75th Annual Meeting; 6 March 2008, San Francisco.

60. Kuhn JE. A new classification system for shoulder instability. Br J Sports Med. 2010;44(5):341–6.

61. Browe DP, Voycheck CA, McMahon PJ, Debski RE. Changes to the mechanical properties of the glenohumeral capsule during anterior dislocation. J Biomech. 2014;47(2):464–9.

62. Bigliani LU, Pollock RG, Soslowsky LJ, Flatow EL, Pawluk RJ, Mow VC. Tensile properties of the inferior glenohumeral ligament. J Orthop Res. 1992;10(2):187–97.

63. Rowe CR, Zarins B, Ciullo JV. Recurrent anterior dislocation of the shoulder after surgical repair. Apparent causes of failure and treatment. J Bone Joint Surg Am. 1984;66(2):159–68.

64. Rockwood Jr CA. Subluxation and dislocations about the shoulder. In: Rockwood Jr CA, Green DP, editors. Fractures in adults. Philadelphia: JB Lippincott; 1984. p. 722–950.

65. Wischer TK, Bredella MA, Genant HK, Stoller DW, Bost FW, Tirman PF. Perthes lesion (a variant of the Bankart lesion): MR imaging and MR arthrographic findings with surgical correlation. AJR Am J Roentgenol. 2002;178(1):233–7.

66. Baker CL, Uribe JW, Whitman C. Arthroscopic evaluation of acute initial anterior shoulder dislocations. Am J Sports Med. 1990;18(1):25–8.

67. Taylor DC, Arciero RA. Pathologic changes associated with shoulder dislocations. Arthroscopic and physical examination findings in first-time, traumatic anterior dislocations. Am J Sports Med. 1997;25(3):306–11.

68. Speer KP, Deng X, Borrero S, Torzilli PA, Altchek DA, Warren RF. Biomechanical evaluation of a simulated Bankart lesion. J Bone Joint Surg Am. 1994;76(12):1819–26.

69. Neviaser TJ. The anterior labroligamentous periosteal sleeve avulsion lesion: a cause of anterior instability of the shoulder. Arthroscopy. 1993;9(1):17–21.

70. Burkhart SS, Morgan CD. The peel-back mechanism: its role in producing and extending posterior type II SLAP lesions and its effect on SLAP repair rehabilitation. Arthroscopy. 1998;14(6):637–40.

71. Pagnani MJ, Deng XH, Warren RF, Torzilli PA, Altchek DW. Effect of lesions of the superior portion of the glenoid labrum on glenohumeral translation. J Bone Joint Surg Am. 1995;77(7):1003–10.

72. Martetschläger F, Ames JB, Millett PJ. HAGL and reverse HAGL lesions. In: Milano G, Grasso A, editors. Shoulder arthroscopy: principles and practice, Chap. 33. Springer: London. 2014.

73. Ames JB, Millett PJ. Combined posterior osseous Bankart lesion and posterior humeral avulsion of the glenohumeral ligaments: a case report and pathoanatomic subtyping of "floating" posterior inferior glenohumeral ligament lesions. J Bone Joint Surg Am. 2011;93(20):e118(1)–(4).

74. Boileau P, Villalba M, Héry JT, Balg F, Ahrens P, Neyton L. Risk factors for recurrence of shoulder instability after arthroscopic Bankart repair. J Bone Joint Surg Am. 2006;88(8):1755–63.

75. Itoi E, Lee SB, Berglund LJ, Berge LL, An KN. The effect of a glenoid defect on anteroinferior stability of the shoulder after Bankart repair: a cadaveric study. J Bone Joint Surg Am. 2000;82(1):35–46.

76. Yamamoto N, Itoi E, Abe H, Kikuchi K, Seki N, Minagawa H, Tuoheti Y. Effect of an anterior glenoid defect on anterior shoulder stability: a cadaveric study. Am J Sports Med. 2009;37(5):949–54.

77. Kaar SG, Fening SD, Jones MH, Colbrunn RW, Miniaci A. Effect of humeral head defect size on glenohumeral stability: a cadaveric study of simulated Hill–Sachs defects. Am J Sports Med. 2010;38(3):594–9.

78. Murray IR, Ahmed I, White NJ, Robinson CM. Traumatic anterior shoulder instability in the athlete. Scand J Med Sci Sports. 2013;23(4):387–405.

79. Sekiya JK, Jolly J, Debski RE. The effect of a Hill–Sachs defect on glenohumeral translations, in situ capsular forces, and bony contact forces. Am J Sports Med. 2012;40(2):388–94.

80. Friedman RJ, Hawthorne KB, Genez BM. The use of computerized tomography in the measurement of glenoid version. J Bone Joint Surg Am. 1992;74(7):1032–7.

81. Gerber C, Ganz R, Vinh TS. Glenoplasty for recurrent posterior shoulder instability. An anatomic reappraisal. Clin Orthop Relat Res. 1987;216:70–9.

82. Randelli M, Gambrioli PL. Glenohumeral osteometry by computed tomography in normal and unstable shoulders. Clin Orthop Relat Res. 1986;208:151–6.

83. O'Driscoll SW, Evans DC. Contralateral shoulder instability following anterior repair. An epidemiological investigation. J Bone Joint Surg Br. 1991;73(6):941–6.

84. Rodeo SA, Suzuki K, Yamauchi M, Bhargava M, Warren RF. Analysis of collagen and elastic fibers in shoulder capsule in patients with shoulder instability. Am J Sports Med. 1998;26(5):634–43.

85. Dewing CB, McCormick F, Bell SJ, Solomon DJ, Stanley M, Rooney TB, Provencher MT. An analysis of capsular area in patients with anterior, posterior, and multidirectional shoulder instability. Am J Sports Med. 2008;36(3):515–22.

86. Hsu YC, Pan RY, Shih YY, Lee MS, Huang GS. Superior-capsular elongation and its significance in atraumatic posteroinferior multidirectional shoulder instability in magnetic resonance arthrography. Acta Radiol. 2010;51(3):302–8.

87. Lee HJ, Kim NR, Moon SG, Ko SM, Park JY. Multidirectional instability of the shoulder: rotator interval dimension and capsular laxity evaluation using MR arthrography. Skeletal Radiol. 2013;42(2):231–8.

88. Borsa PA, Jacobson JA, Scibek JS, Dover GC. Comparison of dynamic sonography to stress radiography for assessing glenohumeral joint laxity in asymptomatic shoulders. Am J Sports Med. 2005;33(5):734–41.

89. Harryman 2nd DT, Sidles JA, Harris SL, Matsen 3rd FA. Laxity of the normal glenohumeral joint: a quantitative in vivo assessment. J Shoulder Elbow Surg. 1992;1(2):66–76.

90. McFarland EG, Campbell G, McDowell J. Posterior shoulder laxity in asymptomatic athletes. Am J Sports Med. 1996;22(4):264–72.

91. Hawkins RJ, Koppert G, Johnston G. Recurrent posterior instability (subluxation) of the shoulder. J Bone Joint Surg Am. 1984;66(2):169–74.

92. Altchek DW, Warren RF, Skyhar MJ, Ortiz G. T-plasty modification of the Bankart procedure for multidirectional instability of the anterior and inferior types. J Bone Joint Surg Am. 1991;73(1):105–12.

93. Hawkins RJ, Schutte JP, Janda DH, Huckell GH. Translation of the glenohumeral joint with the patient under anesthesia. J Shoulder Elbow Surg. 1996;5(4):286–92.

94. Levy AS, Lintner S, Kenter K, Speer KP. Intra- and interobserver reproducibility of the shoulder laxity examination. Am J Sports Med. 1999;27(4):460–3.

95. Silliman JF, Hawkins RJ. Classification and physical diagnosis of instability of the shoulder. Clin Orthop Relat Res. 1993;291:7–19.

96. Cofield RH, Irving JF. Evaluation and classification of shoulder instability. With special reference to examination under anesthesia. Clin Orthop Relat Res. 1987;223:32–43.

97. Maki NJ. Cineradiographic studies with shoulder instabilities. Am J Sports Med. 1988;16(4):362–4.

98. Norris TR. Diagnostic techniques for shoulder instability. Instr Course Lect. 1985;34:239–57.

99. Papilion JA, Shall LM. Fluoroscopic evaluation for subtle shoulder instability. Am J Sports Med. 1992;20(5):548–52.

100. Hawkins RJ, Bokor DJ. Clinical evaluation of shoulder problems. In: Rockwood Jr CA, Matsen III FA, editors. The shoulder. 2nd ed. Philadelphia: WB Saunders; 1998. p. 164–97.

101. McFarland EG, Jobe FW, Perry JP, Glousman R, Pink M. Electromyographic analysis of recurrent posterior instability of the shoulder. In: Post M, Morrey BF, Hawkins RJ, editors. Surgery of the shoulder. Chicago: Mosby; 1990. p. 112–6.

102. Lin HT, Hsu AT, Chang GL, Chien JC, An KN, Su FC. Determining the resting position of the glenohumeral joint in subjects who are healthy. Phys Ther. 2007;87(12):1669–82.

103. McFarland EG. Instability and laxity. In: McFarland EG, editor. Examination of the shoulder: the complete guide. New York: Thieme Medical Publishers, Inc; 2006.

104. McFarland EG, Kim TK, Park HB, Neira CA, Gutierrez MI. The effect of variation in definition on the diagnosis of multidirectional instability of the shoulder. J Bone Joint Surg Am. 2003;8-A(11):2138–44.

105. Lin CH, Chou LW, Wei SH, Lieu FK, Chiang SL, Sung WH. Validity and reliability of a novel device for bilateral upper extremity functional measurements. Comput Methods Programs Biomed. 2014;114(3):315–23.

106. Reis MT, Tibone JE, McMahon PJ, Lee TQ. Cadaveric study of glenohumeral translation using electromagnetic sensors. Clin Orthop Relat Res. 2002;400:88–92.

107. Sauers EL, Borsa PA, Herling DE, Stanley RD. Instrumented measurement of glenohumeral joint laxity: reliability and normative data. Knee Surg Sports Traumatol Arthrosc. 2001;9(1):34–41.

108. Lam MH, Fong DT, Yung PS, Ho EP, Chan WY, Chan KM. Knee stability assessment on anterior cruciate ligament injury: clinical and biomechanical approaches. Sports Med Arthrosc Rehabil Ther Technol. 2009;1(1):20.

109. Lippitt SB, Harris SL, Harryman 2nd DT, Sidles J, Matsen 3rd FA. In vivo quantification of the laxity of normal and unstable glenohumeral joints. J Shoulder Elbow Surg. 1994;3(4):215–23.

110. Tzannes A, Paxinos A, Callanan M, Murrell GA. An assessment of the interexaminer reliability of tests for shoulder instability. J Shoulder Elbow Surg. 2004;13(1):18–23.

111. Emery RJH, Mullaji AB. Glenohumeral joint instability in normal adolescents. Incidence and significance. J Bone Joint Surg Br. 1991;7(3):406–8.
112. Gerber C, Ganz R. Clinical assessment of instability of the shoulder: with special reference to anterior and posterior drawer tests. J Bone Joint Surg Br. 1984;66(4):551–6.
113. Cyriax JH, Cyriax PJ. Illustrated manual of orthopaedic medicine. London: Butterworth; 1993.
114. Debski RE, Wong EK, Woo SLY, Sakane M, Fu FH, Warner JJP. In situ force distribution in the glenohumeral joint capsule during anterior-posterior loading. J Orthop Res. 1999;17(5):769–76.
115. Hsu AT, Chang JG, Chang CH. Determining the resting position of the glenohumeral joint: a cadaver study. J Orthop Sports Phys Ther. 2002;32(12): 605–12.
116. Kaltenborn FM. Manual mobilization of the joints. Oslo: Olaf Norlis Bokhandel; 2002.
117. Magee D. Orthopedic physical examination, vol. 1. Philadelphia: Saunders; 2002.
118. McFarland EG, Torpey BM, Curl LA. Evaluation of shoulder laxity. Sports Med. 1996;22(4):264–72.
119. Neer 2nd CS, Foster CR. Inferior capsular shift for involuntary inferior and multidirectional instability of the shoulder. A preliminary report. J Bone Joint Surg Am. 1980;62(6):897–908.
120. Ferrari DA. Capsular ligaments of the shoulder: anatomical and functional study of the anterior superior capsule. Am J Sports Med. 1990;18(1):20–4.
121. Gagey OJ, Gagey N. The hyperabduction test. J Bone Joint Surg Br. 2001;83(1):69–74.
122. van Kampen DA, van den Berg T, van der Woude HJ, Vastelein RM, Terwee CB, Willems WJ. Diagnostic value of patient characteristics, history, and six clinical tests for traumatic anterior shoulder instability. J Shoulder Elbow Surg. 2013;22(10): 1310–9.
123. Rowe CR, Zarins B. Recurrent transient subluxation of the shoulder. J Bone Joint Surg Am. 1981; 63(6):863–72.
124. Lo IK, Nonweiler B, Woolfrey M, Litchfield R, Kirkley A. An evaluation of the apprehension, relocation, and surprise tests for anterior shoulder instability. Am J Sports Med. 2004;32(2):301–7.
125. Bushnell BD, Creighton RA, Herring MM. The bony apprehension test for instability of the shoulder: a prospective pilot analysis. Arthroscopy. 2008;24(9):974–82.
126. Huxel KC, Swanik CB, Swanik KA, Bartolozzi AR, Hillstrom HJ, Sitler MR, Moffit DM. Stiffness regulation and muscle-recruitment strategies of the shoulder in response to external rotation perturbations. J Bone Joint Surg Am. 2008;90(1):154–62.
127. Jia X, Petersen SA, Khosravi AH, Almareddi V, Pannirselvam V, McFarland EG. Examination of the shoulder: the past, the present, and the future. J Bone Joint Surg Am. 2009;91 Suppl 6:10–8.
128. Speer KP, Hannafin JA, Altchek DW, Warren RF. An evaluation of the shoulder relocation test. Am J Sports Med. 1994;22(2):177–83.
129. Jobe FW, Kvitne RS, Giangarra CE. Shoulder pain in the overhand or throwing athlete. The relationship of anterior instability and rotator cuff impingement. Orthop Rev. 1989;18(9):963–75.
130. Davidson PA, ElAttrache NS, Jobe CM, Jobe FW. Rotator cuff and posterior-superior glenoid labrum injury associated with increased glenohumeral motion: a new site of impingement. J Shoulder Elbow Surg. 1995;4(5):384–90.
131. Jobe CM. Posterior superior glenoid impingement: expanded spectrum. Arthroscopy. 1995;11(5):530–6.
132. Paley KJ, Jobe FW, Pink MM, Kvitne RS, ElAttrache NS. Arthroscopic findings in the overhand throwing athlete: evidence for posterior internal impingement of the rotator cuff. Arthroscopy. 2000;16(1):35–40.
133. Gross ML, Distefano MC. Anterior release test. A new test for occult shoulder instability. Clin Orthop Relat Res. 1997;339:105–8.
134. Kessel L. Clinical disorders of the shoulder, vol. 1. Edinburgh: Churchill Livingstone; 1982.
135. Rowe CR. Dislocations of the shoulder. In: Rowe CR, editor. The shoulder. New York: Churchill Livingstone; 1988. p. 165–291.
136. Matsen III FA, Thomas SC, Rockwood CA, Wirth MA. Glenohumeral instability. In: Rockwood CA, Matsen III FA, editors. The shoulder. Philadelphia: Saunders; 1990. p. 611–755.
137. Kim SH, Ha KI, Park JH, Kim YM, Lee YS, Lee JY, Yoo JC. Arthroscopic posterior labral repair and capsular shift for traumatic unidirectional recurrent posterior subluxation of the shoulder. J Bone Joint Surg Am. 2003;85-A(8):1479–87.
138. Kim SH, Park JS, Jeong WK, Shin SK. The Kim test: a novel test for posteroinferior labral lesion of the shoulder – a comparison to the jerk test. Am J Sports Med. 2005;33(8):1188–92.
139. Neer CS. Dislocations. In: Neer CS, editor. Shoulder reconstruction. Philadelphia: Saunders; 1990. p. 273–362.
140. Imerci A, Gölcük Y, Uğur SG, Ursavaş HT, Savran A, Sürer L. Inferior glenohumeral dislocation (luxatio erecta humeri): report of six cases and review of the literature. Ulus Travma Acil Cerrahi Derg. 2013;19(1):41–4.
141. Kelley C, Quimby T, MacVane CZ. Unusual shoulder injury from a motorcycle crash. Luxatio erecta. J Fam Pract. 2013;62(5):255–7.
142. Patel DN, Zuckerman JD, Egol KA. Luxatio erecta: case series with review of diagnostic and management principles. Am J Orthop (Belle Mead NJ). 2011;40(11):566–70.
143. Ellanti P, Davarinos N, Connolly MJ, Khan HA. Bilateral luxation erecta humeri with a unilateral brachial plexus injury. J Emerg Trauma Shock. 2013;6(4):308–10.
144. Frank MA, Laratta JL, Tan V. Irreducible luxation erecta humeri caused by an aberrant position of the axillary nerve. J Shoulder Elbow Surg. 2012;21(7): e6–9.
145. Iakovlev M, Marchand JB, Poirier P, Bargoin K, Gouëffic Y. Posttraumatic axillary false aneurysm

after luxatio erecta of the shoulder: case report and literature review. Ann Vasc Surg. 2014;28(5):1321.e13-8.

146. Lev-El A, Adar R, Rubinstein Z. Axillary artery injury in erect dislocation of the shoulder. J Trauma. 1981;21(4):323–5.

147. Nho SJ, Dodson CC, Bardzik KF, Brophy RH, Domb BG, MacGillivray JD. The two-step maneuver for closed reduction of inferior glenohumeral dislocation (luxation erecta to anterior dislocation to reduction). J Orthop Trauma. 2006;20(5):354–7.

148. Yanturali S, Aksay E, Holliman CJ, Duman O, Ozen YK. Luxatio erecta: clinical presentation and management in the emergency department. J Emerg Med. 2005;29(1):85–9.

149. Neer 2nd CS. Involuntary inferior and multidirectional instability of the shoulder: etiology, recognition, and treatment. Instr Course Lect. 1985;34:232–8.

150. Ogston JB, Ludewig PM. Differences in 3-dimensional shoulder kinematics between persons with multidirectional instability and asymptomatic controls. Am J Sports Med. 2007;35(8):1361–70.

151. Czaprowski D, Kotwicki T, Pawłowska P, Stoliński L. Joint hypermobility in children with idiopathic scoliosis: SOSORT award 2011 winner. Scoliosis. 2011;6:22.

152. Pande P, Hawkins R, Peat M. Electromyography in voluntary posterior instability of the shoulder. Am J Sports Med. 1989;17(5):644–8.

The Acromioclavicular Joint

7.1 Introduction

When compared to other areas of the shoulder, physical examination of the AC joint is more straightforward given its subcutaneous location—a factor that facilitates inspection, palpation and, in some cases, pain localization. In addition, many of the provocative maneuvers used to diagnose AC joint pathologies are more reliable due to the limited potential for confounding variables. However, even if the AC joint is the most likely source for the patient's pain, the inciting etiology is not always clear-cut. A thorough understanding of the anatomy, biomechanics, radiographic features, and relevant physical examination findings related to the AC joint will ultimately contribute to the generation of an accurate diagnosis, an effective treatment plan, and a successful clinical outcome.

7.2 Anatomy and Biomechanics

The AC joint represents a complex articulation between the distal clavicle and the anteromedial aspect of the acromion and plays an important role in the coordination shoulder motion and force transmission between the shoulder girdle and the axial skeleton (Fig. 7.1) [1, 2]. Because the clavicle is linked to the acromion, three-dimensional scapular motion requires that the clavicle also be capable of three-dimensional

motion (Fig. 7.2) [3]. Therefore, the AC joint must be flexible enough to allow for acromioclavicular motion while also being stiff enough to confer stability. Unconstrained osseous anatomy, capsular and extra-capsular ligamentous structures, and dynamic muscle contraction function in harmony to maintain the balance between mobility and stability across the AC joint throughout the entire range of shoulder motion.

7.2.1 Osseous Anatomy

The clavicle is an S-shaped bone that develops from three separate ossification centers via an intramembranous ossification mechanism beginning during the fifth gestational week [4]. Complete ossification of the clavicle does not occur until at least 25 years of age and physeal fusion may be delayed until 31 years of age [5–7]. Similarly, the acromion has four centers of ossification which fuse together by approximately 18 years of age [8]. The fusion sites of these ossification centers are referred to as the preacromion, mesoacromion, and meta-acromion (Fig. 7.3). In approximately 7 % of individuals, one or more of these ossifications centers may fail to fuse, producing a defect known as os acromiale which is primarily diagnosed with radiographs (Fig. 7.4) [9]. Bone scans can also be used to detect increased metabolism of the bony fragment which is closely correlated with the presence of pain (Fig. 7.5). Because the symptoms related to

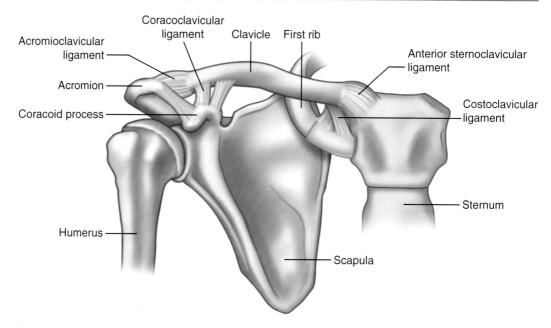

Coracoclavicular
ligament   Clavicle   First rib

Acromioclavicular
ligament

Anterior sternoclavicular
ligament

Acromion

Coracoid process

Costoclavicular
ligament

Sternum

Humerus

Scapula

Fig. 7.1 Illustration showing the basic osseoligamentous anatomy of the shoulder girdle. The AC joint is the central coordinator of three-dimensional shoulder motion and is responsible for the transmission of forces between the axial skeleton and the glenohumeral joint.

Fig. 7.2 Illustration highlighting the spatial relationship between the scapula, clavicle, and sternum. Note that scapular motion in any plane requires a coordinated motion to occur across both the AC and SC joints.

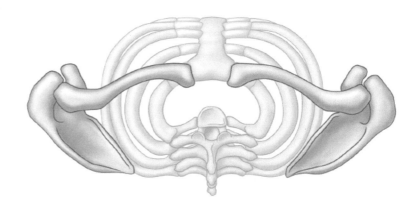

os acromiale can mimic those of other painful AC joint pathologies, patients who present with pain at the top of the shoulder should always be evaluated for the possibility of os acromiale [8]. Os acromiale is also frequently associated with rotator cuff impingement since the deltoid muscle can pull the loosely attached bone downward with arm elevation, thus decreasing the volume of the subacromial space (Fig. 7.6) [8].

Overall, the mean size of the AC joint is approximately 9 mm × 19 mm [10]. However, the size and shape of the distal clavicle and acromion can vary widely across the population [11, 12].

The inclination of the joint surfaces may also be highly variable [13]. When viewed from anteriorly, the joint line can range from a vertical orientation to nearly 50° of angulation where the articular surface of the distal clavicle overrides that of the acromion (Fig. 7.7) [14, 15]. Some AC joints may have an "ellipsoid" shape that may limit internal and external scapular rotation, thus elevating the risk for subacromial impingement [16]. In most cases, the articular surface of the acromion is concave whereas the articular surface of the distal clavicle is convex [13]; both of these surfaces are initially covered in hyaline

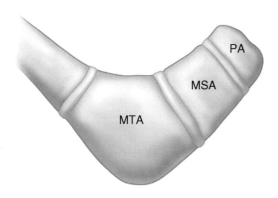

Fig. 7.3 Illustration showing the fusion sites for each ossification center of the acromion. The preacromion, mesoacromion, and meta-acromion are shown. Os acromiale occurs when two of the ossification centers fail to fuse together, sometimes leading to a pseudarthrosis.

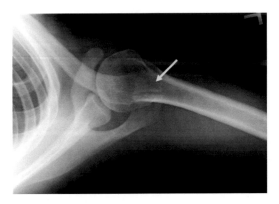

Fig. 7.4 Axillary radiograph of a left shoulder in a patient with symptomatic os acromiale.

cartilage (either completely or partially [17]) followed by a slow transformation to fibrocartilage beginning in adolescence [18]. Rockwood et al. [19] stated that this transition to fibrocartilage is completed by ages 17 and 24 on the acromial and clavicular joint surfaces, respectively.

7.2.2 Intra-Articular Disk

An intra-articular disk (i.e., meniscal homologue) of widely variable shapes and sizes attaches firmly to the acromial side of the joint (Fig. 7.8). The disk functions to disperse the forces associated with joint loading and corrects for any joint incongruency. The upper portion of the disk is made up of fibrocartilage whereas the lower portion of the disk is primarily made up of dense fibrous tissue, possibly reflecting differential load-bearing across the AC joint [16, 20]. Normal degeneration of the intra-articular disk begins during adolescence and progresses through the fourth decade, at which point the disk has become a vestigial structure [21–23]. Degeneration of the intra-articular disk has been associated with osteoarthritis of the AC joint; however, this finding is inevitable since disk degeneration appears to be nearly universal in normal adults.

7.2.3 Capsular and Extra-Capsular Ligaments

The AC joint is surrounded by a fibrous joint capsule with inward-facing synovial tissue that facilitates joint mobility by providing adequate lubrication (see Figs. 7.1 and 7.8). The joint capsule inserts between approximately 3 and 5 mm lateral to the acromial articular surface and between approximately 3 and 6 mm medial to the clavicular articular surface [24]. This capsule is reinforced by closely integrated and confluent AC joint ligaments (superior, inferior, anterior, and posterior), the combined actions of which primarily resist horizontal displacement, accounting for up to 50 and 90 % of anterior and posterior stability of the distal clavicle, respectively [25–27]. More specifically, the superior AC ligament is thought to contribute up to 90 % of the overall strength of the AC joint capsule [82]. In addition, the fibers of the deltotrapezial fascia merge and coalesce with those of the superior AC ligament, thus providing even more structural reinforcement. In contrast, the anterior, posterior, and inferior AC ligaments have significantly less tensile strength [28]. In general, the AC joint capsular ligaments are responsible for resisting relatively small horizontal translations of the distal clavicle relative to the acromion [26].

On the other hand, the coracoclavicular (CC) ligaments are primarily responsible for preventing large translations of the distal clavicle relative to the acromion [26]. The CC ligaments include the conoid (centromedial) and the trapezoid

Fig. 7.5 Positron emission tomography (PET) scan in a patient with symptomatic os acromiale of the right shoulder. (**a**) The coronal sequence demonstrates increased uptake of the radioactive tracer at the site of the os acromiale, suggesting that the patient's pain was most likely related to the os acromiale itself instead of another underlying pathology. (**b**) The axial sequence confirms that the increased uptake did, in fact, involve the mesoacromion.

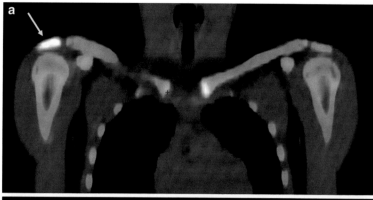

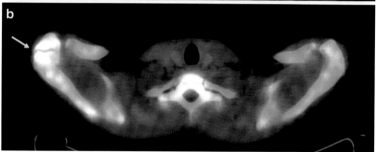

Fig. 7.6 Illustration depicting a possible mechanism of rotator cuff impingement in patients with os acromiale. The downward pull that the deltoid imparts upon the acromion displaces the unfused bony fragment downward, thus decreasing the space available for the rotator cuff tendons to pass beneath the acromion as the humerus is elevated.

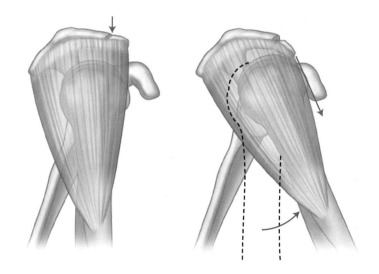

(anterolateral) ligaments which travel between the inferior surface of the distal clavicle and the base of the coracoid process (Fig. 7.9). The conoid and trapezoid ligaments insert approximately 32.1 and 14.7 mm medial to the articular surface of the distal clavicle, respectively [24].

The conoid ligament is the primary restraint to excessive superior translation and rotation of the distal clavicle whereas the trapezoid ligament helps prevent excessive anterior–posterior translation of the distal clavicle and compression of the AC joint [17, 26, 27]. The CC ligaments

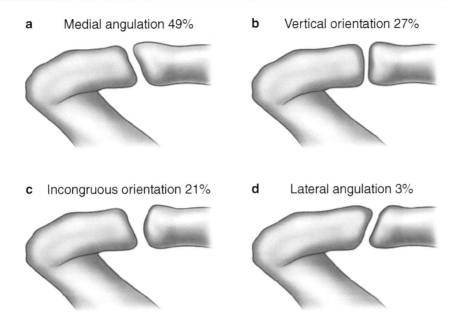

a Medial angulation 49%

b Vertical orientation 27%

c Incongruous orientation 21%

d Lateral angulation 3%

Fig. 7.7 Illustrations showing the variable angulation of the AC joint surfaces when viewed from anteriorly. (**a**) Medial angulation occurs in approximately 50 % of cases, (**b**) a vertical joint line occurs in approximately 25 % of cases, (**c**) an incongruent joint occurs in approximately 25 % of cases, and (**d**) lateral angulation occurs in approximately 5 % of cases.

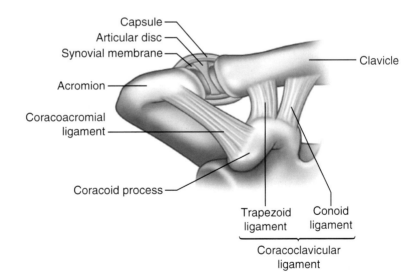

Fig. 7.8 Illustration highlighting the intra-articular structure of the AC joint. The intra-articular disk typically adheres to the acromial side of the joint. The AC joint capsule inserts between 3 and 5 mm lateral to the acromial articular surface and between 3 and 6 mm medial to the clavicular articular surface [24].

Capsule
Articular disc
Synovial membrane
Clavicle
Acromion
Coracoacromial ligament
Coracoid process
Trapezoid ligament
Conoid ligament
Coracoclavicular ligament

assume complete responsibility for both horizontal and vertical stability when the AC joint capsule has been disrupted [26, 29]. Therefore, dislocation of the AC joint is not possible unless disruption of the CC ligaments has occurred [18].

7.2.4 Dynamic Stability

Dynamic stability of the distal clavicle is provided by the serratus anterior, upper trapezius, and anterior deltoid (see Chap. 3 for a more

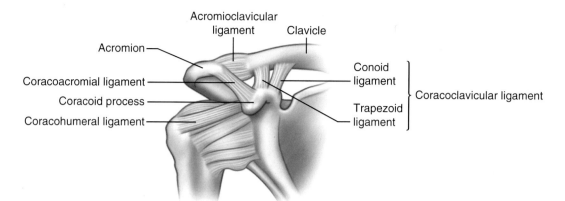

Fig. 7.9 The coracoclavicular (CC) ligaments are composed of the conoid and trapezoid ligaments. The conoid ligament travels between the coracoid base and the conoid tubercle which is centrally located on the inferior aspect of the clavicle. The trapezoid ligament runs anterolateral to the conoid ligament and inserts approximately 15 mm medial to the articular surface of the distal clavicle. The CC ligaments are responsible for preventing large displacements of the distal clavicle relative to the acromion.

detailed anatomic description of these muscles). Of note, the upper trapezius inserts into the posterosuperior aspect of the distal clavicle and the medial acromion and its fibers blend into those of the superior AC joint ligament. The serratus anterior and upper trapezius function in synchrony to optimize the three-dimensional position of the scapula which facilitates glenohumeral stability and supports a large arc of motion. The deltoid primarily functions to support the weight of the arm, thus reducing articular shear forces and reducing tension across the AC joint capsuloligamentous structures [30].

7.2.5 Neurovascular Anatomy

The AC joint capsule receives its blood supply from small branches derived from the suprascapular and thoracoacromial arteries. The joint is innervated by the suprascapular nerve just before it passes beneath the transverse scapular ligament (the suprascapular artery travels with the nerve and passes above the transverse scapular ligament). Branches of the lateral pectoral nerve which travel with the thoracoacromial artery also provide some joint innervation (Fig. 7.10).

7.2.6 Joint Motion

To achieve normal shoulder motion, the AC joint must be able of coordinating the unique three-dimensional motion planes of both the scapula and the clavicle (Fig. 7.11) [1, 2]. Shoulder elevation requires long-axis rotation (up to 50° [31–34]), elevation (up to 15° [35]), and posterior angulation (i.e., retraction.; up to 30° [35]) of the clavicle relative to its resting position; however, the AC joint itself may only be responsible for a portion of this motion where sternoclavicular (SC) joint motion makes up the majority of this difference [35]. More specifically, Ludewig et al. [35] found that approximately 31° of posterior longitudinal rotation of the clavicle occurred at the SC joint whereas about 19° of posterior scapular tilt was allowed across the AC joint. Disruption of the AC joint following an acute injury can therefore result in uncoordinated scapular motion and global shoulder dysfunction (scapular dyskinesis following an AC joint injury is discussed in further detail in Chap. 9).

Relative positional changes of the scapula and the clavicle also require a small amount of joint translation—up to 6 mm of translation in any direction [29, 36]. Given the small articular

Fig. 7.10 Illustration of the neurovascular anatomy that supplies the AC joint. The suprascapular nerve and lateral pectoral nerve provide the innervation while the suprascapular artery and thoracoacromial artery provide the blood supply.

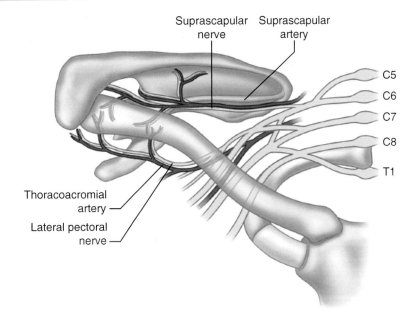

surface area and the high compressive and shear forces that are applied to the joint with daily activities, the AC joint is susceptible to locally elevated contact stresses which may favor the development of osteoarthritis [13].

7.3 Instability of the Acromioclavicular Joint

7.3.1 Pathogenesis

The vast majority of injuries to the AC joint occur during contact sports following an impact to the lateral shoulder with the arm in an adducted position (Fig. 7.12). Although much less common, other types of injury mechanisms such as a direct blow to the distal clavicle or a fall onto an outstretched hand (driving the humeral head into the acromion and producing an inferior dislocation) are also possible.

7.3.2 Physical Examination

7.3.2.1 Acute AC Joint Injuries

Patients with acute AC joint injuries will complain of pain at the top of the shoulder following a significant impact-type injury to the lateral shoulder. Examination of the patient in the sitting or standing position allows the weight of the arm to pull the scapula downward, thus exaggerating the deformity (if present). Inspection of the shoulder usually reveals swelling surrounding the area of the AC joint. In cases of higher-grade injuries, an obvious step-off deformity may be present (Fig. 7.13). Patency of the deltotrapezial fascia can be assessed by having the patient shrug their shoulders—spontaneous joint reduction with this maneuver indicates that the deltotrapezial fascia is intact (discussed below for grades III and V injuries). The clinician should assess for a concomitant clavicle fracture by palpating the entire length of the clavicle, beginning at the SC joint and moving towards the AC joint.

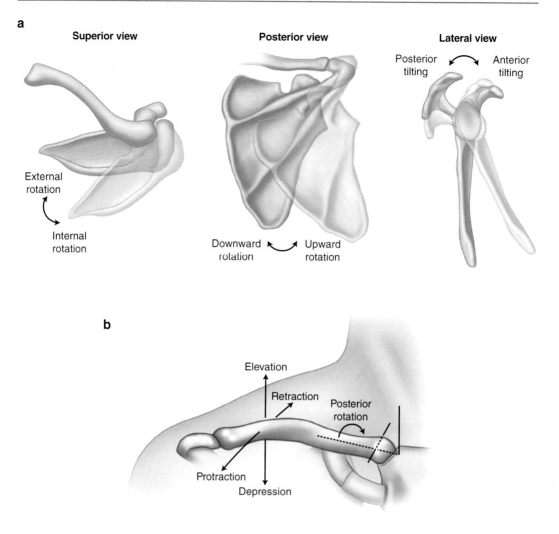

Fig. 7.11 Illustrations highlighting the three-dimensional movements of the clavicle and the scapula. Note that any scapular motion requires force transmission through the AC joint, leading to clavicular motion and, therefore, SC joint motion. (**a**) The three-dimensional motion planes of the scapula. The kinetic energy from these motions travels through the AC joint thus resulting in clavicular motion. (**b**) The three-dimensional motion planes of the clavicle that are closely coordinated with scapular motion through both mechanical and neuromuscular stimuli.

In most cases, these general physical findings lie along a spectrum of severity that are closely related to radiographic findings. The Zanca view is most often used to evaluate injuries to the AC due to its accuracy, excellent diagnostic utility, and its ability to identify concomitant clavicle fractures which can sometimes mimic an AC joint dislocation, especially in younger patients with open physes [37, 38]. To obtain this view, the X-ray beam is centered on the AC joint and tilted 10–15° cephalad [39]. It is recommended to decrease the X-ray penetrance by approximately 50 % to improve visibility of the coracoid, distal clavicle, and other surrounding structures [17]. Many practitioners prefer to obtain a Zanca view that includes both shoulders in order to compare the amount of distal clavicle displacement between the injured and non-injured shoulders (Fig. 7.14). To objectively assess the amount of distal clavicle displacement, the CC distance can be measured and compared between shoulders. Using the same Zanca radiograph, the CC distance is determined by the length of a vertical line that begins from the most superior point of the coracoid and ends at the most inferior point of the clavicle (Fig. 7.15). Although "normal" CC distances have

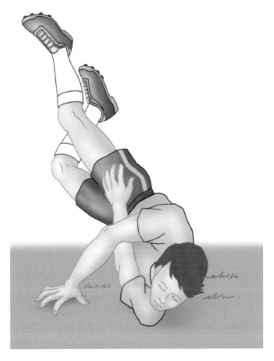

Fig. 7.12 Illustration of the most common injury mechanism resulting in acute AC joint dislocations. Direct impact to the superolateral aspect of the shoulder forces the acromion inferiorly leading to rupture of the AC joint capsule and CC ligaments, thus allowing the distal clavicle to translate superiorly.

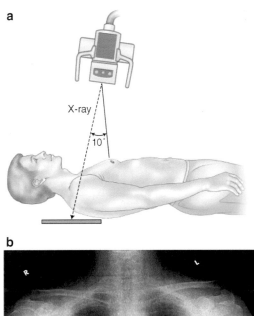

Fig. 7.14 (**a**) Illustration of the technique used to obtain a Zanca radiograph. The X-ray beam is aimed directly towards the AC joint with 10–15° of cephalad angulation. The X-ray beam can also be centered on the midline with cephalad angulation to obtain an image that includes the bilateral AC joints. (**b**) Example of a Zanca radiograph in a patient with an acute grade III AC joint dislocation of the left shoulder.

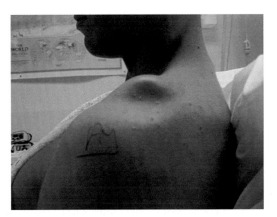

Fig. 7.13 Clinical photograph of a patient's left shoulder following an acute AC joint dislocation. This patient had a grade V injury.

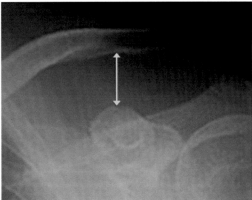

Fig. 7.15 Measurement of the CC distance using a Zanca radiograph. A *vertical line* is drawn connecting the most superior point of the coracoid to the most inferior point of the distal clavicle. The length of the vertical line represents the CC distance.

been reported, these raw measurements are highly variable between individuals due to variations in anatomy. Therefore, comparisons should be made using a ratio in which the CC distance of the injured shoulder is compared to that of the non-injured shoulder. Bearden et al. [40] suggested that a 25 % increase in the CC distance of the injured shoulder probably represents complete disruption of the CC ligaments. Pre- and postoperative Zanca radiographs of the same patient are helpful to ensure maintenance of joint reduction following operative management of an AC joint injury. Of importance, a normal-appearing CC distance in a patient with signs, symptoms, and historical features characteristic of an AC joint dislocation should generate suspicion of a concomitant fracture of the coracoid with superior displacement. When a coracoid fracture is suspected, a Stryker notch view should also be obtained. In this radiographic view, the patient lies supine, places the hand of the affected extremity on top of the head, and the technician directs the X-ray beam towards the coracoid process with approximately 10° of cephalad angulation (Fig. 7.16).

Although less common, posterior dislocations of the AC joint can also occur and may appear normal on standard Zanca radiographs in some cases. Therefore, in all cases of AC joint instability, clinicians should also obtain an axillary view (or Velpeau axillary view) of the shoulder to identify posterior displacement of the distal clavicle relative to the acromion (Figs. 7.17 and 7.18).

Tossy et al. [41] and Rockwood [42] developed a classification system for AC joint injuries based on anteroposterior (AP), Zanca or axillary radiographs (types I–VI, described below [Fig. 7.19]). This classification system is closely related to injury severity which, in turn, is closely related to physical examination findings. However, it should be noted that up to 30 % of patients with an acute AC joint injury are likely to have concomitant intra-articular injuries [43–45]. Therefore, the clinical examination should involve an evaluation of the entire shoulder girdle in all cases to identify potentially treatable concomitant injuries.

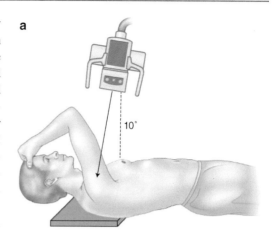

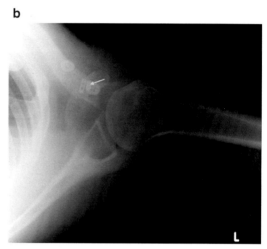

Fig. 7.16 (**a**) Illustration of the technique used to obtain a Stryker notch view. With the patient supine and the hand of the affected extremity placed on top of the head, the X-ray beam is aimed towards the coracoid process with approximately 10° of cephalad angulation. (**b**) Example of a Stryker notch view obtained in a patient with a suspected coracoid fracture following AC reconstruction. The patient presented with loss of reduction following a skiing fall. The image demonstrates displacement of a cortical fixation button that was placed through a drill hole in the coracoid to reduce the initial dislocation (*arrow*).

Type I Injuries

Patients with type I injuries typically present with mild to moderate pain and swelling over the AC joint following a traumatic injury; however, there are no visible or palpable deformities of the

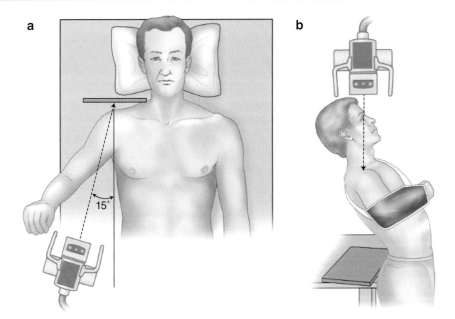

Fig. 7.17 (**a**) The axillary view is obtained with the patient supine (or standing) and the X-ray cassette positioned above the injured shoulder. The shoulder must be sufficiently abducted to allow the X-ray beam to pass between the humerus and the thorax. The X-ray tube is positioned inferior to the shoulder and aimed directly towards the glenohumeral joint at approximately half the angle of abduction (e.g., an abduction angle of 30° would require the X-ray tube to be positioned approximately 15° lateral to the midline). This method ensures that the axillary radiograph is obtained within the plane of the glenoid. (**b**) The Velpeau axillary view is used when the patient cannot adequately abduct the arm to obtain the standard axillary view. While wearing a sling (e.g., Velpeau dressing), the patient is asked to lean backwards to approximately 30° over the X-ray table and cassette. The X-ray beam is directed vertically downward towards the cassette.

AC joint on clinical examination. In these cases, shoulder motion does not consistently generate increased pain at the AC joint. Radiographically, although some soft-tissue swelling may be present, the distal clavicle appears aligned with the acromion without any significant increase in the measured CC distance when compared to the contralateral shoulder (Fig. 7.20). According to the original classification, type I injuries represent a sprain of the capsuloligamentous structures without disruption of any associated structural ligaments.

Type II Injuries
Type II injuries are characterized by moderate to severe pain over the AC joint which usually increases when shoulder motion is initiated. Palpation of the AC joint often reveals moderate swelling and slight superior migration of the distal clavicle relative to the acromion. Horizontal instability, which can be detected by manually grasping the clavicle and applying an anterior–posterior pressure, may be present in some type II injuries. AP or Zanca radiographs may show slight superior displacement of the distal clavicle; however, there is no significant difference in CC distances between the injured and non-injured shoulders (Fig. 7.21). In type II injuries, the AC capsuloligamentous structures are torn which allows the clavicle to migrate superiorly; however, the CC ligaments remain intact.

Type III Injuries
Patients with type III injuries usually present in moderate to severe pain with the arm in an adducted position and the weight of the arm supported either by a sling or the uninjured arm to help provide pain relief. The joint is tender to

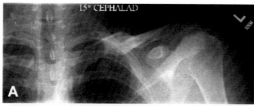

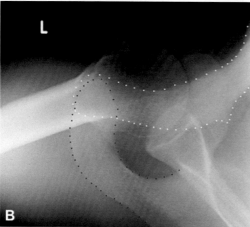

Fig. 7.18 (**a**) Normal-appearing Zanca radiograph of the left AC joint in a patient with pain at the top of the shoulder following an acute injury. Note the normal alignment between the distal clavicle and the acromion. (**b**) Axillary radiograph of the same shoulder demonstrating posterior displacement of the distal clavicle (outlined in *white*) relative to the acromion (outlined in *red*) that was not detectable on the Zanca view.

palpation and an obvious deformity is usually present which represents significant superior displacement of the distal clavicle. Manipulation of the clavicle would reveal both horizontal and vertical instability although significant guarding is usually present in the clinical setting. Radiographically, the clavicle will appear superiorly displaced relative to the acromion by approximately 100 % the width of the distal clavicle (Fig. 7.22). It should be recognized that the distal clavicle actually does not translate superiorly by a large amount—much of this superior displacement is related to the weight of the arm which pulls the acromion inferiorly relative to the clavicle. This injury pattern requires complete disruption of both the AC joint capsule and the CC ligaments while the deltotrapezial fascia remain intact. A shrug test has been described to differentiate type III and V injuries. In this test, reduction of

the injured AC joint by having the patient shrug their shoulders indicates that the deltotrapezial fascia is intact. If shrugging does not reduce the joint, the deltotrapezial fascia has been ruptured which usually signifies a type V injury [17].

Type IV Injuries

Type IV injuries are characterized by complete posterior dislocation of the distal clavicle which typically pierces or punctures the fascia of the trapezius muscle. Patients with type IV injuries often present with severe swelling and pain localized to an area posterior to the medial acromion. In some cases, the distal clavicle may also produce skin tenting posteriorly. Evaluation of Zanca radiographs may reveal mild superior displacement whereas the axillary view will show significant displacement of the distal clavicle posteriorly, possibly making contact with the anterior aspect of the scapular spine (Fig. 7.23). Although infrequent, type IV AC joint injuries can occur in combination with an anterior dislocation of the medial clavicle at the SC joint, thus producing a "floating clavicle" (Fig. 7.24). Therefore, the clinician should also examine the SC joint for any signs of instability in cases where a type IV AC joint injury is suspected (details regarding examination of the SC joint are presented in Chap. 8).

Type V Injuries

Patients with type V injuries present similarly to those with type III injuries; however, the degree of pain, swelling, and deformity are markedly more severe. Type V injuries are characterized by >100 % superior displacement of the distal clavicle on Zanca radiographs, increased scapular protraction and more severe soft-tissue injuries when compared to type III injuries (Fig. 7.25). Disruption of the deltotrapezial fascia is a hallmark for type V dislocations and may generate radiating pain towards the side of the neck along the superior margin of the trapezius muscle.

Type VI Injuries

Type VI AC joint injuries are inferior dislocations in which the distal clavicle may end up in the subacromial space or beneath the coracoid

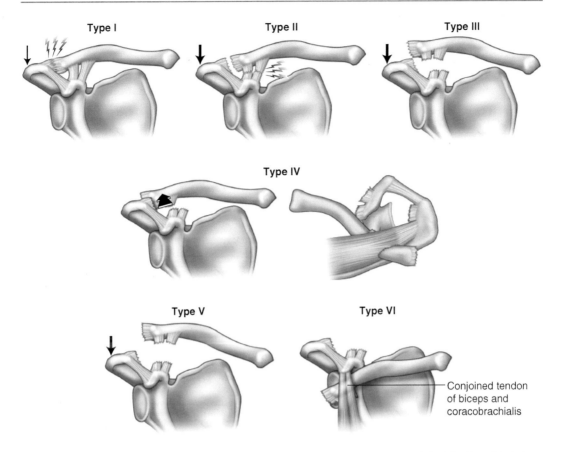

Fig. 7.19 Rockwood classification of AC joint injuries. *Type I* = sprain of the AC joint capsule; *Type II* = rupture of the AC joint capsule with possible sprain of the CC ligaments; *Type III* = rupture of the CC ligaments (i.e., dislocation) with superior displacement equal to approximately 100 % the width of the distal clavicle; *Type IV* = dislocation with posterior displacement that often punctures the trapezial fascia; *Type V* = dislocation with superior displacement of >100 % of the width of the distal clavicle; *Type VI* = subcoracoid dislocation.

Fig. 7.20 Zanca radiograph demonstrating a right type I AC joint injury.

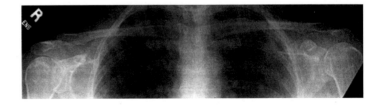

process following a severe hyperabduction injury (see Fig. 7.19). These dislocations are infrequently encountered in clinical practice, although they can be observed following polytraumatic events such as high-speed motor vehicle accidents [46–50]. Subcoracoid dislocations may also involve neurovascular symptoms given the proximity of the brachial plexus and surrounding vessels; however, symptoms usually resolve following joint reduction.

7.3.2.2 Chronic AC Joint Injuries

Although controversy exists regarding the precise definition of "chronic" following an AC joint injury (usually ranges between 30 and 90 days post-injury), we prefer to assign the term "chronic" to injuries in which inflammation, tenderness, and disability have begun to subside as the patient returns to their normal activities. Based on anecdotal evidence and clinical experience, we estimate that 20–30 % of patients who are treated nonoperatively for an acute AC joint injury will experience continued symptoms and seek further treatment at some point, although the timing is generally unpredictable. Patients with chronic AC joint injuries who return for clinical evaluation should be thoroughly evaluated for possible sequelae such as scapular dyskinesis (see Chap. 9), rotator cuff disease (see Chap. 3), and osteoarthritis of the AC joint (discussed below). In addition, concomitant injuries such as labral tears and superior labral anterior to posterior (SLAP) tears may occur in up to 30 % of acute high-grade AC joint dislocations [43, 44, 51]—the symptoms related to these injuries may have never resolved through nonoperative treatment or non-treatment. In all of these cases, the distal clavicle should be evaluated for occult instability which can exacerbate the progression of AC joint degeneration (discussed below).

Distal Clavicle Manipulation

Although the technique has only been described in patients who underwent previous distal clavicle excision (i.e., no traumatic AC joint injuries involved) [52], manipulation of the distal clavicle can be performed to evaluate increased anterior–posterior or superior–inferior translation of the distal clavicle relative to the acromion in cases of chronic AC joint instability. To perform this maneuver, the clinician places one hand on the lateral shoulder for stability and uses the fingers and thumb of the other hand to grasp the mid-shaft of the clavicle. From this position, the distal clavicle can be translated anteriorly, posteriorly, superiorly, and inferiorly when AC joint instability is present (Fig. 7.26). The test should be repeated on the contralateral shoulder for direct comparison. Although there is no precise definition of what constitutes a "positive" test, the original investigators did find that increased translational distances were highly correlated with increased pain. This finding suggests that the pain related to increased distal clavicle translation may be a primary contributor to poor operative and nonoperative outcomes in some patients. This technique is only useful in the setting of a chronic AC joint injury, prior AC reconstruction, or prior distal clavicle excision since those with acute injuries usually exhibit significant apprehension and guarding due to pain and swelling. In addition, manipulating the clavicle in the acute setting could displace a previously unidentified clavicle fracture.

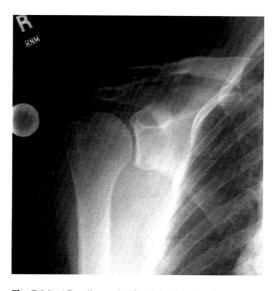

Fig. 7.21 AP radiograph of a right shoulder in a patient with an acute type II AC joint injury.

Fig. 7.22 Zanca radiograph demonstrating a left type III AC joint dislocation.

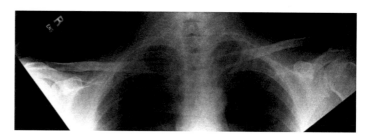

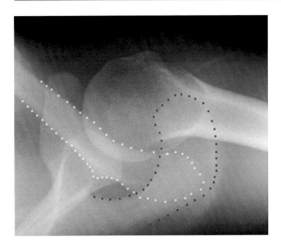

Fig. 7.23 Axillary radiograph demonstrating posterior displacement of the left distal clavicle (outlined in *white*) relative to the acromion (outlined in *red*). This image is diagnostic for a type IV AC joint dislocation.

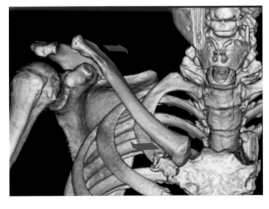

Fig. 7.24 CT scan with 3-D reconstruction of the right shoulder demonstrating a type IV AC joint dislocation with a concomitant anterior SC joint dislocation (commonly referred to as a "floating clavicle").

7.4   Osteoarthritis of the Acromioclavicular Joint

7.4.1   Pathogenesis

7.4.1.1 Post-traumatic Osteoarthritis

Although many patients become asymptomatic with the passage of time, symptoms related to a previous AC joint injury may reappear in the form of post-traumatic osteoarthritis many years after the initial injury. It is presumed that nonoperative treatment of the initial injury (or non-treatment when patients do not seek medical attention) allows repetitive micromotion and elevated shear stresses to occur across articular surfaces during shoulder motion until joint destruction leads to the development of pain (Fig. 7.27) [53]. In addition, many patients with chronic AC joint dislocations display evidence of scapular dyskinesis [54–56] which may increase the risk for other conditions such as rotator cuff impingement. Therefore, these patients should also undergo a complete evaluation of scapular motion throughout the course of their treatment, especially in those with chronic dislocations who complain non-AC joint-related shoulder pain (scapular dyskinesis is discussed in Chap. 9).

7.4.1.2 Repetitive Microtrauma

Repetitive microtrauma is also an important cause of chronic AC joint degeneration and, similar to post-traumatic osteoarthritis, is mostly attributed to abnormally high stresses placed upon the distal

Fig. 7.25 Zanca radiograph demonstrating a left type V AC joint dislocation.

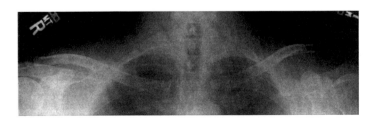

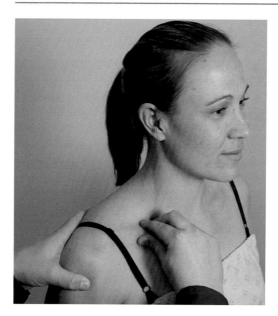

Fig. 7.26 Distal clavicle manipulation. The examiner places one hand over the lateral shoulder to stabilize the upper torso and uses the fingers and thumb of the other hand to grasp the mid-shaft of the clavicle. When instability is present, the distal clavicle can then be translated anteriorly, posteriorly, superiorly, and/or inferiorly.

clavicle which increases the rate of bone turnover in the area. As a result of this remodeling process, joint surfaces become incongruent and the articular cartilage degenerates due to abnormally elevated contact stresses and shear forces. Distal clavicle osteolysis most commonly occurs in those who regularly perform bench press exercises [57], possibly as a result of repeated maximal contraction of the clavicular head of the pectoralis major muscle which may lead to the development of small stress fractures within the subchondral bone of the distal clavicle and subsequent bony remodeling [58, 59]. Although this diagnosis is difficult to distinguish from post-traumatic osteoarthritis due to similar symptomatology, physical examination findings, and imaging findings [60–62], surgical resection of the AC joint is usually indicated for either case when non-operative treatment fails to relieve the patient's symptoms.

7.4.1.3 Advancing Age
Osteoarthritis of the AC joint can also develop as an atraumatic, age-related phenomenon that is most often associated with degeneration of the

intra-articular disk which occurs with normal aging. Several authors have suggested that the intra-articular disk is almost always non-functional beyond 40 years of age [21–23]. Symptomatic disk degeneration is usually observed in patients over 50 years of age; however, the degenerative process may begin during adolescence [21] and it is unknown when symptoms begin to occur, if they occur at all [63]. In fact, a study by Stein et al. [64] found that up to 93 % of asymptomatic patients over 30 years of age had MRI evidence of AC joint osteoarthritis. Similar results were found by Needell et al. [65] in which 75 % of asymptomatic volunteers had AC joint osteoarthritis as evidenced by MRI (Fig. 7.28).

7.4.1.4 Inflammatory Arthropathies
Similar to other synovialized joints, the AC joint is also susceptible to inflammatory arthropathies such as rheumatoid arthritis [66] and psoriatic arthritis [67] along with crystal deposition diseases such as gout and pseudogout [68, 69]. Patients with inflammatory arthropathies typically present with pain over the AC joint in the presence of warmth, redness, swelling, and fever. Infectious etiologies related to the AC joint, such as osteomyelitis and septic arthritis, can occur due to hematogenous spread or direct inoculation (such as during a joint injection) and may be related to immunocompromised [70, 71]. Infection should always be ruled out before any treatment interventions are undertaken.

7.4.1.5 Synovial Cysts
Synovial cysts can occur near the AC joint and may be associated with various AC and glenohumeral joint arthritides along with massive rotator cuff tears (Fig. 7.29) [72]. Although painless, these cysts can be alarming for some patients since the lesion may enlarge very rapidly. According to Hiller et al. [72], a type 1 cyst is isolated to the AC joint and probably involves overproduction of synovial fluid in response to degenerative changes. Type 2 cysts occur as a result of anterosuperior humeral head migration (as in some cases of massive rotator cuff tears) which produces damage to the posteroinferior aspect of the AC joint capsule and the anterosuperior glenohumeral joint capsule. With concomitant synovial fluid overproduction

Close-up view of joint

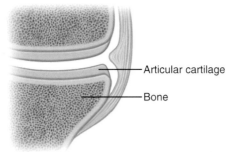

- Articular cartilage
- Bone

During injury

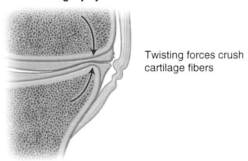

Twisting forces crush cartilage fibers

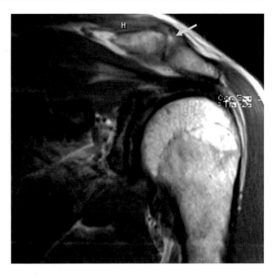

Fig. 7.28 MRI of the right shoulder in a 30-year-old male with posterior glenohumeral instability. In this case, degeneration of the AC joint (*arrow*) was an incidental finding. The patient's AC joint was painless throughout the physical examination.

Post-traumatic arthritis

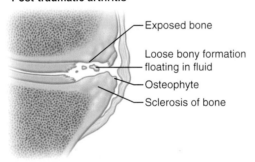

- Exposed bone
- Loose bony formation floating in fluid
- Osteophyte
- Sclerosis of bone

Fig. 7.27 Illustration showing the progression of post-traumatic degenerative osteoarthritis of the AC joint. The initial articular cartilage injury creates a catabolic biochemical environment that is exacerbated by repetitive micromotion. Uneven articular surfaces create stress risers that are subjected to elevated shear stresses when motion occurs, thus accelerating cartilage degeneration. The joint may eventually become eburnated with characteristic radiographic findings of osteoarthritis such as a narrowed joint space, subchondral cysts, subchondral sclerosis, and osteophytosis.

by the glenohumeral joint as a result of cuff arthropathy, synovial fluid can then transfer between glenohumeral and AC joint compartments, thus potentially producing an AC joint synovial cyst. Lesions should be illuminated to confirm its cystic appearance before aspiration since solid tumors in this area have been reported in the literature [73, 74]. These painless cysts may fluctuate in size over a period of time and, especially in cases of cuff arthropathy, cysts may reappear after aspiration since due to the existence of a persistent communication tract between the AC and glenohumeral joints.

7.4.2   Physical Examination

In contrast to acute injuries, chronic pain related to the AC joint can have numerous etiologies and determining the correct diagnosis can sometimes be difficult. The spectrum of AC joint disease can produce symptoms that often overlap with other common shoulder conditions. While some patients may present with global, diffuse shoulder pain and dysfunction, others may only have mild point tenderness located precisely at the AC joint. In addition, physical examination findings can also be confusing since many provocative testing maneuvers designed for other types of pathologies can induce AC joint pain. However, motion-dependent AC joint pain is mostly

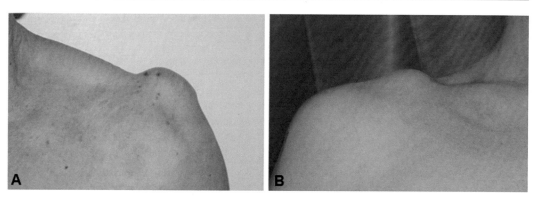

Fig. 7.29 (**a**) Synovial cyst involving the AC joint. (**b**) Distal clavicle hypertrophy. These entities can be differentiated by palpation and illumination.

induced by scapular motion when the humerus is either extended or elevated above approximately 90° (see Chap. 2 for further details regarding isolated glenohumeral versus combined glenohumeral and scapulothoracic motion). Thus, patients who experience pain mostly during simultaneous scapular motion are more likely to have AC joint pathology than patients who experience pain throughout the entire range of motion. Possible exceptions include those with inflammatory or infectious conditions in which AC joint pain is not motion-dependent.

Perhaps one of the more important methods used in the physical diagnosis of AC joint pathologies is simple observation of the patient's shoulders. Although there is a wide range of variation in AC joint anatomy, comparison of the overall contour of each AC joint can often provide a helpful hint (Fig. 7.30). Although not diagnostic, relative prominence of one AC joint relative the other may direct the clinicians towards a more thorough examination of the AC joint, especially if the prominence is located on the symptomatic side. As mentioned above, there are numerous potential causes of a prominent AC joint such as osteoarthritis, synovial cysts, tumors, chronic dislocations, and many others and therefore may necessitate full examination and diagnostic imaging.

Before making the physical diagnosis of a chronic AC joint pathology, it is important to rule in or out other potentially coexistent conditions that may contribute to the patient's pain and dysfunction. This step is important since other shoulder conditions may actually be identified as primary symptomatic lesions. Pain associated with rotator cuff disease is perhaps the most common contributor and may be perceived by the patient as involving the superior aspect of the shoulder. Impingement signs may also be positive since all of these tests involve overhead motion which requires motion to occur across the AC joint. While pain related to rotator cuff disease and the AC joint often occur simultaneously, it is important to determine which condition is the primary instigator since the treatment options for each can vary significantly. SLAP tears are also commonly identified in patients with AC joint-related pain and may be related to a previous traumatic injury, such as an AC joint dislocation, for which the patient has developed symptomatic post-traumatic osteoarthritis [43, 44, 51]. The quality and distribution of pain related to SLAP tears frequently overlaps that of AC joint pain which can therefore complicate the diagnosis. Patients with cervical spine diseases, such as zygoapophyseal joint degeneration and/ or nerve root irritation, may also complain of superior shoulder pain—however, this type of pain is often dependent on the position of the neck and is usually localized to the superior border of the trapezius muscle. Spurling's test, among other provocative cervical spine maneuvers, can be used to successfully differentiate between shoulder pain and neck pain and is discussed in Chap. 10.

7.4.2.1 Distal Clavicle Manipulation

As mentioned above, the clavicle can be manipulated by simply using one's thumb and fingers to grasp the mid-shaft of the clavicle and translate the joint anteroposteriorly and superoinferiorly (see Fig. 7.26) [52]. This can be a useful method to help solidify the diagnosis of occult AC joint instability. In addition, the clavicular motion produced by the examiner may induce a certain degree of painful sheer across the joint when chronic instability has led to post-traumatic osteoarthritis. This technique has not been evaluated for its diagnostic utility; however, we find it is helpful to determine the nature and mechanism of the patient's pain.

7.4.2.2 Paxinos Test

The Paxinos test was first described by Walton et al. [75] in 2004 and is functionally similar to clavicle manipulation when evaluating the joint for osteoarthritis. In this test, the examiner places their hand over the top of the symptomatic shoulder with the thumb overlying posterior aspect of the acromion and the fingers resting over the anterior aspect of the distal clavicle. The examiner then squeezes the top of the shoulder which essentially forces the distal clavicle posteriorly and the acromion anteriorly (Fig. 7.31). Pain in the area of AC joint with this technique is considered a positive test and may indicate joint degeneration. The original investigators calculated a sensitivity of 82 % and a specificity of 50 %; however, the presence of a positive bone scan significantly increased the post-test probability of AC joint-related pain. Yelland [76] obtained similar results when bone scans were used to help solidify the diagnosis. A potential variation of this test involves the clinician using the heels of their clasped hands to squeeze the clavicle posteriorly and the scapular spine anteriorly (Fig. 7.32). Although no studies have evaluated this modified technique, we suspect that the sensitivity and specificity values are similar to those for the Paxinos test which requires ancillary maneuvers to confirm the suspected diagnosis.

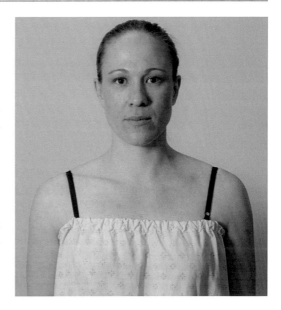

Fig. 7.30 Observation of both shoulders is important to identify any evidence of asymmetry.

7.4.2.3 Cross-Body Adduction Test

In 1951, McLaughlin [77] noted that many patients with AC joint pathologies developed a sharp pain at the top of the shoulder when the arm was actively adducted across the chest and towards the contralateral shoulder. The clinician may also palpate the AC joint during this maneuver to localize the source of the patient's pain. To confirm the diagnosis of AC joint-related pain, McLaughlin then injected the joint with local anesthetic—when repetition of the test following this injection was painless, it was determined that AC joint compression was causative and distal clavicle excision was recommended to alleviate the patient's symptoms.

Several years later, Moseley [78] described a modified version of this test in which the patient was asked to actively place the arm in a position of adduction as described by McLaughlin [77]. The clinician would then apply an additional passive force to the patient's elbow which effectively increased the amount of adduction and AC joint compression (Fig. 7.33). Although this version of the test has not been validated by any study, it may be a useful adjunct to detect more subtle

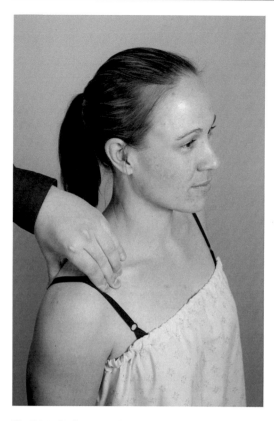

Fig. 7.31 Paxinos test. The examiner places one hand over the patient's shoulder with the thumb over the scapular spine and the fingers over the distal clavicle. The scapula and the clavicle are gently squeezed together, thus translating the clavicle posteriorly relative to the acromion.

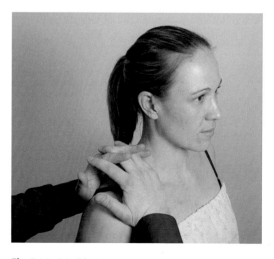

Fig. 7.32 Modified technique to produce AC joint shearing. The examiner places the heels of their clasped hands over the distal clavicle anteriorly and the spine of the scapula posteriorly. The clavicle and the scapula are squeezed together to produce joint shearing.

forms of AC joint-related pain when the diagnosis is unclear.

While there are many studies that have used the cross-body adduction test as a method of diagnosis, very few studies have been conducted with the purpose of evaluating the diagnostic utility of the cross-body adduction test in patients with and without AC joint pain. Maritz and Oosthuizen [79] studied the test in a series of 22 patients with AC joint pain and calculated a sensitivity of 100 % using joint injection as the diagnostic standard. Chronopoulos et al. [80] evaluated the clinical efficacy of the test in 35 patients who later underwent distal clavicle excisions. In that study, the sensitivity was 77 %, the specificity was 79 %, the positive predictive value (PPV) was 20 %, and the negative predictive value (NPV) was 98 %.

7.4.2.4 Active Compression Test

The active compression test was first described by O'Brien et al. [11] in 1998 as a method to detect either SLAP tears or AC joint pathologies. To detect AC joint pain, the test is performed exactly as described for SLAP tears in Chap. 5 although the resulting pain is primarily localized to the superior shoulder near the AC joint (the resulting pain in patients with SLAP tears is usually located "deep inside" the glenohumeral joint). Briefly, the patient's arm is flexed to approximately 90°, adducted 10–20° and internally rotated until the thumb points towards the floor. The clinician first applies a downward force to the top of the forearm while the patient resists. The patient then turns the palm upward and the clinician applies the same downward force in this position (Fig. 7.34). Pain with the first maneuver that is relieved by the second maneuver signifies a positive test although, as mentioned, the pain distribution in those with SLAP tears is primarily deep within the glenohumeral joint whereas pain related to AC joint pathology would be localized to the top of the shoulder. The original investigators studied the test in 318 patients (62 of which had AC joint pain) and found a sensitivity of 100 %, a specificity of 96.6 %, a PPV of 89 %, and an NPV of 100 %. On the other hand, the more recent independent study by Chronopoulos et al. [80] calcu-

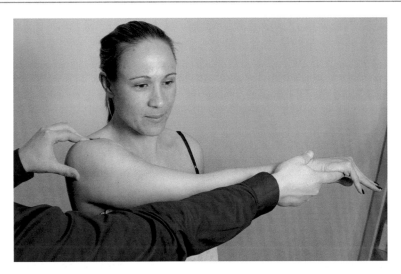

Fig. 7.33 Cross-body adduction test. The patient's arm is placed in a position of 90° of forward flexion. With the palm facing downward, the arm is slowly horizontally adducted towards the contralateral shoulder. Palpation of the AC joint can also be performed. This test should be avoided in patients with known subscapularis pathology as this position may also produce pain related to subscapularis impingement beneath the coracoid process.

lated a sensitivity of 41 %, a specificity of 95 %, a PPV of 29 %, and an NPV of 97 %. Therefore, combination of the test with other provocative maneuvers may be helpful in the diagnosis of AC joint pathology. As with any other clinical maneuver, the results of this test can be confounded by other concomitant pathologies which may produce similar pain distributions.

7.4.2.5 Resisted Arm Extension Test

The resisted arm extension test was first described by Jacob and Sallay [81] in 1997 as a method to detect pain within the AC joint. In this test, the humerus is flexed to 90°, the elbow is flexed 90°, and the arm is internally rotated such that the forearm is positioned along the horizontal plane. The clinician places one hand over the posterior scapula to stabilize the torso and uses the other hand to apply a medially directed force to the elbow at the olecranon while the patient provides resistance (Fig. 7.35). The test is considered positive when pain is produced at the top of the shoulder near the AC joint when resistance is applied by the patient. Chronopoulos et al. [80] calculated a sensitivity of 72 %, a specificity of 85 %, a PPV of 20 %, and an NPV of 98 %. Similar to the active compression test, it is recommended to use this test in combination with other maneuvers to help improve diagnostic accuracy. We are unaware of any other studies that have evaluated the clinical utility of this test in the diagnosis of AC joint pain.

7.5 Conclusion

An understanding of the anatomy and biomechanics of the AC joint is required to arrive at the correct diagnosis. This knowledge, in addition to a thorough history, will guide the clinician towards the selection of high-yield diagnostic tests such as provocative physical examination maneuvers and appropriate imaging modalities. An evidence-based approach improves the likelihood that an accurate diagnosis and effective treatment plan will be produced.

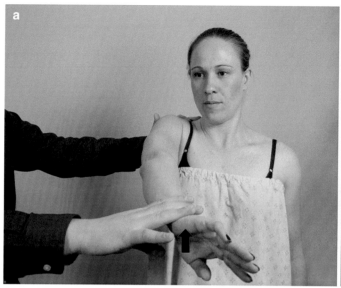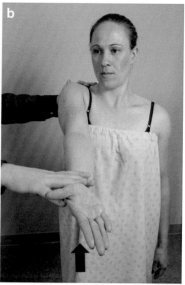

Fig. 7.34 Active compression test. (**a**) With the patient standing, the humerus is forward flexed to 90° with approximately 10° of horizontal adduction and the thumb pointed downward. The examiner then applies a downward force to the distal arm while the patient provides resistance. (**b**) The test is repeated with the palm facing upward. Characteristic pain with the first maneuver that is relieved by the second maneuver indicates a positive test.

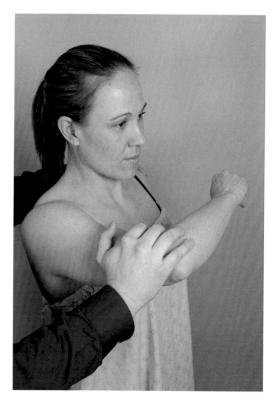

Fig. 7.35 Resisted arm extension test. The patient's arm is positioned at 90° of forward flexion with the elbow flexed 90° in the direction of the contralateral shoulder. The patient is then asked to extend the humerus laterally while the examiner provides resistance.

References

1. Oki S, Matsumura N, Iwamoto W, Ikegami H, Kiriyama Y, Nakamura T, Toyama Y, Nagura T. Acromioclavicular joint ligamentous system contributing to clavicular strut function: a cadaveric study. J Shoulder Elbow Surg. 2013;22(10):1433–9.
2. Oki S, Matsumura N, Iwamoto W, Ikegami H, Kiriyama Y, Nakamura T, Toyama Y, Nagura T. The function of the acromioclavicular and coracoclavicular ligaments in shoulder motion: a whole-cadaver study. Am J Sports Med. 2012;40(11): 2617–26.
3. Branch TP, Burdette HL, Shahriari AS, Carter II FM, Hutton WC. The role of the acromioclavicular ligaments and the effect of distal clavicle resection. Am J Sports Med. 1996;24(3):293–7.
4. Ogata S, Uhthoff HK. The early development and ossification of the human clavicle – an embryologic study. Acta Orthop Scand. 1990;61(4):330–4.
5. Iannotti JP, Williams GR. Disorders of the shoulder: diagnosis and management. Philadelphia: Lippincott Williams & Wilkins; 1999. p. 765–813.
6. Koch MJ, Wells L. Proximal clavicle physeal fracture with posterior displacement: diagnosis, treatment, and prevention. Orthopedics. 2012;35(1):e108–11.
7. Webb PA, Schuey JM. Epiphyseal union of the anterior iliac crest and medial clavicle in a modern multiracial sample of American males and females. Am J Phys Anthropol. 1985;68:457–66.
8. Warner JJP, Beim GM, Higgins L. The treatment of symptomatic os acromiale. J Bone Joint Surg Am. 1998;80(9):1320–6.

9. Yammine K. The prevalence of os acromiale: a systematic review and meta-analysis. Clin Anat. 2014;27(4):610–21.

10. Bosworth BM. Complete acromioclavicular dislocation. N Engl J Med. 1949;241(6):221–5.

11. O'Brien SJ, Pagnani MJ, Fealy S, McGlynn SR, Wilson JB. The active compression test: a new and effective test for diagnosing labral tears and acromioclavicular joint abnormality. Am J Sports Med. 1998;26(5):610–3.

12. Rios CG, Arciero RA, Mazzocca AD. Anatomy of the clavicle and coracoid process for reconstruction of the coracoclavicular ligaments. Am J Sports Med. 2007; 35(5):811–7.

13. Colegate-Stone T, Allom R, Singh R, Elias DA, Standring S, Sinha J. Classification of the morphology of the acromioclavicular joint using cadaveric and radiological analysis. J Bone Joint Surg Br. 2010; 92(5):743–6.

14. DePalma AF. Surgery of the shoulder. 2nd ed. Philadelphia: LB Lippincott; 1973.

15. Urist MR. Complete dislocation of the acromioclavicular joint: the nature of the traumatic lesion and effective methods of treatment with an analysis of 41 cases. J Bone Joint Surg. 1946;28:813–37.

16. Emura K, Arakawa T, Miki A, Terashima T. Anatomical observations of the human acromioclavicular joint. Clin Anat. 2014;27(7):1046–52.

17. Bontempo NA, Mazzocca AD. Biomechanics and treatment of acromioclavicular and sternoclavicular joint injuries. Br J Sports Med. 2010;44(5):361–9.

18. Collins DN. Disorders of the acromioclavicular joint. In: Rockwood Jr CA, Matsen 3rd FA, Wirth MA, Lippitt SB, editors. The shoulder, vol. 2. 4th ed. Philadelphia: Saunders; 2009. p. 453–526.

19. Rockwood Jr CA, Williams GR, Young D. Disorders of the acromioclavicular joint. In: Rockwood Jr CA, Matsen F, editors. The Shoulder. Philadelphia: Saunders; 1998. p. 483–553.

20. Heers G, Götz J, Schubert T, Schachner H, Neumaier U, Grifka J, Hedtmann A. MR imaging of the intraarticular disk of the acromioclavicular joint: a comparison with anatomical, histological and in-vivo findings. Skeletal Radiol. 2007;36(1):23–8.

21. DePalma AF. The role of the discs of the sternoclavicular and acromioclavicular joints. Clin Orthop Relat Res. 1959;13:7–12.

22. Petersson CJ. Degeneration of the acromioclavicular joint: a morphological study. Acta Orthop Scand. 1983;54(3):434–8.

23. Salter Jr EG, Nasca RJ, Shelley BS. Anatomical observations on the acromioclavicular joint and supporting ligaments. Am J Sports Med. 1987;15(3): 199–206.

24. Stine IA, Vangsness Jr CT. Analysis of the capsule and ligament insertions about the acromioclavicular joint: a cadaveric study. Arthroscopy. 2009;25(9): 968–74.

25. Corteen DP, Teitge RA. Stabilization of the clavicle after distal resection: a biomechanical study. Am J Sports Med. 2005;33(1):61–7.

26. Fukuda K, Craig EV, An KN, Cofield RH, Chao EY. Biomechanical study of the ligamentous system of the acromioclavicular joint. J Bone Joint Surg Am. 1986;68(3):434–40.

27. Klimkiewicz JJ, Williams GR, Sher JS, Karduna A, Des Jardins J, Iannotti JP. The acromioclavicular capsule as a restraint to posterior translation of the clavicle: a biomechanical analysis. J Shoulder Elbow Surg. 1999;8:119–24.

28. Lee KW, Debski RE, Chen CH, Woo SL, Fu FH. Functional evaluation of the ligaments at the acromioclavicular joint during anteroposterior and superoinferior translation. Am J Sports Med. 1997; 25(6):858–62.

29. Debski RE, Parsons II IM, Fenwick J, Vangura A. Ligament mechanics during 3 degree-of-freedom motion at the acromioclavicular joint. Ann Biomed Eng. 2000;28(6):612–8.

30. Mazzocca AD, Arciero RA, Bicos J. Evaluation and treatment of acromioclavicular joint injuries. Am J Sports Med. 2007;35(2):316–29.

31. Flatow EL. The biomechanics of the acromioclavicular, sternoclavicular, and scapulothoracic joints. Instr Course Lect. 1993;42:237–45.

32. Giphart JE, van der Meijden OA, Millett PJ. The effects of arm elevation on the 3-dimensional acromiohumeral distance: a biplane fluoroscopy study with normative data. J Shoulder Elbow Surg. 2012; 21(11):1593–600.

33. Inman VT, Saunders JB, Abbott LC. Observations on the function of the shoulder joint. J Bone Joint Surg. 1944;26:1–30.

34. Kennedy JC. Complete dislocation of the acromioclavicular joint: 14 years later. Trauma. 1968;8(3): 311–8.

35. Ludewig PM, Phadke V, Braman JP, Hassett DR, Cieminski CJ, LaPrade RF. Motion of the shoulder complex during multiplanar humeral elevation. J Bone Joint Surg Am. 2009;91(2):378–89.

36. Sahara W, Sugamoto K, Murai M, Tanaka H, Yoshikawa H. 3D kinematic analysis of the acromioclavicular joint during arm abduction using vertically open MRI. J Orthop Res. 2006;24(9):1823–31.

37. Rashid A, Christofi T, Thomas M. Surgical treatment of physeal injuries of the lateral aspect of the clavicle: a case series. Bone Joint J. 2013;95-B(5):664–7.

38. Richards DP, Howard A. Distal clavicle fracture mimicking type IV acromioclavicular joint injury in the skeletally immature athlete. Clin J Sports Med. 2001; 11(1):57–9.

39. Zanca P. Shoulder pain: involvement of the acromioclavicular joint. (Analysis of 1,000 cases). Am J Roentgenol Radium Ther Nucl Med. 1971;112(3):493–506.

40. Bearden JM, Hughston JC, Whatley GS. Acromioclavicular dislocation: method of treatment. J Sports Med. 1973;1(4):5–17.

41. Tossy JD, Mead NC, Sigmond HM. Acromioclavicular separations: useful and practical classification for treatment. Clin Orthop Relat Res. 1963;28:111–9.

42. Rockwood CA. Injuries to the acromioclavicular joint. In: Rockwood CA, Green DP, editors. Fractures

in adults, vol. 1. 2nd ed. Philadelphia: JB Lippincott Co; 1984.

43. Pauly S, Gerhardt C, Haas NP, Scheibel M. Prevalence of concomitant intraarticular lesions in patients treated operatively for high-grade acromioclavicular joint separations. Knee Surg Sports Traumatol Arthrosc. 2009;17(5):513–7.

44. Pauly S, Kraus N, Greiner S, Scheibel M. Prevalence and pattern of glenohumeral injuries among acute high-grade acromioclavicular joint instabilities. J Shoulder Elbow Surg. 2013;22(6):760–6.

45. Tischer T, Salzmann GM, El-Azab H, Vogt S, Imhoff AB. Incidence of associated injuries with acute acromioclavicular joint dislocations types III through V. Am J Sports Med. 2009;37(1):136–9.

46. Canbora KM, Tüzüner T, Yanik SH, Görgeç M. Subcoracoid dislocation of the acromioclavicular joint. Acta Orthop Traumatol Turc. 2011;45(6):463–5.

47. Gerber C, Rockwood Jr CA. Subcoracoid dislocation of the lateral end of the clavicle. A report of three cases. J Bone Joint Surg Am. 1987;69(6):924–7.

48. McPhee IB. Inferior dislocation of the outer end of the clavicle. J Trauma. 1980;20(8):709–10.

49. Patterson WR. Inferior dislocation of the distal end of the clavicle. A case report. J Bone Joint Surg Am. 1967;49(6):1184–6.

50. Schwarz N, Kuderna H. Inferior acromioclavicular separation. Report of an unusual case. Clin Orthop Relat Res. 1988;234:28–30.

51. Arrigoni P, Brady PC, Zottarelli L, Barth J, Narbona P, Huberty D, Koo SS, Adams CR, Parten P, Denard PJ, Burkhart SS. Associated lesions requiring additional surgical treatment in grade 3 acromioclavicular joint dislocations. Arthroscopy. 2014;30(1):6–10.

52. Blazar PE, Iannotti JP, Williams GR. Anteroposterior instability of the distal clavicle after distal clavicle resection. Clin Orthop Relat Res. 1998;348:114–20.

53. Simovitch R, Sanders B, Ozbaydar M, Lavery K, Warner JJ. Acromioclavicular joint injuries: diagnosis and management. J Am Acad Orthop Surg. 2009;17(4):207–19.

54. Carbone S, Postacchini R, Gumina S. Scapular dyskinesis and SICK syndrome in patients with a chronic type III acromioclavicular dislocation. Results of rehabilitation. Knee Surg Sports Traumatol Arthrosc. 2014 (in press).

55. Gumina S, Carbone S, Postacchini F. Scapular dyskinesis and SICK scapular syndrome in patients with chronic type III acromioclavicular dislocation. Arthroscopy. 2009;25(1):40–5.

56. Murena L, Canton G, Culcano E, Cherubino P. Scapular dyskinesis and SICK scapular syndrome following surgical treatment of type III acute acromioclavicular dislocations. Knee Surg Sports Traumatol Arthrosc. 2013;21(5):1146–50.

57. Charron KM, Schepsis AA, Voloshin I. Arthroscopic distal clavicle resection in athletes: a prospective comparison of the direct and indirect approach. Am J Sports Med. 2007;35(1):53–8.

58. Kassarjian A, Llopis E, Palmer WE. Distal clavicular osteolysis: MR evidence for subchondral fracture. Skeletal Radiol. 2007;36(1):17–22.

59. Schwarzkopf R, Ishak C, Elman M, Gelber J, Strauss DN, Jazrawi LM. Distal clavicular osteolysis: a review of the literature. Bull NYU Hosp Jt Dis. 2008;66(2):94–101.

60. de la Puente R, Boutin RD, Theodorou DJ, Hooper A, Schweitzer M, Resnick D. Post-traumatic and stress-induced osteolysis of the distal clavicle: MR imaging findings in 17 patients. Skeletal Radiol. 1999;28(4):202–8.

61. Fiorella D, Helms CA, Speer KP. Increased T2 signal intensity in the distal clavicle: incidence and clinical implications. Skeletal Radiol. 2000;29(12):697–702.

62. Patten RM. Atraumatic osteolysis of the distal clavicle: MR findings. J Comput Assist Tomogr. 1995;19(1):92–5.

63. Shaffer BS. Painful conditions of the acromioclavicular joint. J Am Acad Orthop Surg. 1999;7(3):176–88.

64. Stein BE, Wiater JM, Pfaff HC, Bigliani LU, Levine WN. Detection of acromioclavicular joint pathology in asymptomatic shoulders with magnetic resonance imaging. J Shoulder Elbow Surg. 2001;10(3):204–8.

65. Needell SD, Zlatkin MB, Sher JS, Murphy BJ, Uribe JW. MR imaging of the rotator cuff: peritendinous and bone abnormalities in an asymptomatic population. AJR Am J Roentgenol. 1996;166(4):863–7.

66. Mease PJ. Disease-modifying anti-rheumatic drug therapy for spondyloarthropathies: advances in treatment. Curr Opin Rheumatol. 2003;15(3):205–12.

67. Day MS, Nam D, Goodman S, Su EP, Figgie M. Psoriatic arthritis. J Am Acad Orthop Surg. 2012;20(1):28–37.

68. Huang GS, Bachmann D, Taylor JA, Marcelis S, Haghighi P, Resnick D. Calcium pyrophosphate dehydrate crystal deposition disease and pseudogout of the acromioclavicular joint: radiographic and pathologic features. J Rheumatol. 1993;20(12):2077–82.

69. Parperis K, Carrera G, Baynes K, Mutz A, Dubois M, Cerniglia R, Ryan LM. The prevalence of chondrocalcinosis (CC) of the acromioclavicular (AC) joint on chest radiographs and correlation with calcium pyrophosphate dehydrate (CPPD) crystal deposition disease. Clin Rheumatol. 2013;32(9):1383–6.

70. Hong MJ, Kim YD, Ham HD. Acute septic arthritis of the acromioclavicular joint caused by Haemophilus parainfluenzae: a rare causative origin. Clin Rheumatol. 2015;34(4):811–4.

71. Noh KC, Chung KJ, Yu HS, Koh SH, Yoo JH. Arthroscopic treatment of septic arthritis of acromioclavicular joint. Clin Orthop Surg. 2010;2(3):186–90.

72. Hiller AD, Miller JD, Zeller JL. Acromioclavicular joint cyst formation. Clin Anat. 2010;23(2):145–52.

73. Kontakis GM, Karantanas AH, Pasku D, Alpantaki K, Katonis P, Hadjipavlou AG. Delayed diagnosis of a symptomatic osteochondroma of the distal clavicle. Orthopedics. 2006;29(8):734–6.

74. Sugi MT, Fedenko AN, Menendez LR, Allison DC. Clavicular eosinophilic granuloma causing adult shoulder pain. Rare Tumors. 2013;5(1):e8.

75. Walton J, Mahajan S, Paxinos A, Marshall J, Bryant C, Shnier R, Quinn R, Murrell GA. Diagnostic values of tests for acromioclavicular joint pain. J Bone Joint Surg Am. 2004;86-A(4):807–12.

76. Yelland M. A positive result on both the Paxinos test and bone scan ruled in a diagnosis of acromioclavicular joint pain. Evid Based Med. 2005;10(1):27.

77. McLaughlin HL. On the frozen shoulder. Bull Hosp Joint Dis. 1951;12(2):383–93.

78. Moseley HF. Athletic injuries to the shoulder region. Am J Surg. 1959;98:401–22.

79. Maritz NG, Oosthuizen PJ. Diagnostic criteria for acromioclavicular joint pathology. J Bone Joint Surg Br. 2002;78 Suppl 1:78.

80. Chronopoulos E, Kim TK, Park HB, Ashenbrenner D, McFarland EG. Diagnostic value of physical tests for isolated chronic acromioclavicular lesions. Am J Sports Med. 2004;32(3):655–61.

81. Jacob AK, Sallay PI. Therapeutic efficacy of corticosteroid injections in the acromioclavicular joint. Biomed Sci Instrum. 1997;34:380–5.

82. Dawson PA, Adamson GJ, Pink MM, Kornswiet M, Lin S, Shankwiler JA, Lee TQ. Relative contribution of acromioclavicular joint capsule and coracoclavicular ligaments to acromioclavicular stability. J Shoulder Elbow Surg. 2009;18(2):237–44.

The Sternoclavicular Joint

8.1 Introduction

The sternoclavicular (SC) joint is a complex articulation that can have significant anatomic variations within individuals, between individuals, and
throughout a population. Nevertheless, the inherent stability and biomechanics of the SC joint
remain relatively unchanged. While an acute traumatic injury can lead to an anterior or posterior
SC joint dislocation, repetitive micromotion and
shear can lead to degenerative changes which
may produce chronic symptomatology. Clinicians
should be familiar with the anatomy, biomechanics, and process of diagnostic evaluation in
patients with pain or disability related to the SC
joint such that an accurate diagnosis and effective
treatment modality can be chosen.

8.2 Relevant Anatomy and Biomechanics

8.2.1 Osseous Anatomy

Although the clavicle is the first bone to ossify
(fifth gestational week), the medial clavicular
physis typically does not close until at least 25
years of age. In fact, some studies have shown
that physeal closure may not actually occur until
31 years of age in some patients [1, 2]. Therefore,
patients younger than 31 years of age who present with possible SC joint dislocations should be
evaluated for both ligamentous integrity and
patency of the medial clavicular physis.

The SC joint is a diarthrodial joint lined with
synovium that primarily functions to connect the
shoulder girdle to the axial skeleton (Fig. 8.1).
Because the articular surface of the medial clavicle is highly incongruent with the manubrium,
joint stability is maintained primarily by strong
ligamentous attachments. Specifically, the articular surface of the medial clavicle is much larger
than that of the manubrium and has been described
as having a "saddle-like" configuration (i.e., concave in the axial plane and convex in the coronal
plane) which biomechanically functions similarly
to a ball-and-socket joint (Fig. 8.2) [4, 5].

Both the manubrium and the medial clavicle
can have a variety of different anatomic configu-
rations which may vary across populations,
between genders and, potentially, within the same
patient [6, 7]. Tuscano et al. [7] quantified this
asymmetry in a series of 104 patients who had
previously undergone a computed tomography
(CT) scan of the chest for other reasons. In their
study, the investigators measured joint spaces and
the maximum diameter of the medial clavicular
head in each patient. Overall, joint spaces ranged
from 0.2 to 1.37 cm across the study population
and medial clavicular head diameters ranged
from 1.2 to 3.7 cm. Interestingly, some patients
displayed differences in medial clavicular head
diameters between their right and left clavicles
(range, 0.0–1.0 cm difference). Other authors
have found that the manubrium may also be sub-

R.J. Warth and P.J. Millett, *Physical Examination of the Shoulder: An Evidence-Based Approach*,
DOI 10.1007/978-1-4939-2593-3_8, © Springer Science+Business Media New York 2015

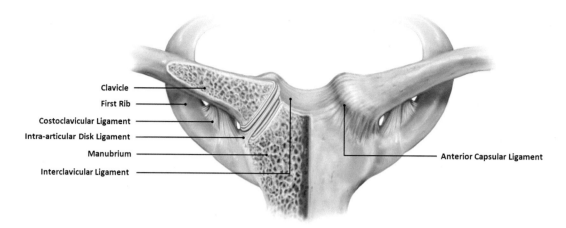

Fig. 8.1 Illustration highlighting the important structural components of the SC joint. (From Martetschläger et al. [3]; with permission).

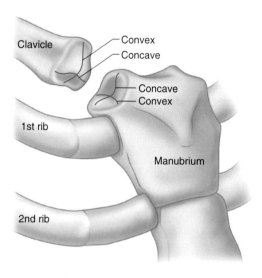

Fig. 8.2 The articular surfaces of the sternum and medial clavicle are incongruent, although the medial clavicle typically exists in a "saddle" configuration (i.e., concave in the axial plane and convex in the coronal plane).

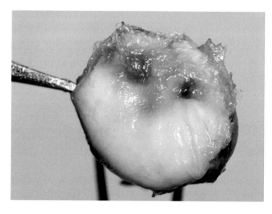

Fig. 8.3 Approximately two-thirds of the medial clavicle is covered with articular cartilage. The forceps point to the pectoralis ridge which may be an important landmark for surgical orientation. (From Warth RJ, Lee JT, Millett PJ. Anatomy and biomechanics of the sternoclavicular joint. Oper Tech Sports Med. 2014;22(3):248–52; with permission).

ject to significant anatomic variation [8]. As a result, osseous asymmetry of the SC joint should be expected in the clinical setting to prevent misdiagnoses and unnecessary surgery.

8.2.2 Chondral Surfaces

The articular surfaces of the medial clavicle and the manubrium are covered with hyaline cartilage that eventually become fibrocartilage with increasing age [9]. Recent dissections performed at this institution revealed that only approximately two-thirds of the medial clavicle was covered with articular cartilage: the majority of this cartilage was found anteriorly and inferiorly where the medial clavicle was devoid of capsuloligamentous attachments (Fig. 8.3). This finding has also been confirmed by others [10]. We also identified a previously undescribed ridge that traveled along the superior aspect of the clavicular head of the pectoralis major insertion site [11]. This "pectoralis ridge" may prove to be

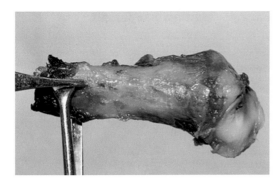

Fig. 8.4 The forceps point to the pectoralis ridge of the medial clavicle. The ridge extends from the tip of the forceps medially towards the articular surface.

an important landmark for orientation during arthroscopy or rotational alignment during open reconstructive procedures (see Figs. 8.3 and 8.4).

8.2.3   Ligamentous Anatomy

As mentioned above, the articular surfaces of the SC joint are highly incongruent and rely primarily on the patency of static capsuloligamentous structures to maintain stability. These structures include the capsular ligaments, costoclavicular ligament, interclavicular ligament, and the intra-articular disc ligament.

8.2.3.1   Capsular Ligaments

Integrated within the SC joint capsule are discrete thickenings that represent the anterior and posterior capsular ligaments. The anterior capsular ligament runs from an area just superior to the articular cartilage of the medial clavicle to an area just superior to the articular cartilage of the manubrium. The posterior capsular ligament is essentially a thickening of the entire posterior capsule and spans between the posterosuperior aspect of the medial clavicle to the posterior aspect of the manubrium. Several studies have shown that the posterior capsule is most important for the maintenance of horizontal stability, thus preventing anterior and posterior translation of the medial clavicle [12, 13]. The anterior capsular ligament most likely plays a secondary role in the maintenance of horizontal stability.

8.2.3.2   Costoclavicular Ligament

The costoclavicular ligament is a thick, robust fibrous band that inserts across the costochondral junction of the first rib and travels towards the inferior aspect of the medial clavicle to insert on the costoclavicular tubercle (see Fig. 8.1) [11]. The ligament is commonly described as being composed of two separate fascicles (anterior and posterior) oriented in a "twisted" configuration with an interposed bursa spanning between the first rib and the medial clavicle [14]. However, our recent cadaveric dissections revealed that the costoclavicular ligament may actually exist as a single ligament since we were unable to identify or separate the previously described anterior and posterior fascicles [11]. The costoclavicular ligament may be the most important ligamentous stabilizer of the SC joint in both the vertical and the horizontal axes [14, 15].

8.2.3.3   Interclavicular Ligament

The interclavicular ligament is a thick, fibrous band that lies over the superior aspect of the manubrium as it runs between the superomedial aspect of each SC joint capsule (see Fig. 8.1) [11]. Despite its anatomic position and thickness, the interclavicular ligament actually does not significantly contribute to vertical stability of the SC joint. Although we were able to identify the ligament in all of our recent cadaveric dissections, its attachments to the manubrium and the SC joint capsules are quite weak and could potentially be removed during the reflection of overlying soft tissues [11].

8.2.3.4   Intra-Articular Disc Ligament

The intra-articular disc ligament attaches near the chondral junction of the first rib, passes through the SC joint (thus creating two separate joint spaces), and inserts along the superior margin of the articular cartilage of the medial clavicle (see Fig. 8.1). This ligament does not confer joint stability. Rather, it probably functions to diminish the force transmission between the manubrium and the medial clavicle which is thought to decrease the detrimental effects of bony incongruity on the health of the articular surfaces [9,

16, 17]. The morphology of the intra-articular disc has also been shown to vary considerably between individuals. Although DePalma [9] found the intra-articular disc to be complete in 97 % of his specimens, others have found that as many was 52 % of specimens may have disc degeneration which is often clinically associated with symptomatic osteoarthritis of the SC joint [10, 13, 17, 18].

8.2.4   Mediastinal Vessels

Traumatic injuries to the SC joint can result in severe complications due to the proximity of the mediastinal vessels, especially in those with posterior SC joint dislocations. These mediastinal vessels include the subclavian vessels, the right and left brachiocephalic veins, the brachiocephalic artery and the left carotid artery (Fig. 8.5).

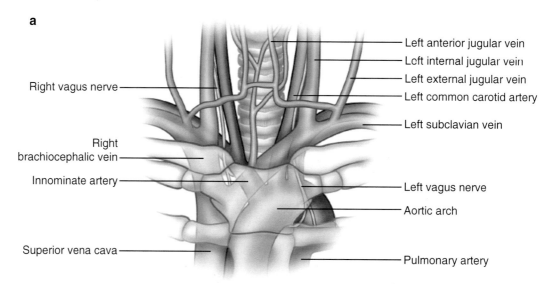

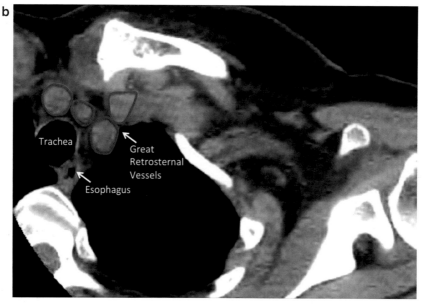

Fig. 8.5 (**a**) Illustration showing the important structures that are situated posterior to the SC joint. (**b**) CT scan showing the orientation of these structures in the axial plane.

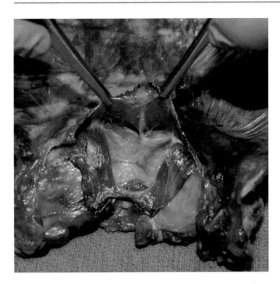

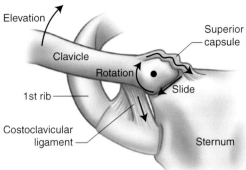

Fig. 8.7   Anterior view showing the motion across the SC joint as the humerus is elevated above 90°.

Fig. 8.6 Cadaveric dissection photograph showing the fascial raphe between the sternohyoid and sternothyroid muscles which is thought to provide some protection to the mediastinal vessels.

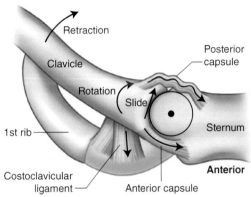

Fig. 8.8   Axial view showing the motion across the SC joint as the shoulder is protracted and retracted.

According to Ponce et al. [6], the closest vessel lies approximately 6.6 mm deep to the posterior SC joint capsule (left or right brachiocephalic vein). In some cases, the subclavian vein may actually cross over the first rib along the posterolateral aspect of the costoclavicular ligament before merging with the brachiocephalic vein [14].

In our cadaveric dissections, the fascial raphe between the sternohyoid and sternothyroid muscles was found to provide some protection to the mediastinal vessels since it forms a physical barrier between the medial clavicle and the mediastinal vessels (Fig. 8.6). We also noted a "safe zone" for posterior dissection in the interval between the sternothyroid muscle and area directly posterior to the manubrium and the medial clavicle [11]. However, in the event of posterior dislocation, the sternohyoid and sternothyroid muscle bellies may become disrupted, placing the posterior vessels at an increased risk for iatrogenic injury during posterior surgical dissection of the SC joint. Disruption of the sternohyoid and sternothyroid muscle bellies can easily be identified on diagnostic axial MRI scans.

8.2.5   Biomechanics

For every 10° of humeral elevation, the SC joint contributes approximately 4° of rotation (Fig. 8.7) [19]. The SC joint also contributes approximately 50° of posterior rotation with every 35° of elevation, flexion and extension of the humerus (Fig. 8.8) [20, 21]. Therefore, surgical procedures involving rigid fixation of the SC joint have largely been abandoned due to the potential for poor functional outcomes in addition to the high reported incidence of hardware failure. Large resections of the medial clavicle have also been reported; however, this can result in uncontrollable scapulothoracic motion and, therefore, may require subsequent scapulothoracic fusion [22].

In a biomechanical study performed to evaluate the structures involved in resisting vertical displacement of the medial clavicle, Bearn [12] applied a downward force to the distal clavicle and determined the structures providing the most resistance to upward migration of the medial clavicle after sequential ligament sectioning. In that study, the posterosuperior capsule was found to be the primary restraint to superior migration of the medial clavicle while the interclavicular ligament, the intra-articular disc ligament, and the anterior joint capsule provided little resistance to vertical displacement. More recently, Spencer et al. [13] evaluated the ligamentous restraints to horizontal translation of the medial clavicle. In their study, 24 cadaveric SC joints were dissected and sub-failure horizontal loads were applied to the medial clavicle to measure anteroposterior joint translation. They found that the costoclavicular and interclavicular ligaments did not significantly contribute to the resistance of horizontal translation of the medial clavicle. However, transection of posterior capsule resulted in an increased posterior translation of 106 % and an increased anterior translation of 41 % relative to an intact control specimen. Division of the anterior capsule resulted in an increased anterior translation of 25 %; however, this degree of anterior translation was less than that which was observed after sectioning of the posterior capsule. The results of these studies indicate that the posterior capsule is important for both vertical and horizontal stability and restoring its function should be the primary goal of ligamentous reconstruction.

8.3 Acute Sternoclavicular Joint Dislocation

8.3.1 Pathogenesis

Injuries to the SC joint are uncommon and account for less than 3 % of all injuries to the shoulder girdle [23, 24]. Due to the strength of its ligamentous stabilizers, subluxation or dislocation of the SC joint typically requires high-energy

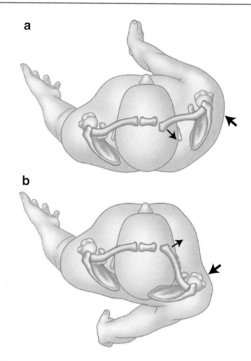

Fig. 8.9 Most common mechanisms that result in acute SC joint dislocations. (**a**) A blow to the shoulder from the posterolateral direction can force the medial clavicle posteriorly relative to the sternum. (**b**) A blow to the shoulder from the anterolateral direction can force the medial clavicle anteriorly relative to the sternum (more common).

trauma (Fig. 8.9) [25, 26]. In fact, many patients who present with these injuries often sustain other, more dramatic injuries that require more immediate attention [27, 28]. As a result, the diagnosis can be missed which can have devastating consequences, especially in some cases of posterior SC joint dislocation where disruption of the mediastinal vessels may have occurred. Injury to the mediastinal vessels is much more likely when a posterior dislocation results in disruption of the sternohyoid and sternothyroid muscles as evidenced by axial imaging studies [11].

Instability of the SC joint is typically classified according to etiology (traumatic versus atraumatic), chronicity (acute versus chronic, direction (anterior versus posterior), and severity (sprain, subluxation or complete dislocation) [26, 29, 30]. The most referenced classification system for SC joint instability, developed by Allman in 1967, accounts for the degree of ligamentous disruption [29]. Type I injuries represent a simple sprain of the SC capsuloligamentous structures without evidence of increased medial clavicular mobility. Type II injuries involve a partial disruption of the SC capsuloligamentous structures and results in anterior or posterior subluxation of the medial clavicle. Type III injuries are the most severe and represent a complete rupture of all supporting ligaments which leads to complete anterior or posterior dislocation of the medial clavicle. It is important to remember that an apparent SC joint injury in a patient younger than 31 years of age may actually represent fracture of the medial clavicular physis (e.g., Salter–Harris type 1 or 2 injury) rather than injury to the capsuloligamentous structures of the SC joint (i.e., "pseudodislocation") [1, 2, 30, 31].

8.3.2 Physical Examination

In most cases, patients with acute injuries to the SC joint typically complain of pain and swelling in the vicinity of the medial clavicle after a traumatic event. While anterior dislocations are usually evident due to the prominence of the medial clavicle with scapulohumeral motion (Fig. 8.10), posterior dislocations are less obvious since the medial clavicle has migrated posteriorly and, thus, does not produce an anterior prominence despite the possibility of extensive swelling. These injuries may be more difficult to recognize in patients with multiple trauma (especially in narcotized and ventilated patients) since other, more dramatic injuries may mask the SC joint injury. Thorough inspection and palpation of the entire clavicle is necessary to rule out concomitant fractures and the possibility of acromioclavicular (AC) joint dislocation ("floating clavicle") [32–34]. In patients with Allman type I or II injuries, severe anterior chest and shoulder pain is often exacerbated by arm motion and supine repositioning [30].

In acute anterior SC joint dislocations, closed reduction is usually attempted in the emergency room [30, 35, 36]. In most cases, the medial clavicle will reduce when a firm posteriorly directed pressure is applied by the clinician with the patient supine and a thick pad placed beneath the thoracic spine to retract the scapulae. However,

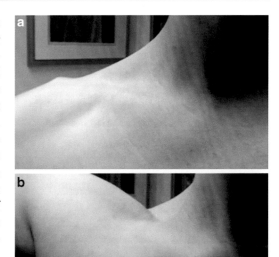

Fig. 8.10 Anterior subluxation of the medial clavicle with humeral elevation. (**a**) The medial clavicle remains in a reduced position when the humerus is at the side. (**b**) The medial clavicle subluxates anteriorly (arrow) as the humerus is elevated above the horizontal plane. Note that this particular patient presented with chronic instability. Pain and swelling over the SC joint with additional guarding is generally present in cases of acute traumatic instability.

spontaneous re-dislocation may occur immediately after the clinician removes this pressure [30]. When maintenance of reduction cannot be safely achieved, outpatient reconstruction of the SC joint may be needed to restore shoulder function, to maintain joint stability and to prevent the progression of post-traumatic osteoarthritis [3].

Acute posterior SC joint dislocations should always be considered an emergency since up to 30 % of these injuries result in compromise of the mediastinal vasculature [37]. These patients may display evidence of venous congestion in the neck or ipsilateral arm in addition to coughing, dyspnea, hoarseness, or dysphagia which may suggest disruption of airway patency. Standard anteroposterior (AP) radiographs (including a Serendipity view [26]) and a computed tomographic (CT) scan of the chest should always be obtained in the setting of any acute SC joint dislocation (Figs. 8.11 and 8.12). In the case of a posterior dislocation, a

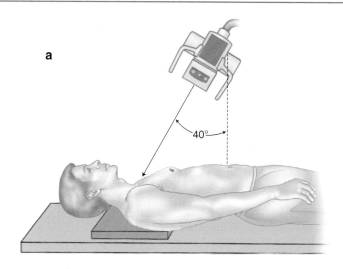

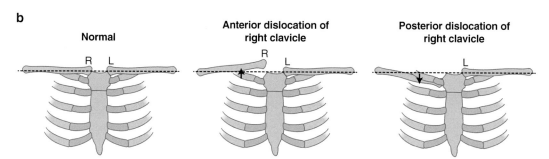

Fig. 8.11 (**a**) The technique used to obtain a Serendipity view of the SC joint. With the patient supine, the X-ray beam is centered over the SC joint with approximately 40° of cephalad angulation. (**b**) Illustration showing the interpretation of the resulting Serendipity view.

Fig. 8.12 Axial CT scan demonstrating a left posterior SC joint dislocation. This patient presented with dysphagia and underwent urgent reconstruction.

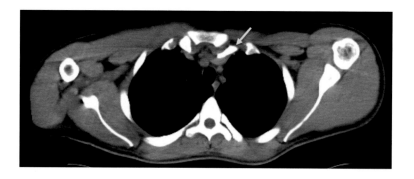

CT angiogram should also be obtained and the on-call cardiothoracic surgeon should be made aware of the situation [27, 30]. Closed reduction of a posterior SC joint dislocation should never be performed in the emergency room without prior consultation with a cardiothoracic surgeon.

8.4 Osteoarthritis of the Sternoclavicular Joint

8.4.1 Pathogenesis

Progressive articular cartilage degeneration of the SC joint most commonly occurs following an acute injury to surrounding capsuloligamentous structures, especially in cases that were initially treated nonoperatively [35, 38]. On the other hand, osteoarthritis of the SC joint can also have atraumatic etiologies such as SAPHO syndrome (*s*ynovitis, *a*cne, *p*ustulosis, *h*yperostosis, *o*steitis), avascular necrosis, tumors, septic arthritis, and rheumatoid arthritis, among other potential causes. The indications for surgical treatment of these conditions are case-based [3].

8.4.2 Physical Examination

Patients with degenerative conditions involving the SC joint will generally present with pain and swelling over the medial clavicle in the absence of a recent traumatic injury. The clinician should palpate the SC joint to detect crepitus or microinstability while the shoulder is placed through a range of motion. However, shoulder range of motion is often inhibited due to significant pain, swelling, and crepitation that can often be relieved following injection of local anesthetic and/or corticosteroids. Although nonoperative treatment is typically the modality of choice, some patients with recalcitrant symptoms may require open [39] or arthroscopic [40] resection arthroplasty of the SC joint to alleviate their symptoms.

8.5 Voluntary Instability of the Sternoclavicular Joint

Voluntary subluxation or dislocation of the SC joint is an extremely rare condition that is most often seen in young patients with multiligamentous laxity. The ability to subluxate the joint with specific positions and movements of the arm is usually discovered during adolescence. Although the condition is mostly asymptomatic, some patients may develop symptoms related to instability or chondral degeneration due to the high frequency of subluxation, especially in those involved in overhead sports or manual labor.

8.6 Summary

Unfortunately, pathologies related to the SC joint have been less well studied when compared to other areas of the shoulder girdle. However, the clinician is still charged to make accurate and rapid diagnoses and treatment decisions. Knowledge of basic anatomy and biomechanics along with pertinent radiographic features and physical examination findings will allow clinicians to successfully evaluate and treat patients with SC joint pathologies in an efficient manner.

References

1. Koch MJ, Wells L. Proximal clavicle physeal fracture with posterior displacement: diagnosis, treatment, and prevention. Orthopedics. 2012;35(1):e108–11.
2. Webb PA, Schuey JM. Epiphyseal union of the anterior iliac crest and medial clavicle in a modern multiracial sample of American males and females. Am J Phys Anthropol. 1985;68(4):457–66.
3. Martetschläger F, Warth RJ, Millett PJ. Instability and degenerative arthritis of the sternoclavicular joint: a current concepts review. Am J Sports Med. 2014; 42(4):999–1007.
4. Hobbs DW. Sternoclavicular joint: a new axial radiographic view. Radiology. 1968;90:801.
5. Lowman CL. Operative correction of old sternoclavicular dislocation. J Bone Joint Surg. 1928;10:740–1.
6. Ponce BA, Kundukulam JA, Pflugner R, McGwin G, Meyer R, Carroll W, Minnich DJ, Larrison MC. Sternoclavicular joint surgery: how far does danger lurk below? J Shoulder Elbow Surg. 2013;22(7): 993–9.
7. Tuscano D, Banerjee S, Terk MR. Variations in normal sternoclavicular joints; a retrospective study to quantify SCJ asymmetry. Skeletal Radiol. 2009; 38(10):997–1001.
8. Wijertna MD, Turmezei TD, Tytherleigh-Strong G. Novel assessment of the sternoclavicular joint with computed tomography for planning interventional approach. Skeletal Radiol. 2013;42(4):473–8.
9. DePalma AF. Surgical anatomy of the acromioclavicular and sternoclavicular joints. Surg Clin North Am. 1963;43:1541–50.

10. van Tongel A, van Hoof T, Pouliart N, Debeer P, D'Herde K, De Wilde L. Arthroscopy of the sternoclavicular joint: an anatomic evaluation of structures at risk. Surg Radiol Anat. 2014;36(4):375–81.
11. Lee JT, Campbell K, Michalski M, Wilson K, Spiegl U, Wijdicks C, Millett PJ. Surgical anatomy of the sternoclavicular joint: a qualitative and quantitative anatomical study. J Bone Joint Surg. 2014; 96(19):e166.
12. Bearn JG. Direct observations on the function of the capsule of the sternoclavicular joint in the clavicular support. J Anat. 1967;101(Pt 1):159–70.
13. Spencer EE, Kuhn JE, Huston LJ, Carpenter JE, Hughes RE. Ligamentous restraints to anterior and posterior translation of the sternoclavicular joint. J Shoulder Elbow Surg. 2002;11(1):43–7.
14. Cave AJ. The nature and morphology of the costoclavicular ligament. J Anat. 1961;95:170–9.
15. Tubbs RS, Shah NA, Sullivan BP, Marchase ND, Cömert A, Acar HI, Tekdemir I, Loukas M, Shoja MM. The costoclavicular ligament revisited: a functional and anatomic study. Rom J Morphol Embryol. 2009;50(3):475–9.
16. Brossman J, Stäbler A, Preidler K, Trudell D, Resnick D. Sternoclavicular joint: MR imaging–anatomic correlation. Radiology. 1996;198(1):193–8.
17. Emura K, Arakawa T, Terashima T, Miki A. Macroscopic and histological observations on the human sternoclavicular joint disc. Anat Sci Int. 2009; 84(3):182–8.
18. Barbaix E, Lapierre M, Van Roy P, Clarijs JP. The sternoclavicular joint: variants of the discus articularis. Clin Biomech (Bristol, Avon). 2000;15 Suppl 1:S3–7.
19. Renfree KJ, Wright KW. Anatomy and biomechanics of the acromioclavicular and sternoclavicular joints. Clin Sports Med. 2003;22:219–37.
20. Inman VT, Saunders DM, Abbott LC. Observations on the function of the shoulder joint. J Bone Joint Surg. 1944;26:1–30.
21. Rockwood CA, Williams GR, Young DC. Disorders of the acromioclavicular joint. In: Rockwood Jr CA, Mattson FA, editors. The shoulder. 2nd ed. Philadelphia: WB Saunders; 1998.
22. Elhassan B, Chung ST, Ozbaydar M, Diller D, Warner JJ. Scapulothoracic fusion for clavicular insufficiency. A report of two cases. J Bone Joint Surg Am. 2008;90(4):875–80.
23. Groh GI, Wirth MA. Management of traumatic sternoclavicular joint injuries. J Am Acad Orthop Surg. 2011;19(1):1–7.
24. Panzica M, Zeichen J, Hankemeier S, Gaulke R, Krettek C, Jagodzinski M. Long-term outcome after joint reconstruction or medial resection arthroplasty

for anterior SCJ instability. Arch Orthop Trauma Surg. 2010;130(5):657–65.
25. de Jong KP, Sukul DM. Anterior sternoclavicular dislocation: a long term follow-up study. J Orthop Trauma. 1990;4(4):420–3.
26. Wirth MA, Rockwood CA. Disorders of the sternoclavicular joint. In: Rockwood Jr CA, Matsen III FA, Wirth MA, Lippitt SB, editors. The shoulder. 4th ed. Philadelphia: Saunders; 2009. p. 527–60.
27. Chaudhry FA, Killampalli VV, Chowdhry M, Holland P, Knebel RW. Posterior dislocation of the sternoclavicular joint in a young rugby player. Acta Orthop Traumatol Turc. 2011;45(5):376–8.
28. Perron AD. Chest pain in athletes. Clin Sports Med. 2003;22:37–50.
29. Allman Jr FL. Fractures and ligamentous injuries of the clavicle and its articulation. J Bone Joint Surg Am. 1967;49(4):774–84.
30. Iannotti JP, Williams GR. Disorders of the shoulder: diagnosis and management. Philadelphia: Lippincott Williams & Wilkins; 1999. p. 765–813.
31. El Mekkaoui MJ, Sekkach N, Bazeli A, Faustin JM. Proximal clavicle physeal fracture-separation mimicking an anterior sterno-clavicular dislocation. Orthop Traumatol Surg Res. 2011;97(3):349–52.
32. Eni-Olotu DO, Hobbs NJ. Floating clavicle – simultaneous dislocation of both ends of the clavicle. Injury. 1997;28(4):319–20.
33. Sanders JO, Lyons FA, Rockwood Jr CA. Management of dislocations of both ends of the clavicle. J Bone Joint Surg Am. 1990;72(3):399–402.
34. Thomas Jr CB, Friedman RJ. Ipsilateral sternoclavicular dislocation and clavicle fracture. J Orthop Trauma. 1989;3(4):355–7.
35. Lunseth PA, Chapman KW, Frankel VH. Surgical treatment of chronic dislocations of the sterno-clavicular joint. J Bone Joint Surg Br. 1975;57(2):193–6.
36. Yeh GL, Williams Jr GR. Conservative management of sternoclavicular injuries. Orthop Clin North Am. 2000;31(2):189–203.
37. Bicos J, Nicholson GP. Treatment and results of sternoclavicular joint injuries. Clin Sports Med. 2003; 22(2):359–70.
38. Eskola A, Vainionpaa S, Vastamaki M, Slatis P, Rokkanen P. Operation for old sternoclavicular dislocation: results in 12 cases. J Bone Joint Surg Br. 1989;71(1):63–5.
39. Rockwood CA, Groh GI, Wirth MA, Grassi FA. Resection arthroplasty of the sternoclavicular joint. J Bone Joint Surg Am. 1997;79(3):387–93.
40. Warth RJ, Lee JT, Campbell KJ, Millett PJ. Arthroscopic sternoclavicular joint resection arthroplasty: a technical note and illustrated case report. Arthrosc Tech. 2014;3(1):e165–73.

Scapular Dyskinesis

9

9.1 Introduction

The scapula is a complex osseous structure that plays a critical role in the maintenance of glenohumeral stability throughout the entire range of motion of the shoulder. Therefore, an evaluation of scapular motion should be performed in each patient to prevent the development or progression of various shoulder conditions such as rotator cuff disease and glenohumeral instability. Specific physical exam findings and observations related to scapular motion can have a significant effect on the approach to either operative or nonoperative management in patients who present with shoulder pain. As an example, increased upward rotation of the scapula may be a compensatory mechanism to *prevent* pain related to shoulder pathology whereas increased downward rotation may be factor associated with the *production* of shoulder pathology [1]. An understanding of the pertinent anatomy and biomechanics of scapular motion is required before any diagnosis can be made regarding scapular motion.

9.2 Anatomy and Biomechanics

The primary function of the scapula is to provide a stable fulcrum against which humeral elevation and rotation can occur. This is achieved through dynamic positioning of the glenoid to maximize glenohumeral contact through all planes of shoulder motion (see Chap. 3 for a detailed explanation of normal three-dimensional scapular motion). A complete understanding of the osseous, muscular, bursal, and neurovascular anatomy along with the biomechanics of normal scapular motion is critical to the evaluation of any patient with shoulder pathology.

9.2.1 Osseous Anatomy

The scapula is a large, flat, triangular-shaped bone positioned over the posterior thorax between the second and seventh ribs. The scapula has three borders (superior, medial, and lateral) and two important angles (superomedial and inferomedial) that primarily serve as sites for muscle attachment (Fig. 9.1). According to Lewitt [2], the three-dimensional resting position of the scapula is defined as being tilted anteriorly between 10° and 20° and medially rotated in the coronal plane between 30° and 40° (in other words, the glenoid faces more in the superior direction). As discussed in Chap. 2, the scapula is also angled anteriorly between 10° and 20° from the coronal plane. This position of anterior angulation is often referred to as the "scapular plane" when evaluating the shoulder.

While the general shape of the scapula is fairly consistent across the population, there exist several known topographical variations that may predispose some individuals to certain pathologic conditions (such as scapulothoracic bursitis

Fig. 9.1 Posterior view of a normal scapula. The superior, medial, and lateral borders along with the superomedial and inferomedial angles are labeled.

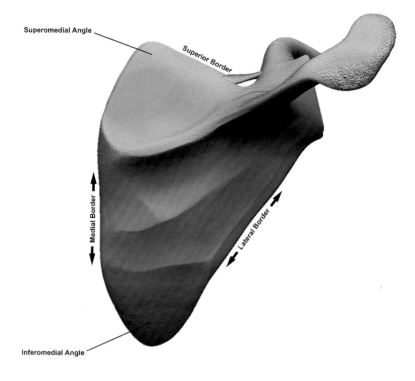

or snapping scapula syndrome). For example, Aggarwal et al. [3] performed measurements in 92 dried scapulae and found that the costal (anterior) surface of the scapula "undulated" and also varied in depth between 10.5 and 26.5 mm. The investigators noted that the thickness of the superomedial angle ranges between 2 and 4 mm whereas the inferomedial angle had a thickness between 5 and 8 mm. Anterior angulation of the superomedial angle also varied between 124° and 162° in the majority of their specimens. In addition, the investigators also identified an anterior "horn-like" projection along the lateral border of at least one scapula. Several researchers have described other osseous abnormalities that may predispose some individuals to painful scapular snapping. These include the superomedial "bare area," [4] the "Luschka tubercle" (bony protuberance at the superomedial angle) [5], the teres major tubercle (located at the insertion of this muscle) [6], and anterior "hooking" of the superomedial angle [7].

The suprascapular notch is located near the junction of the lateral third of the superior scapular border, just medial to the confluence of the coracoid process with the scapular body [8]. The anatomy of the suprascapular notch is also known to have various morphological features that may predispose some individuals to suprascapular nerve entrapment [9–12]. The transverse scapular ligament travels mediolaterally between the crests of the suprascapular notch. In most cases, the suprascapular nerve is found below the ligament and within the notch whereas the suprascapular artery is found above the ligament and outside of the notch (Fig. 9.2). The transverse scapular ligament is also known to have significant anatomic variations that can also generate symptoms related to suprascapular nerve entrapment [13, 14].

9.2.2 Muscular Anatomy

The scapulothoracic articulation is unique in that its motion is not dictated by osseous constraints. Rather, the scapula is positioned through the dynamic, coordinated action of surrounding periscapular muscles (see Chap. 3). Therefore, disruption or dysfunction of any one of these muscles can result in scapular malposition or dyskinetic motion which can lead to disordered shoulder function.

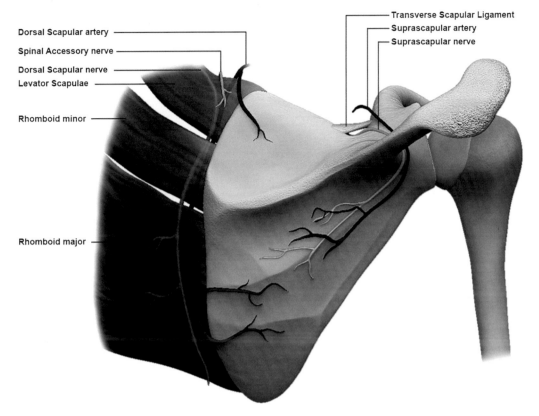

Dorsal Scapular artery

Spinal Accessory nerve

Dorsal Scapular nerve

Levator Scapulae

Rhomboid minor

Rhomboid major

Transverse Scapular Ligament
Suprascapular artery
Suprascapular nerve

Fig. 9.2 Posterior view of a normal scapula with important neurovascular structures highlighted. The dorsal scapular nerve and artery lie approximately 2 cm medial to the medial scapular border. The suprascapular nerve travels below the transverse scapular ligament whereas the suprascapular artery passes above the ligament.

9.2.3   Bursal Anatomy

Bursae are fluid-filled sacs lined with synovial-like cells that facilitate gliding of opposing surfaces over one another. In the case of the scapula, there are several periscapular bursae that allow the scapula to glide smoothly over interposed muscle layers. These bursae are commonly defined as either "anatomic" or "adventitial" bursae, depending on their propensity to cause periscapular pain [15]. Anatomic bursae are typically thought to represent normal, physiologic bursae that allow smooth gliding over the posterior thorax. The infraserratus and supraserratus bursae lie on either side of the serratus anterior muscle along the medial scapular border and are the most frequently recognized anatomic bursae [15, 16]. Adventitial bursae are most often located at the superomedial or inferomedial scapular

angles and are thought to be significant pathological pain generators [17, 18]. Some researchers have suggested that pain near the superomedial angle can be due to pathologic infraserratus or supraserratus bursal tissue [19, 20], pain near the inferomedial angle is most likely the result of pathologic infraserratus bursal tissue [21, 22], and pain near the confluence of the scapular spine may be caused by a pathologic scapulotrapezial bursa which is most commonly located deep to the trapezius and superficial to the scapular spine (Fig. 9.3) [23].

9.2.4   Neurovascular Anatomy

Knowledge of pertinent neurovascular anatomy around the scapula is necessary to fully evaluate any patient with a condition related to disordered

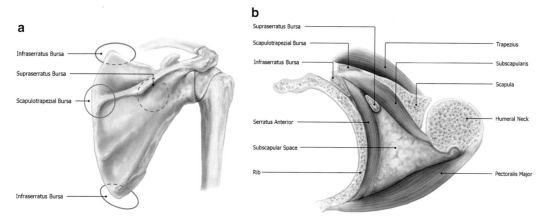

Fig. 9.3 Illustrations demonstrating the positions of the pertinent periscapular bursae. (**a**) Positions of the periscapular bursae relative to the scapular body. (**b**) Axial view showing the positions of the periscapular bursae relative to the surrounding musculature from [23].

shoulder motion (see Chap. 3). The spinal accessory nerve, which innervates the levator scapulae muscle, travels with the transverse cervical artery along the levator scapulae muscle which is situated deep to the trapezius muscle. In some cases, the spinal accessory nerve may penetrate through the central portion of the levator scapulae [24]. As the transverse cervical artery travels distally, it becomes the dorsal scapular artery which, in turn, travels with the dorsal scapular nerve beneath the rhomboid musculature a few fingerbreadths medial to the medial scapular border (see Fig. 9.2) [25]. The long thoracic nerve is relatively protected as it travels along the anterior aspect of the serratus anterior muscle. The suprascapular nerve arises from the superior trunk of the brachial plexus and courses towards the suprascapular notch with the suprascapular artery. As mentioned above, the suprascapular nerve passes beneath the transverse scapular ligament whereas the suprascapular artery travels above the ligament (see Fig. 9.2).

9.2.5 Biomechanics

With respect to normal shoulder kinematics, the scapula has several important functions that should be considered before evaluating any patient with a complaint related to the shoulder. First, the scapula provides a stable fulcrum against which glenohumeral motion can occur through the dynamic action of the periscapular musculature, including the rotator cuff and deltoid muscles. In fact, several authors have shown that external stabilization of the scapula may improve the contraction strength of the rotator cuff [26, 27]. Smith et al. [27] found that stabilizing the scapula in a position of retraction substantially increased external rotation strength in 20 normal subjects when compared to external rotation strength with the scapula protracted. Similarly, in a series of 20 patients with shoulder pain (but without rotator cuff tears) and ten healthy controls, Kibler et al. [26] demonstrated a 13–24 % increase in supraspinatus strength when the "empty can" test was performed with the scapulae in a retracted position (see Chap. 4 for details regarding Jobe's "empty can" test). In 29 overhead athletes with scapular dyskinesis, Merolla et al. [28] measured significantly increased contraction forces of both the supraspinatus and the infraspinatus muscles following the completion of specially designed rehabilitation protocols designed to improve periscapular muscle balance. The same group published similar results in a series of volleyball players who also demonstrated scapular dyskinesis upon initial presentation [29]. Second, accurate positioning of the scapula through coordinated muscle contractions facilitates glenohumeral articular congruency by maintaining alignment of opposing force couples, thus preserving the so-called concavity compression mechanism of dynamic stability (concavity compression is discussed more thoroughly in Chaps. 4 and 6). Third, the scapula plays an important role in the transmission of force through the kinetic chain. In short, the scapula facilitates the transfer of kinetic and potential energy from the largest muscles of the core and trunk towards site of action [30]. Dynamic scapular stability, which is facilitated by adequate core and trunk strength, is necessary to optimize the efficiency of this complex system [31]. Perhaps one of the most well-known examples of this concept is the classic pitching motion most often utilized to deliver a high-velocity pitch in baseball.

9.3   Scapular Dyskinesis

Although most established sports medicine clinicians (both generalists and upper extremity subspecialists) evaluate and treat patients with some form of scapular dyskinesis on a regular basis, the disorder is still an understudied, underappreciated, and often overlooked category of shoulder dysfunction, especially in novice examiners. The knowledge deficiency in this area may be caused by the relatively infrequent need for surgical intervention, by the lack of sufficient education on the topic or, perhaps, by generational differences in examination and treatment philosophies (such as the gradual transition from primarily experience-based practice to primarily evidence-based practice). In addition to these potential challenges, the precise cause of the condition is often unknown, the risk for secondary injury is often unknown and its effect on shoulder mechanics is probably very complex. In most cases, we prefer to view this problem as a manifestation of some underlying condition rather than an isolated disorder, regardless of whether the pathology is academically defined as "primary" or "secondary" (described below), since appropriate treatment of the underlying condition (ranging from a specific physical therapy protocol to surgical excision of a space-occupying mass) typically resolves the

issue altogether. Once scapular dyskinesis has been detected by the initial screening examination, the remainder of the patient encounter should focus on the evaluation and treatment of its potential causes and effects.

9.3.1   Possible Etiologies of Scapular Dyskinesis

There are numerous potential etiologies responsible for the development of scapular dyskinesis, most of which can be divided into primary and secondary causes.

9.3.1.1 Primary Causes of Scapular Dyskinesis

Primary causes of scapular dyskinesis are most commonly related to mechanical or neurogenic defects. Mechanical problems may be associated with a decrease in the scapulothoracic space, such as kyphoscoliosis, rib fracture callus or hypertrophic nonunion, shortened clavicle as a result of fracture malunion and enlarging soft-tissue or skeletal masses, among several other potential defects, can produce symptoms such as scapulothoracic crepitation with shoulder motion (caused by any abnormality that results in a decreased scapulothoracic space) or clinical findings such as the gradual appearance of scapular malposition (caused by the presence of an enlarging mass within the scapulothoracic space which can push the scapular body away from the posterior thorax, thus producing the appearance of scapular winging and dyskinesis). In addition to disordered scapular motion, many of these mechanical issues manifest as periscapular bursitis, crepitus, or so-called scapular "snapping" and are discussed later in this chapter (see the Sect. 9.3.3.7 below).

9.3.1.2 Secondary Causes of Scapular Dyskinesis

Many patients with shoulder pain develop compensatory periscapular muscle contraction (or relaxation) that functions to limit the pain associated with shoulder motion. This abnormal firing pattern produces disordered scapular motion that, in some cases, may exacerbate the inciting injury.

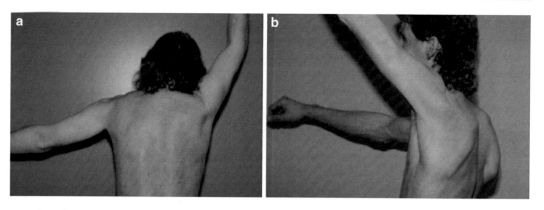

Fig. 9.4 (**a**) Scapular winging due to trapezius muscle weakness. (**b**) Scapular winging due to serratus anterior muscle weakness.

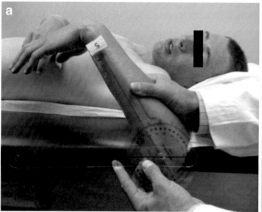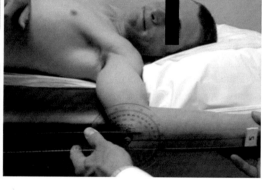

Fig. 9.5 Clinical photographs showing a patient with GIRD. (**a**) Measurement of passive internal rotation with a goniometer revealed decreased internal rotation capacity. (**b**) Measurement of passive external rotation with a goniometer revealed increased external rotation capacity. Because the total arc of motion was decreased, the loss of internal rotation was deemed pathologic (Courtesy of Craig Morgan, MD).

In at least one study, the amplitude of activation and the contraction strength of the serratus anterior muscle was significantly decreased in patients with subacromial impingement. This produced an abnormal scapular resting position (increased anterior tilt and downward rotation) and subsequent scapular dyskinesis due to the unbalanced opposing force couple between the serratus anterior muscle (weaker muscle) and the trapezius muscle (stronger muscle). Other potential etiologies of scapular dyskinesis include AC joint instability and/or degenerative osteoarthritis, some forms of glenohumeral instability and neurogenic causes such as cervical radiculopathy and the oft-cited palsies involving the long thoracic nerve (results in prominence of the medial scapular border) and the spinal accessory nerve (results in more subtle scapular winging with difficulty in abduction) (Fig. 9.4).

Currently, most forms of scapular dyskinesis are attributed to underlying defects related to soft-tissue structures around the shoulder. For example, many overhead athletes display physical evidence of a *glenohumeral internal rotation deficit* (GIRD) which generally is not considered pathologic unless there is an associated range of motion loss relative to the total arc of motion (Fig. 9.5). However, posterior capsular contractures are often found in these same athletes due to repeated throwing [32]. These contractures essentially "stiffen" the posterior capsule such that glenohumeral adduction and internal rotation causes the scapula to internally rotate (or "windup") without input from the periscapular musculature [1]. In this example, the scapula can no longer be placed in a position of maximal glenohumeral contact when the arm is adducted and internally rotated, potentially leading to subsequent injuries if not clinically addressed (often related to the SICK scapula syndrome). Other common findings in patients (most commonly athletes) with scapular dyskinesis are tightness of the short head of the biceps tendon and the pectoralis minor tendon [33]. Because each of their tendons forms an attachment to the coracoid process, tightness of either muscle (or both) can result in scapular malposition and disordered scapular motion.

Overall, many of the above-mentioned etiologies (except for the specific nerve palsies) result in the same general pattern of scapular malposition and dyskinesis—that is, a protracted resting position and further protraction with arm motion. This is the most common manifestation of scapular dyskinesis which can lead to subacromial impingement (due to a decreased volume within the subacromial space), diminished rotator cuff contraction strength (due to alterations in the length-force relationship of each muscle [discussed in Chap. 3]) [26–28], and chronic overuse injuries such as symptomatic internal impingement in throwing athletes (due to repeated supraphysiologic scapulohumeral angulation) and superior labral anterior to posterior (SLAP) tears (due to the "peel back" mechanism proposed by Burkhart et al. [34] [discussed in Chap. 6] and/or repeated maximal tension placed on the anterior capsule). These common secondary effects, which are often at least partially attributed to scapular dyskinesis, can also lead to tertiary pathologies, thus initiating a so-called vicious cycle. The most commonly encountered cascade of events occurs in the following sequence: (1) primary or secondary dyskinesis, which leads to (2) submaximal supraspinatus contraction, which leads to (3) gradual superior humeral head migration, which leads to (4) a gradual decrease in subacromial space, which leads to (5) subacromial impingement and supraspinatus tears, which lead to (6) pain, which leads to (7) compensatory, asymmetric muscle firing patterns, which lead to (8) worsening of scapular malposition, dyskinesis, superior humeral head migration, and so on.

Regardless of the precise cause, recognition and correct interpretation of disordered scapular motion is an extremely important part of the clinical examination that should never be overlooked in any patient who presents with a shoulder complaint. It is important to remember that the scapula also plays an important role in force transmission through the kinetic chain. Therefore, in most athletic (i.e., non-sedentary) individuals with secondary scapular dyskinesis, a thorough, yet efficient assessment of scapular motion can be considered a reflection of muscular symmetry and the overall health of the kinetic chain.

9.3.2 Physical Examination

Scapular dyskinesis is usually diagnosed by simple palpation of the relevant scapular landmarks while also observing both scapulae during movement of the shoulder through the various motion planes. The condition is most often characterized by prominence of the inferomedial angle and the medial scapular border (as a result of protraction in the resting position), early upward rotation of the scapula during arm elevation and/or early downward rotation of the scapula when lowering the arm back to the side (variations in dyskinetic patterns are described below for specific conditions). Recent evidence suggests that increased upward rotation may be associated with symptom *compensation* whereas increased downward rotation may be associated with symptom *causation*. Regardless, any abnormal scapular motion can compromise normal shoulder function by reducing glenohumeral articular congruency, reducing the acromiohumeral distance, increasing tension and strain across the AC joint capsule, decreasing the strength of rotator cuff contraction (which can also reduce glenohumeral stability) and shifting the arc of glenohumeral motion as which commonly occurs in overhead athletes. In addition to these changes, scapular dyskinesis can also mask or enhance the symptoms related to other concomitant shoulder pathologies, such as rotator cuff tears and labral tears, thus complicating the physical diagnosis and subsequent treatment decisions.

Clinical examination of the scapulae should begin with an assessment of posture and symmetry. In many overhead athletes, the dominant

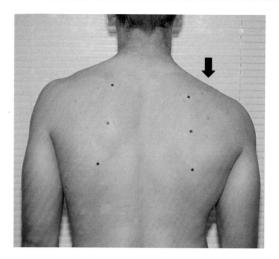

Fig. 9.6 Clinical photograph of right-handed overhead throwing athlete with a depressed right shoulder (Courtesy of Craig Morgan, MD).

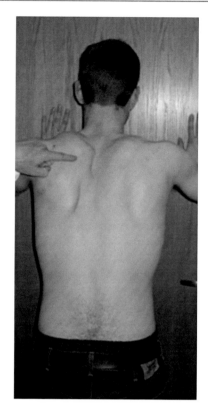

Fig. 9.7 Clinical photograph of a patient performing a wall push-up (also discussed in Chap. 3). Note the prominence of the medial scapular border of the left shoulder, a common finding in patients with scapular dyskinesis.

shoulder will appear to rest in a slightly lower, or depressed, position relative to the contralateral shoulder (Fig. 9.6). This abnormality often occurs in conjunction with SICK scapula syndrome (*s*capular malposition, *i*nferomedial angle prominence, *c*oracoid pain, and scapular dys*k*inesis) which can often be corrected by a focused rehabilitation program. As necessary components of scapular motion, AC and SC joints should also be evaluated for any evidence of pain and/or instability (see Chaps. 7 and 8 for details regarding the AC and SC joints, respectively). The clavicle should also be palpated to confirm adequate length and to identify any abnormal angulation or malrotation.

In most cases, the clinician can identify dyskinetic scapular motion by simple observation, palpation and compression of the medial scapular border as the patient elevates and lowers the affected arm (forward flexion, horizontal abduction, and scaption). Specifically, the appearance of a visible prominence of the medial scapular border with any of these motions can be considered dyskinetic motion (Fig. 9.7) [35]. Weights (e.g., 3 or 5 pounds) can also be used to increase the visibility of medial border prominence with shoulder motion (also known as the scapular dyskinesis test). Similarly, resisted external rotation can also produce same pattern of scapular dyskinesis as that which is observed during humeral

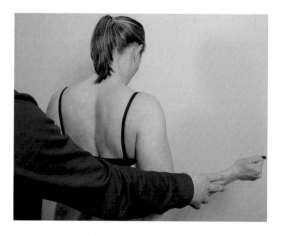

Fig. 9.8 Flip test. Resisted external rotation can often elicit signs of scapular dyskinesis when the examiner is positioned behind the patient in order to visualize both scapulae from posteriorly.

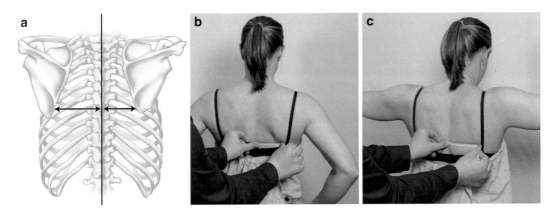

Fig. 9.9 Lateral scapular slide test. (**a**) This test is meant to identify a difference in the medial-lateral positioning of the scapula relative to the thoracic spine. (**b**) With the patient standing and their arms at the side, the examiner uses measuring tape to measure the distance between the inferomedial scapular angle and the midline, typically marked by the spinous processes (be wary of patients with abnormal spinal curvature, such as those with scoliosis). The measurement is repeated for the contralateral scapula. (**c**) The measurement is repeated with the hands on the iliac crests and/or with the arms abducted.

elevation (i.e., a positive "flip test"; Fig. 9.8). Pain with compression of the scapular body against the thoracic wall with shoulder motion may also be an indicator of snapping scapula syndrome.

9.3.2.1 Lateral Scapular Slide Test
The lateral scapular slide test was originally developed by Kibler [36] in 1991 as a method to detect asymmetric scapular resting positions with the arms in various degrees of abduction. According to the original description, the distance from the inferomedial scapular angle to the corresponding spinous process along the same horizontal plane was measured bilaterally with both arms (1) at the side, (2) abducted to approximately 30° and slightly internally rotated (i.e., hands on hips), and (3) abducted to 90° in the coronal plane (Fig. 9.9). Kibler [36] suggested that the latter two testing positions required substantial muscular activation involving the upper and lower trapezius and the serratus anterior muscle—weakness of any of these muscles would therefore produce increased lateral deviation of the scapular body. Thus, a difference in bilateral measurements in any of the three testing positions was considered a positive test. Kibler [37] more recently proposed that this cut-off point be increased to 1.5 cm based on experiences within clinical practice combined with other unpublished work involving scapular mal-

position. However, a study by Odom et al. [38] found no improvement in sensitivity or specificity for the detection of scapular dyskinesis with any of the three testing positions or when the threshold for diagnosis was increased from 1.0 to 1.5 cm. Another study by Shadmehr et al. [39] found that the test was unreliable. However, it should be noted that any study that evaluates the accuracy of a physical examination test for the detection of a specific pathology or defect, the findings on examination should always be coupled with the findings obtained from the diagnostic gold standard. In the case of scapular dyskinesis, there currently does not exist a diagnostic gold standard and, thus, inhibits study interpretation.

9.3.2.2 Scapular Assistance Test
The scapular assistance test was first described by Kibler et al. [26] in 2006 and is typically used to assess the effect of scapular malposition on rotator cuff impingement. In this test, the examiner applies an anterior and superior force to the inferomedial scapular angle to assist upward rotation and posterior tilt of the scapula while the patient flexes and/or abducts the arm (Fig. 9.10). A positive test occurs when the patient reports relief of impingement-like symptoms as the scapula of the affected extremity is manipulated. Acceptable inter-rater reliability has been

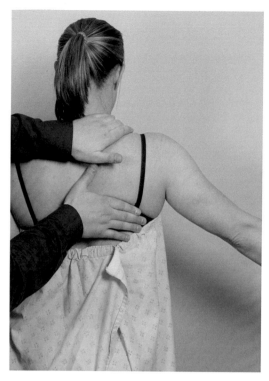

Fig. 9.10 Scapular assistance test. With the patient standing, the examiner places on hand over the superior aspect of the involved scapula with the fingers resting on the anterior clavicle. The examiner's other hand is placed on the inferomedial scapular angle with the fingers pointed towards the lateral thorax. The patient is then asked to slowly abduct the humerus (scapular plane or sagittal plane). During the process of abduction, the examiner facilitates upward rotation of the scapula by pushing upward and laterally on the inferomedial angle. This maneuver encourages increased posterior scapular tilt and may relieve symptoms of rotator cuff impingement during humeral elevation.

reported when the test was performed during elevation in either the scapular plane (scaption) or the sagittal plane (forward flexion) [40].

9.3.2.3 Scapular Retraction Test

The scapular retraction test, described by Kibler et al. [41] in 2009, is often used in conjunction with the dynamic labral shear test (discussed in Chap. 6) or the Jobe test (discussed in Chap. 4) to evaluate the potential role of scapular dyskinesis on supraspinatus strength and labral injuries. In this maneuver, the scapula is first positioned and stabilized in a fully retracted position. With the scapula in this position, the examiner performs the dynamic labral shear test to evaluate the gle-

noid labrum followed by the Jobe test to evaluate supraspinatus strength (empty- or full-can position; however, it is advisable to use the full-can position in the setting of a positive scapular assistance test to minimize symptoms of impingement which can decrease strength measurements) (Fig. 9.11). The test is considered positive when the above-described scapular manipulation decreases the symptoms associated with labral injury or rotator cuff impingement. A similar test has been described for the evaluation of infraspinatus strength in overhead athletes with scapular dyskinesis [42].

9.3.2.4 Scapular Reposition Test

The scapular reposition test was first described in 2008 by Tate et al. [43] as a modification of the scapular retraction test. The investigators aimed to decrease the amount of retraction while also emphasizing increased posterior tilt and external rotation of the scapula. In their study, the Neer sign, Hawkins–Kennedy test, and Jobe's empty can test (these maneuvers are described in Chap. 4) were performed in 142 collegiate-level asymptomatic athletes. If any of the above-mentioned tests were positive, each maneuver was repeated with the addition of manual scapular repositioning. Manual scapular repositioning was performed by first manually grasping the top of the shoulder with the fingers over the AC joint and the thumb resting along the scapula spine. The examiner's forearm was then obliquely positioned over the scapular body. The examiner then applied a moderate force to the scapula using both their hand and forearm to encourage increased posterior tilt and external rotation without achieving full retraction (Fig. 9.12). Following scapular manipulation, the Neer sign and Hawkins–Kennedy test were repeated to assess for any change in shoulder symptoms and the Jobe test was repeated to assess for any change in rotator cuff strength. The intra-class correlation coefficients for the evaluation of rotator cuff strength (using Jobe's empty can test) were above 0.95 when the scapula was in its original resting position and during manual repositioning. No other studies have evaluated the clinical utility of this test.

Fig. 9.11 Scapular retraction test. With the patient standing, the examiner manipulates the involved scapula into a position of full retraction. The patient then actively abducts the arm within the scapular plane while the examiner continues to apply a stabilizing pressure to the scapula. This posterior stabilization is maintained while the examiner performs both the dynamic labral shear test and Jobe test to assess for pathology involving the labrum or the rotator cuff, respectively [109].

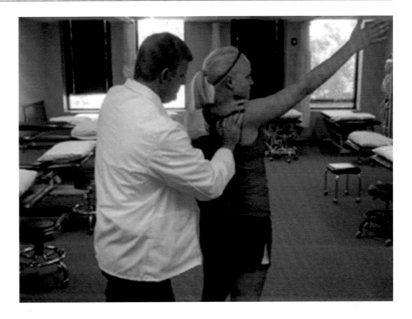

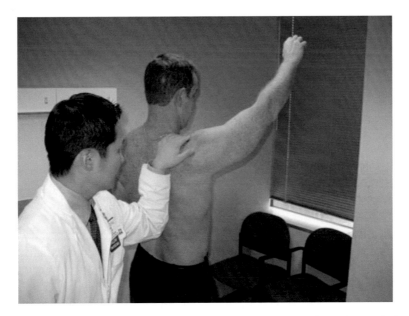

Fig. 9.12 Scapular reposition test. With the patient standing, the examiner positions their forearm obliquely across the scapular body such that the fingers rest over the anterior shoulder. The patient is then asked to abduct the humerus in the scapular plane. During humeral elevation, the examiner's elbow is used to push the inferomedial angle anterolaterally while the fingers are used to pull the scapula posteriorly. This posterior stabilization is maintained while the examiner performs the rotator cuff impingement signs [110].

9.3.3 Selected Conditions Associated with Scapular Dyskinesis

As mentioned above, there are many shoulder disorders that may have an association with scapular dyskinesis. However, we have chosen to focus on several of the more common conditions that we believe are closely related to scapular dyskinesis. The purpose of this section is to highlight the most important concepts related to disordered scapular motion that can subsequently be applied to other, less common shoulder pathologies that are not specifically mentioned below.

9.3.3.1 Subacromial Impingement and Rotator Cuff Disease

Numerous studies have documented the presence of scapular dyskinesis in patients with subacromial impingement and rotator cuff tears [44–48]. The precise abnormality in scapular motion that predisposes individuals to rotator cuff disease appears to vary significantly; however, these studies have generally found decreased upward rotation, decreased posterior tilt, and increased internal rotation of the scapula in patients with rotator cuff tears or impingement. Although these associations exist, it is not known whether scapular dyskinesis is the cause or the result (or both) of rotator cuff disease. If scapular dyskinesis is causative, decreased upward rotation and decreased posterior tilt would most likely be implicated since these factors would also decrease the functional acromiohumeral distance leading to mechanical impingement of the superior cuff tendons. Scapular dyskinesis could also be the result of rotator cuff disease via alterations in periscapular muscle firing patterns that function to either decrease the pain associated with impingement or to compensate for rotator cuff weakness during arm elevation.

Both the serratus anterior and the lower portion of the trapezius have been suggested as major points of periscapular muscle weakness in patients with rotator cuff disease and should be the primary focus of the clinical examination. The techniques commonly used for individual strength testing of each of these muscles are presented in

Chap. 3. With specific regard to scapular dyskinesis, maneuvers such as the scapular assistance test [26] and the scapular retraction test [41] have been developed as diagnostic methods that reposition the scapula during humeral elevation (discussed above). Scapular malposition with secondary rotator cuff impingement may be causative when the patient's symptoms are relieved with either one of these tests. Periscapular strengthening and proprioceptive training are typical rehabilitation options that are most often successful at providing symptomatic improvement.

9.3.3.2 SLAP Tears

SLAP tears are often seen in combination with scapular dyskinesis, especially in overhead athletes who demonstrate GIRD. This adaptation to repetitive throwing places the scapula in a position of decreased posterior tilt and increased internal rotation, thus increasing the strain across the biceps-labral complex via increased anterior capsular tension, extraphysiologic torsional strain (i.e., the peel-back mechanism as discussed in Chap. 5) and posterosuperior glenoid impingement (i.e., symptomatic internal impingement). The scapular retraction test (discussed below) [41] can be used in conjunction with the dynamic labral shear test (described in Chap. 5) to determine the effect of scapular malposition and dyskinesis on the symptomatology related to SLAP tears. When the test results in symptomatic relief, periscapular weakness is most likely a significant contributor to the patient's symptoms and can probably be alleviated with periscapular strengthening and, in overhead athletes, an additional supervised throwing program that encourages proper throwing mechanics and maintenance of a normal scapulohumeral angle.

9.3.3.3 Multidirectional Instability

Inherited multiligamentous laxity is most commonly implicated in patients who present with evidence of multidirectional instability (MDI) such as a positive sulcus sign, apprehension sign, and relocation sign, among several others (details regarding the testing for glenohumeral instability and laxity are presented in Chap. 6). Importantly, examination of the scapula can also provide important diagnostic and therapeutic information and should be performed in all patients with MDI. Specifically, these patients often demonstrate decreased upward rotation, decreased posterior tilt, and increased internal rotation of the scpaula during humeral elevation [49, 50]. However, in contrast to many other shoulder conditions, the cause of scapular malposition and dyskinesis in patients with MDI is most likely secondary to increased capsular laxity. Several studies by Jerosch et al. [51–53] concluded that both the glenohumeral ligaments and the glenohumeral joint capsule have mechanoreceptors that respond to stretch by inducing a proprioceptive reflex mechanism that alters muscle firing patterns around the shoulder in order to optimize the position of the glenoid in three-dimensional space. A more recent study by Barden et al. [54] found that patients with MDI have a decreased capability of utilizing this proprioceptive mechanism, perhaps as a result of increased capsular laxity which decreases the potential for stretching of capsuloligamentous structures. This hypothesis is supported by anecdotal reports of decreased apprehension during the clinical assessment of patients with known capsular laxity, including those with voluntary or positional instability patterns. The above findings suggest that patients with MDI may develop scapular dyskinesis due to the decreased ability to differentiate between normal and abnormal humeral head translations which, in normal patients, is detected by changes in capsuloligamentous tension. As a result, patients with MDI may have decreased proprioceptive responses to humeral head translation, leading to relative deactivation (and possibly disuse-related weakness) of certain shoulder muscles and producing the observed dyskinetic scapular motion. Specific inhibition of the lower trapezius, the serratus anterior and the subscapularis along with activation of the pectoralis minor and latissimus dorsi may be involved with the development of resting scapular protraction where the inferior pull of the latissimus dorsi and teres major muscles (along with the increased downward rotation of the scapula [50]) may be the primary contributors related to increased inferior humeral head translation in patients with MDI.

9.3.3.4 AC Joint Pathology

Currently, controversy exists regarding whether patients with grade III acromioclavicular (AC) joint injuries should be treated using operative or nonoperative treatment modalities (see Chap. 7 for more details related to the AC joint). However, the high prevalence of scapular dyskinesis following nonoperative treatment may be an important factor that could convince surgeons to operate on these patients more frequently. A study by Gumina et al. [55] in 2009 found that 24 of 34 patients (70.6 %) with chronic grade III AC joint dislocations had clinical evidence of scapular dyskinesis. In a recent cadaveric study, Oki et al. [56] found that disruption of the AC capsular ligaments and the coracoclavicular ligaments delayed long-axis posterior rotation of the clavicle and increased the degree of scapular upward rotation when the humerus was passively abducted in the coronal plane. Therefore, nonoperative treatment for AC joint dislocations may decrease the continuity of force transmission between the scapula and the clavicle through the AC joint, leading to altered muscle firing patterns and dyskinetic scapular motion. This notion is supported by a recent study in which only 4 out of 34 patients (11.7 %) displayed evidence of scapular dyskinesis following surgical management of grade III AC joint injuries [57]. Although scapular dyskinesis related to grade III AC joint dislocations can be treated successfully using a conservative approach, a recent study by Carbone et al. [58] found that approximately 22 % of patients still had scapular dyskinesis despite 12 months of rehabilitation (no improvements were documented in the interval between 6 weeks and 12 months after the injury). In addition, recent data from our institution revealed that more than 30 % of patients with grade III AC joint injuries who were initially treated nonoperatively eventually required surgical management due to the lack of clinical improvement (unpublished data). Taken together, the results of these studies suggest that the combined effects of both pain inhibition and mechanical dysfunction may be the primary contributing factors associated with scapular dyskinesis in patients with injuries to the AC capsuloligamentous structures and/or the coracoclavicular ligaments (including grades II–VI injuries) who are not treated surgically. Therefore, surgeons may be forced to undertake more aggressive treatment strategies for lower-grade AC joint dislocations to help prevent the development of scapular dyskinesis and its associated sequelae. Regardless of whether operative or nonoperative treatment is chosen, scapular motion should be evaluated in all patients at regular intervals during the course of rehabilitation.

9.3.3.5 Clavicle Fractures

Clavicle fractures can produce scapular dyskinesis through a similar mechanism to that which was described above for AC joint dislocations—that is, the inability to adequately (or accurately) transmit forces between the scapula and the sternoclavicular (SC) joint via the clavicular strut. In other words, disruption of the cohesive relationship between the scapula and the axial skeleton (through the clavicle) prevents normal scapulohumeral rhythm. Realistically, any alteration in clavicular anatomy can produce disordered scapular motion. These defects might include fracture malalignment, clavicle shortening as a result of fragment overlap or angulation (especially when shortening exceeds 15 mm [59, 60]), external rotation of the distal fragment or fractures that extend into the AC or SC joint which can lead to chronic pain and abnormal periscapular muscle firing patterns. Specifically, these patients often have clinical evidence of scapular protraction and decreased posterior tilt which can lead to chronic sequelae such as rotator cuff disease. Therefore, scapulothoracic motion should be repeatedly evaluated in all patients with clavicle fractures during the course of rehabilitation, regardless of whether the patient was initially treated operatively or nonoperatively.

9.3.3.6 Shoulder Stiffness
and Adhesive Capsulitis

The relationship between scapular dyskinesis and shoulder stiffness or adhesive capsulitis has become a topic of increased interest in recent years since several studies have noted increased ipsilateral scapular upward rotation in this subgroup of patients [61–64]. It is theorized that this increased upward rotation is a compensatory adaptation that maximizes range of motion in the setting of shoulder stiffness. Lin et al. [62] studied the scapular kinematics in patients with stiff shoulders involving either the anterior or posterior aspects of the glenohumeral joint capsule. When compared to those with predominantly posterior stiffness, those with anterior stiffness demonstrated increased scapular upward rotation and decreased posterior tilt both at rest and during active motion. However, most of these patients were found to have range of motion deficits primarily involving internal and external rotation rather than humeral elevation. Nevertheless, Vermeulen et al. [64] found that a course of physical therapy was particularly helpful in correcting the scapular malposition related to shoulder stiffness and improving overall shoulder function. Therefore, the scapula should be thoroughly evaluated in patients with shoulder stiffness (with or without adhesive capsulitis) in order to optimize rehabilitation and clinical outcomes following both operative and nonoperative treatment modalities.

9.3.3.7 Scapulothoracic Bursitis and
Snapping Scapula Syndrome

In order to achieve smooth scapular motion in three-dimensional space, the concave scapula must glide freely over the convex posterior thorax with the aid of interposed muscle layers (i.e., the serratus anterior and subscapularis) and bursal tissue. Therefore, any disorder or abnormality that produces an anatomic derangement within the scapulothoracic space can lead to altered painful bursitis and/or mechanical crepitation—a condition collectively referred to as scapulothoracic bursitis and/or snapping scapula syndrome.

Scapulothoracic bursitis has numerous potential etiologies, many of which can be divided into categories depending on patient symptomatology. For example, patients who present with periscapular pain in the absence of mechanical crepitus during shoulder motion are more likely to have bursitis which is most often the result of chronic overuse, especially in those who participate in overhead activities. In contrast, patients who present with painful crepitus during shoulder activity are more likely to have an anatomic derangement involving the scapulothoracic space that prevents smooth gliding of the scapula over the posterior chest wall. Potential etiologies include kyphoscoliotic posture [65], space-occupying osseous or soft-tissue masses (such as fracture callus, anomalous musculature, benign or malignant tumors, and fibrotic bursae) or predisposing anatomic variations (such as hyperangulation of the superomedial angle [7], a Luschka tubercle [5], or a teres major tubercle [6], among many other possibilities). However, it is important to recognize that symptomatic bursitis can eventually lead to mechanical crepitus (as a result of bursal fibrosis [5, 18, 21, 22]) while mechanical crepitus can also lead to symptomatic bursitis (as a result of disordered scapular motion) [23]. Therefore, most patients will present with characteristics that suggest both mechanical and nonmechanical etiologies.

Scapular dyskinesis is a common finding in patients with scapulothoracic bursitis and is most likely caused by tightness or weakness of the serratus anterior, upper trapezius, levator scapulae, and/or pectoralis minor. This muscular imbalance can be variable and may be the result of a compensatory mechanism that functions to avoid periscapular pain with shoulder motion. Scapular "pseudowinging" may be present in patients with an enlarging scapulothoracic mass which physically pushes the scapular body away from the posterior chest wall. In cases of symptomatic bursitis, superficial palpation around the scapular margins most often reveals the site of maximal tenderness and inflammation. However, deeper palpation may be necessary in some cases—this typically involves placing the arm in the "chicken wing" position (dorsum of hand placed over lumbosacral junction) which increases downward rotation of the scapula and allows deeper palpation along the medial scapular border [66, 67]. During range of motion testing, the clinician can also apply a compressive force to the posterior scapular body to decrease the scapulothoracic space which may help reproduce the patient's symptoms in the office setting [8].

Clinical management of this entity is difficult because its precise etiology is unknown in the majority of cases. Nevertheless, nonoperative management is the first-line treatment strategy and usually includes non-steroidal anti-inflammatory medications, injection of bursal tissue and periscapular muscle strengthening. Open or arthroscopic management may be indicated in patients who fail a course of nonoperative treatment or those who have an obvious space-encroaching mass that is found on imaging studies.

9.3.3.8 Trapezius Myalgia

Trapezius myalgia is vaguely defined as pain in the region of the trapezius, most frequently involving the superior division of the muscle that travels along the neck between the occiput and the scapular spine [68–70]. However, in reality, the myalgia probably involves other muscles in the area such as the levator scapulae, the rhomboid major and minor, and/or the paraspinal musculature [71]. The condition is often attributed to poor sitting posture and alterations in the neck flexion angle during prolonged periods of desk-related work [71–79]. Patients typically present with a dull ache, tenderness to palpation, and subjective "tightness" along the lateral side of the neck. Several studies have identified muscular imbalances, derangements in upper trapezius muscle firing patterns (mostly increased activity), and decreased maximum contraction strength and endurance in this group of patients (i.e., involvement of both fast- and slow-twitch muscle fibers) [69, 80–83]. As a result, many patients with work-related neck pain have clinically significant scapular malposition such as decreased posterior tilt and increased protraction [78, 84, 85] which may predispose these individuals to secondary rotator cuff impingement as a result of a decreased acromio-humeral distance [86]. A study by Juul-Kristensen et al. [68] confirmed these findings and also noted that patients with trapezius myalgia demonstrated a statistically significant increased capacity for passive glenohumeral internal rotation (due to increased scapular protraction) when compared to normal controls. In addition, those patients who reported the greatest work-related disability associated with trapezius myalgia also demonstrated a 20° increase in passive glenohumeral internal rotation capacity when compared to the rest of the cohort.

Given the very high prevalence of neck pain associated with desk-related work, trapezius myalgia is probably much more common than most physicians and researchers have been able to document to this point. This presumed discrepancy between the reported prevalence and the true prevalence of trapezius myalgia is likely present due to multiple factors. Most notably, highly accessible media outlets often misinterpret this work-related neck pain as a manifestation of cervical spine pathology. As a result, many afflicted patients likely seek treatment for pain related to the cervical spine rather than the scapula or the shoulder. This misperception may lead patients to undergo expensive, ineffective, and unnecessary treatments such as cervical spine manipulation, injections, and acupuncture, among many other possibilities. Therefore, it is crucial for clinicians of all specialties to recognize the primary and secondary risk factors for trapezius myalgia in order to minimize the effects of misguided communication on clinical outcomes. Appropriate physical therapy should focus on correcting both the acquired muscular imbalance and the hyperkyphotic sitting posture with the ultimate goals of re-establishing normal scapular motion, preventing secondary sequelae (such as rotator cuff disease) and eliminating the patient's symptoms.

9.3.3.9 Facioscapulohumeral Dystrophy

Facioscapulohumeral dystrophy (FSHD), the third most common type of muscular dystrophy (behind Duchenne muscular dystrophy and myotonic muscular dystrophy) [87] occurring in approximately 1 in 20,000 individuals [88, 89], is an inherited autosomal dominant condition that was first described by Landouzy and Dejerine in the late 1800s [90]. Characteristic features of FSHD include weakness involving the periscapular muscles (e.g., scapular dyskinesis), the facial muscles (e.g., the inability to smile), and the ankle (e.g., difficulty walking due to foot drop) in addition to postural defects related to abdominal weakness (e.g., hyperlordosis). In a retrospective study by Padberg [90], approximately 80 % of

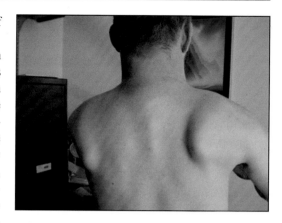

Fig. 9.13 Clinical photograph demonstrating bilateral scapular malposition in a patient with facioscapulohumeral dystrophy (FSHD). Although the scapulae appear asymmetric, they are both in a position of protraction with prominence of the medial scapular border indicating bilateral weakness of the trapezius muscle. Asymmetric periscapular weakness typically differentiates patients with FSHD from patients with other limb-girdle dystrophies.

patients with FSHD initially complained of shoulder girdle weakness, 10 % initially complained of orofacial muscle weakness, and the remaining 10 % initially complained of ankle dorsiflexion weakness (i.e., foot drop). However, physical examination of these patients revealed objective weakness in all three of these muscle groups. Although the recognition of FSHD during infancy and early childhood has been reported on occasion [91], the condition most often goes unrecognized until early adulthood (typically during the second or third decade of life).

With specific reference to the shoulder, patients with FSHD often display evidence of atrophy and/or hypotonia of the middle and lower divisions of the trapezius muscle which forces the scapulae into significant elevation, protraction, upward rotation (Fig. 9.13) [88, 92]. Because the glenoid faces more anteriorly in this type of scapular malposition, the glenohumeral joint almost always assumes a position of increased internal rotation. However, it is important to recognize that although patients with FSHD have bilateral periscapular weakness, the relative amount of weakness between each shoulder is typically asymmetric. In other words, active forward flexion and abduction of the shoulder in patients with FSHD usually reveals *asymmetric* scapular winging—a clinical finding which can be used to differentiate between patients with FSHD and those with other types of limb-girdle muscular dystrophies who most often present with symmetric scapular winging.

Clinical management of this entity is challenging since there is very little evidence to support any possible operative or nonoperative treatment modality. Currently, most treatment strategies involve symptomatic management in order to improve the patient's overall function and quality of life.

9.3.3.10 Medial Scapular Muscle Detachment

Avulsion or detachment of the musculature that inserts along the medial scapular border has only recently been described as a distinct clinical entity with specific physical examination findings [93, 94]. More specifically, the condition is thought to primarily involve detachment of the lower trapezius and rhomboids from the scapular spine and/or the medial scapular border following an acute traumatic injury (especially seatbelt-related motor vehicle accidents). Other possible etiologies include seizure, electrocution, or lifting a heavy object with full elbow extension, among other potential causes (most of which involve a push–pull mechanism of injury). Most patients present with an acute onset of severe pain along the medial scapular border which increases in severity as the humerus is mobilized. Increased activity of the upper trapezius may also produce tension-type headaches in some patients [93, 94].

Physical examination findings are fairly uniform in these patients and are critical to making the correct diagnosis. These findings often include localized tenderness along the medial scapular border with or without a palpable soft-tissue defect, an altered scapular resting position and secondary findings such as rotator cuff impingement, snapping scapula, and symptomatic relief following scapular manipulation procedures during arm elevation (discussed below). Although many of these patients present after having undergone numerous treatments, surgical reattachment is only indicated after a course of appropriate scapular rehabilitation fails to correct the scapular malposition and to relieve the patient's symptoms.

9.3.4 Scapular Dyskinesis in Overhead Athletes

In overhead athletes, the scapula plays a central role in the kinetic chain—muscle contraction forces produced by the trunk are transmitted through the scapula and into the hand where potential energy is converted into kinetic energy [32, 95]. It follows that any disruption of the kinetic chain may lead to disordered scapular motion and inefficient energy transmission.

Most competitive overhead athletes display differences in scapular resting positions between their dominant and non-dominant shoulders as a result of physiologic adaptation [96–99]. These differences typically include increased internal rotation along with alterations in upward rotation and posterior tilt (increased or decreased). However, regardless of the resting position, most overhead athletes display the same pattern of scapular motion when the arm is elevated [100]. During the competitive season, specific abnormalities of scapular motion are only treated when they are found to be associated with an injury; however, during the offseason, efforts should be made to correct scapulohumeral kinematics which can prevent injuries such as SLAP tears [34], symptomatic internal impingement [101], and valgus overload of the medial elbow [102].

Although the scapula is usually found to be internally rotated in overhead athletes, many of these same individuals display seemingly paradoxical evidence of GIRD upon physical examination. Physiologic adaptations such as capsular contractures, muscle inflexibility, and osseous changes (e.g., humeral retrotorsion) which allow the athlete to achieve greater degrees of abduction, extension, and external rotation are responsible for these findings. These changes produce a pattern of scapular dyskinesis characterized by markedly increased protraction and decreased posterior tilt during forward flexion, internal rotation and horizontal adduction which typically occurs during the follow-through phase of the throwing motion.

As mentioned above, untreated scapular dyskinesis in the overhead athlete can lead to secondary injuries that, in some cases, may be severe. However, scapular dyskinesis, along with its many potential sequelae, can be avoided when overhead athletes maintain balanced periscapular strength [103–105], neuromuscular control, and proprioception [104, 106]. For more information regarding injury prevention in overhead athletes, we refer the reader to an excellent two-part review published by Reinold and Gill [107] and Reinold et al. [108] in 2010.

9.4 Conclusion

An understanding of the etiology of disordered scapular motion requires comprehension of the many complex interactions between the static and dynamic components of shoulder motion. Accurate recognition and interpretation of disordered scapular motion is an important skill that should be utilized in any patient with a complaint related to the shoulder. The findings on clinical examination can greatly assist the clinician in the diagnosis and management of scapular dyskinesis.

References

 1. Kibler WB, Sciascia A, Wilkes T. Scapular dyskinesis and its relation to shoulder injury. J Am Acad Orthop Surg. 2012;20(6):364–72.
 2. Lewitt K. Manipulative therapy in rehabilitation of the locomotor system. London, England: Butterworth-Heinemann; 1985.
 3. Aggarwal A, Wahee P, Harjeet, Aggarwal AK, Sahni D. Variable osseous anatomy of costal surface of scapula and its implications in relation to snapping scapula syndrome. Surg Radiol Anat. 2011;33(2):135–40.
 4. Boyle MJ, Misur P, youn SM, Ball CM. The superomedial bare area of the costal scapula surface: a possible cause of snapping scapula syndrome. Surg Radiol Anat. 2013;35(2):95–8.
 5. Milch H. Partial scapulectomy for snapping of the scapula. J Bone Joint Surg Am. 1950;32-A:561–6.
 6. Totlis T, Konstantinidis GA, Karanassos MT, Sofidis G, Anasasopoulos N, Natsis K. Bony structures related to snapping scapula: correlation to gender, side and age. Surg Radiol Anat. 2014;36(1):3–9.
 7. Edelson JG. Variations in the anatomy of the scapula with reference to the snapping scapula. Clin Orthop Relat Res. 1996;322:111–5.
 8. Millett PJ, Gaskill TR, Horan MP, van der Meijden O. Technique and outcomes of arthroscopic bursectomy and partial scapulectomy. Arthroscopy. 2012;28(12):1776–83.
 9. Polguj M, Jędrzejewski K, Podgórski M, Topol M. Correlation between morphometry of the suprascapular notch and anthropometric measurements of the scapula. Folia Morphol (Warsz). 2011;70(2):109–15.
10. Polguj M, Jędrzejewski K, Podgórski M, Topol M. Morphometry study of the suprascapular notch: proposal of classification. Surg Radiol Anat. 2011;33(9):781–7.
11. Rockwood CA, Matsen FA. The shoulder. 2nd ed. Philadelphia, PA: WB Saunders Company; 2000.
12. Wang JH, Chen C, Wu LP, Pan CQ, Zhang WJ, Li YK. Variable morphology of the suprascapular notch: an investigation and quantitative measurements in Chinese population. Clin Anat. 2011;24(1):47–55.
13. Polguj M, Jędrzejewski K, Majos A, Topol M. Variations in bifid superior transverse scapular ligament as a possible factor of suprascapular entrapment: an anatomical study. Int Orthop. 2012;36(10):2095–100.
14. Polguj M, Jędrzejewski K, Podgórski M, Majos A, Topol M. A proposal for classification of the superior transverse scapular ligament: variable morphology and its potential influence on suprascapular nerve entrapment. J Shoulder Elbow Surg. 2013;22(9):1265–73.
15. Ciullo JV. Subscapular bursitis: treatment of "snapping scapula" or "wash-board" syndrome. Arthroscopy. 1992;8:412–3.
16. Kuhne M, Boniquit N, Ghodadra N, Romeo AA, Provencher MT. The snapping scapula: diagnosis and treatment. Arthroscopy. 2009;25(11):1298–311.
17. Cobey MC. The rolling scapula. Clin Orthop Relat Res. 1968;60:193–4.
18. Percy EC, Birbrager D, Pitt MJ. Snapping scapula: a review of the literature and presentation of 14 patients. Can J Surg. 1988;31(4):248–50.
19. Codman E. The shoulder. Malabar, FL: Krieger Publishing; 1984. p. 1–31.
20. Kuhn JE, Plancher KD, Hawkins RJ. Symptomatic scapulothoracic crepitus and bursitis. J Am Acad Orthop Surg. 1998;6(5):267–73.
21. Milch H. Snapping scapula. Clin Orthop. 1961;20:139–50.
22. Sisto DJ, Jobe FW. The operative treatment of scapulothoracic bursitis in professional baseball pitchers. Am J Sports Med. 1986;14(3):192–4.
23. Warth RJ, Spiegl UJ, Millett PJ. Scapulothoracic bursitis and snapping scapula syndrome: a critical review of current evidence. Am J Sports Med. 2015;43(1):236–45.
24. Frank DK, Wenk E, Stern JC, Gottlieb RD, Moscatello AL. A cadaveric study of the motor nerves to the levator scapulae muscle. Otolaryngol Head Neck Surg. 1997;117:671–80.
25. Ruland III LJ, Ruland CM, Matthews LS. Scapulothoracic anatomy for the arthroscopist. Arthroscopy. 1995;11(1):52–6.

26. Kibler WB, Sciascia AD, Dome D. Evaluation of apparent and absolute supraspinatus strength in patients with shoulder injury using the scapular retraction test. Am J Sports Med. 2006;34(10):1643–7.

27. Smith J, Dietrich CT, Kotajarvi BR, Kaufman KR. The effect of scapular protraction on isometric shoulder rotation strength in normal subjects. J Shoulder Elbow Surg. 2006;15(3):339–43.

28. Merolla G, De Santis E, Campi F, Paladini P, Porcellini G. Supraspinatus and infraspinatus weakness in overhead athletes with scapular dyskinesis: strength assessment before and after restoration of scapular musculature balance. Musculoskelet Surg. 2010;94(3):119–25.

29. Merolla G, De Santis E, Sperling JW, Campi F, Paladini P, Porcellini G. Infraspinatus strength assessment before and after scapular muscles rehabilitation in professional volleyball players with scapular dyskinesis. J Shoulder Elbow Surg. 2010;19(8):1256–64.

30. Sciascia A, Thigpen C, Namdari S, Baldwin K. Kinetic chain abnormalities in the athletic shoulder. Sports Med Arthrosc. 2012;20(1):16–21.

31. De May K, Danneels L, Cagnie B, Cools A. Are kinetic chain rowing exercises relevant in shoulder and trunk injury prevention training. Br J Sports Med. 2011;45(4):320.

32. Burkhart SS, Morgan CD, Kibler WB. The disabled throwing shoulder: spectrum of pathology part III: the SICK scapula, scapular dyskinesis, the kinetic chain, and rehabilitation. Arthroscopy. 2003;19(6):641–61.

33. Borstad JD, Ludewig PM. The effect of long versus short pectoralis minor resting length on scapular kinematics in healthy individuals. J Orthop Sports Phys Ther. 2005;35(4):227–38.

34. Burkhart SS, Morgan CD, Kibler WB. The disabled throwing shoulder: spectrum of pathology. Part II: evaluation and treatment of SLAP lesions in throwers. Arthroscopy. 2003;19(5):531–9.

35. Uhl TL, Kibler WB, Gecewich B, Tripp BL. Evaluation of clinical assessment methods for scapular dyskinesis. Arthroscopy. 2009;25(11):1240–8.

36. Kibler WB. Role of the scapula in the overhead throwing motion. Contemp Orthop. 1991;22:525–32.

37. Kibler WB. The role of the scapula in athletic shoulder function. Am J Sports Med. 1998;26(2):325–37.

38. Odom CJ, Taylor AB, Hurd CE, Denegar CR. Measurement of scapular asymmetry and assessment of shoulder dysfunction using the lateral scapular slide test: a reliability and validity study. Phys Ther. 2001;81(2):799–809.

39. Shadmehr A, Bagheri H, Ansari NN, Sarafraz H. The reliability measurements of lateral scapular slide test at three different degrees of shoulder joint abduction. Br J Sports Med. 2010;44(4):289–93.

40. Rabin A, Irrgang JJ, Fitzgerald GK, Eubanks A. The intertester reliability of the scapular assistance test. J Orthop Sports Phys Ther. 2006;36(9):653–60.

41. Kibler WB, Sciascia A, Hester P, Dome D, Jacobs C. Clinical utility of traditional and new tests in the diagnosis of biceps tendon injuries and superior labrum anterior and posterior lesions in the shoulder. Am J Sports Med. 2009;37(9):1840–7.

42. Merolla G, De Santis E, Campi F, Paladini P, Porcellini G. Infraspinatus scapular retraction test: a reliable and practical method to assess infraspinatus strength in overhead athletes with scapular dyskinesis. J Orthop Traumatol. 2010;11(2):105–10.

43. Tate AR, McClure PW, Kareha S, Irwin D. Effect of the scapula reposition test on shoulder impingement symptoms and elevation strength in overhead athletes. J Orthop Sports Phys Ther. 2008;38(1):4–11.

44. Graichen H, Stammberger T, Bonél H, et al. Three-dimensional analysis of shoulder girdle and supraspinatus motion patterns in patients with impingement syndrome. J Orthop Res. 2001;19(6):1192–8.

45. Ludewig PM, Cook TM. Alterations in shoulder kinematics and associated muscle activity in people with symptoms of shoulder impingement. Phys Ther. 2000;80(3):276–91.

46. McClure PW, Michener LA, Karduna AR. Shoulder function and 3-dimensional scapular kinematics in people with and without shoulder impingement syndrome. Phys Ther. 2006;86(8):1075–90.

47. Mell AG, LaScalza S, Guffey P, Ray J, Maciejewski M, Carpenter JE, Hughes RE. Effect of rotator cuff pathology on shoulder rhythm. J Shoulder Elbow Surg. 2005;14((1 Suppl S)):58S–64.

48. Scibek JS, Mell AG, Downie BK, Carpenter JE, Hughes RE. Shoulder kinematics in patients with full-thickness rotator cuff tears after subacromial injection. J Shoulder Elbow Surg. 2008;17(1):172–1281.

49. Ludewig PM, Reynolds JF. The association of scapular kinematics and glenohumeral joint pathologies. J Orthop Sports Phys Ther. 2009;39(2):90–104.

50. Ogston JB, Ludewig PM. Differences in 3-dimensional shoulder kinematics between persons with multidirectional instability and asymptomatic controls. Am J Sports Med. 2007;35(8):1361–70.

51. Jerosch J, Castro WH, Halm H, Drescher H. Does the glenohumeral joint capsule have proprioceptive capability? Knee Surg Sports Traumatol Arthrosc. 1993;1(2):80–4.

52. Jerosch J, Steinbeck J, Clahsen H, Schmitz-Nahrath M, Grosse-Hackmann A. Function of the glenohumeral ligaments in active stabilization of the shoulder joint. Knee Surg Sports Traumatol Arthrosc. 1993;1(3–4):152–8.

53. Jerosch J, Steinbeck J, Schröder M, Westhues M, Reer R. Intraoperative EMG response of the musculature after stimulation of the glenohumeral joint capsule. Acta Orthop Belg. 1997;63(1):8–14.

54. Barden JM, Balyk R, Raso VJ, Moreau M, Bagnall K. Dynamic upper limb proprioception in multidirectional shoulder instability. Clin Orthop Relat Res. 2004;420:181–9.

55. Gumina S, Carbone S, Postacchini F. Scapular dyskinesis and SICK scapular syndrome in patients with chronic type III acromioclavicular dislocation. Arthroscopy. 2009;25(1):40–5.

56. Oki S, Matsumura N, Iwamoto W, Ikegami H, Kiriyama Y, Nakamura T, Toyama Y, Nagura T.

The function of the acromioclavicular and coraco-clavicular ligaments in shoulder motion: a whole-cadaver study. Am J Sports Med. 2012;40(11): 2617–26.

57. Murena L, Canton G, Culcano E, Cherubino P. Scapular dyskinesis and SICK scapular syndrome following surgical treatment of type III acute acro-mioclavicular dislocations. Knee Surg Sports Traumatol Arthrosc. 2013;21(5):1146–50.

58. Carbone S, Postacchini R, Gumina S. Scapular dys-kinesis and SICK syndrome in patients with a chronic type III acromioclavicular dislocation. Results of rehabilitation. Knee Surg Sports Traumatol Arthrosc. 2014 (in press).

59. Ledger M, Leeks N, Ackland T, Wang A. Short mal-unions of the clavicle: an anatomic and functional study. J Shoulder Elbow Surg. 2005;14(4):349–54.

60. Matsumura N, Ikegami H, Nakamichi N, Nakamura T, Nagura T, Imanishi N, Aiso S, Toyama Y. Effect of shortening deformity of the clavicle on scapular kinematics: a cadaveric study. Am J Sports Med. 2010;38(5):1000–6.

61. Fayad F, Roby-Brami A, Yazbeck C, Hanneton S, Fefevre-Colau MM, Gautheron V, Poiraudeau S, Revel M. Three-dimensional scapular kinematics and scapulohumeral rhythm in patients with gleno-humeral osteoarthritis or frozen shoulder. J Biomech. 2008;41(2):326–32.

62. Lin JJ, Lim HK, Yank JL. Effect of shoulder tight-ness on glenohumeral translation, scapular kinemat-ics, and scapulohumeral rhythm in subjects with stiff shoulders. J Orthop Res. 2006;24(5):1044–51.

63. Rundquist PJ. Alterations in scapular kinematics in subjects with idiopathic loss of shoulder range of motion. J Orthop Sports Phys Ther. 2007;37(1):19–25.

64. Vermeulen HM, Stokdijk M, Eilers PH, Meskers CG, Rozing PM, Vliet Vlieland TP. Measurement of three dimensional shoulder movement patterns with an electromagnetic tracking device in patients with fro-zen shoulder. Ann Rheum Dis. 2002;61(2):115–20.

65. Manske RC, Reiman MP, Stovak ML. Nonoperative and operative management of snapping scapula. Am J Sports Med. 2004;32(6):1554–65.

66. Millett PJ, Pacheco I, Gobezie R, Warner JJP. Management of recalcitrant scapulothoracic bursitis: endoscopic scapulothoracic bursectomy and scapulo-plasty. Tech Shoulder Elbow Surg. 2006;7(4):200–5.

67. O'Holleran J, Millett P, Warner JJ. Arthroscopic management of scapulothoracic disorders. In: Miller M, Cole B, editors. Textbook of arthroscopy. Philadelphia: WB Saunders; 2004. p. 277–87.

68. Juul-Kristensen B, Hilt K, Enoch F, Remvig L, Sjøgaard G. Scapular dyskinesis in trapezius myal-gia and intraexaminer reproducibility of clinical tests. Physiother Theory Pract. 2011;27(7):492–502.

69. Juul-Kristensen B, Kadefors R, Hansen K, Byström P, Sandsjö L, Sjøgaard G. Clinical signs and physical function in neck and upper extremities among elderly female computer users: the NEW study. Eur J Appl Physiol. 2006;96(2):136–45.

70. Ohlsson K, Attewell RG, Johnsson B, Ahlm A, Skerfving S. An assessment of neck and upper extremity disorders by questionnaire and clinical examination. Ergonomics. 1994;37(5):891–7.

71. Yoo WG. Changes in pressure pain threshold of the upper trapezius, levator scapular and rhomboid mus-cles during continuous computer work. J Phys Ther Sci. 2013;25(8):1021–2.

72. Bruno Garza JL, Eijckelhof BH, Huysmans MA, Catalano PJ, Katz JN, Johnson PW, van Dieen JH, van der Beek AJ, Dennerlein JT. The effect of over-commitment and reward on trapezius muscle activ-ity and shoulder, head, neck, and toso postures during computer use in the field. Am J Ind Med. 2013;56(10):1190–200.

73. Jensen C. Development of neck and hand-wrist symptoms in relation to duration of computer use at work. Scand J Work Environ Health. 2003;29(3): 197–205.

74. Juul-Kristensen B, Søgaard K, Strøyer J, Jensen C. Computer user's risk factors for developing shoulder, elbow and back symptoms. Scand J Work Environ Health. 2004;30(5):390–8.

75. Laursen B, Jensen BR. Shoulder muscle activity in young and older people during a computer mouse task. Clin Biomech (Bristol, Avon). 2000;15 Suppl 1:S30–3.

76. Park SY, Yoo WG. Effect of sustained typing work on changes in scapular position, pressure pain sensi-tivity and upper trapezius activity. J Occup Health. 2013;55(3):167–72.

77. Sjøgaard G, Rosendal L, Kristiansen J, Blangsted AK, Skotte J, Larsson B, Gerdle B, Saltin B, Søgaard K. Muscle oxygenation and glycolysis in females with trapezius myalgia during stress and repetitive work using microdialysis and NIRS. Eur J Appl Physiol. 2010;108(4):657–69.

78. Szeto GP, Straker L, Raine S. A field comparison of neck and shoulder postures in symptomatic and asymptomatic office workers. Appl Ergon. 2002; 33(1):75–84.

79. Yoo WG. Comparison of upper cervical flexion and cervical flexion angle of computer workers with upper trapezius and levator scapular pain. J Phys Ther Sci. 2014;26(2):269–70.

80. Andersen LL, Holtermann A, Jorgensen MB, Sjøgaard G. Rapid muscle activation and force capacity in conditions of chronic musculoskeletal pain. Clin Biomech (Bristol, Avon). 2008;23(10): 1237–42.

81. Andersen LL, Nielsen PK, Sogaard K, Andersen CH, Skotte J, Sjøgaard G. Torque-EMG-velocity relationship in female workers with chronic neck muscle pain. J Biomech. 2008;41(9):2029–35.

82. Larsson B, Björk J, Elert J, Gerdle B. Mechanical performance and electromyography during repeated maximal isokinetic shoulder forward flexions in female cleaners with and without myalgia of the tra-pezius muscle and in healthy controls. Eur J Appl Physiol. 2000;83(4–5):257–67.

83. Sjøgaard G, Søgaard K, Hermens HJ, Sandsjö L, Läubli T, Thorn S, Vollenbroek-Hutten MM, Sell L, Cristensen H, Klipstein A, Kadefors R, Merletti R. Neuromuscular assessment in elderly workers with and without work related shoulder/neck trouble: the NEW-study design and physiological findings. Eur J Appl Physiol. 2006;96(2):110–21.

84. Finley MA, Lee RY. Effect of sitting posture on 3-dimensional scapular kinematics measured by skin-mounted electromagnetic tracking sensors. Arch Phys Med Rehabil. 2003;84(4):563–8.

85. Kebaetse M, McClure P, Pratt NA. Thoracic position effect on shoulder range of motion, strength, and three-dimensional scapular kinematics. Arch Phys Med Rehabil. 1999;80(8):945–50.

86. Solem-Bertoft E, Thuomas KA, Westerberg CE. The influence of scapular retraction and protraction on the width of the subacromial space. An MRI study. Clin Orthop Relat Res. 1993;296:99–103.

87. Emery AE. Population frequencies of inherited neuromuscular disease–a world survey. Neuromuscul Disord. 1991;1(1):19–29.

88. Flanigan KM, Coffeena CM, Sexton L, Stauffer D, Brunner S, Leppert MF. Genetic characterization of a large, historically significant Utah kindred with FSHD. Neuromuscul Disord. 2001;11(6–7):525–9.

89. Padberg GW, Frants RR, Brouwer OF, Wijmenga C, Bakker E, Sandkuijl LA. Facioscapulohumeral muscular dystrophy in the Dutch population. Muscle Nerve Suppl. 1995;2:S81–4.

90. Padberg GW. Facioscapulohumeral disease [thesis]. Leiden, Netherlands: Leiden University; 1982.

91. Chen TH, Lai YH, Lee PL, Hsu JH, Goto K, Hayashi YK, Nishino I, Lin CW, Shih HH, Huang CC, Liang WC, Wang WF, Jong YJ. Infantile facioscapulohumeral muscaular dystrophy revisited: expansion of clinical phenotypes in patients with a very short EcoRI fragment. Neuromuscul Disord. 2013;23(4):298–305.

92. Tyler FH, Stephens FE. Studies in disorders of muscle. II Clinical manifestations and inheritance of facioscapulohumeral dystrophy in a large family. Ann Intern Med. 1950;32(4):640–60.

93. Kibler WB. Scapular surgery I-IV. In: Reider B, Terry MY, Provencher MT, editors. Sports medicine surgery. Philadelphia: Elsevier Saudners; 2010. p. 237–67.

94. Kibler WB, Sciascia A, Uhl T. Medial scapular muscle detachment: clinical presentation and surgical treatment. J Shoulder Elbow Surg. 2014;23(1):58–67.

95. Lintner D, Noonan TJ, Kibler WB. Injury patterns and biomechanics of the athlete's shoulder. Clin Sports Med. 2008;27:527–52.

96. Laudner KG, Myers JB, Pasquale MR, Bradley JP, Lephart SM. Scapular dysfunction in throwers with pathologic internal impingement. J Orthop Sports Phys Ther. 2006;36(7):385–91.

97. Laudner KG, Stanek JM, Meister K. Differences in scapular upward rotation between baseball pitchers and position players. Am J Sports Med. 2007;35(12): 2091–5.

98. Myers JB, Laudner KG, Pasquale MR, Bradley JP, Lephart SM. Scapular position and orientation in throwing athletes. Am J Sports Med. 2005;33(2): 263–71.

99. Oyama S, Myers JB, Wassinger CA, Daniel Ricci R, Lephart SM. Asymmetric resting scapular posture in healthy overhead athletes. J Athl Train. 2008;43(6): 565–70.

100. Seitz AL, Reinold M, Schneider RA, Gill TJ, Thigpen CA. No effect of scapular position on 3-dimensional scapular motion in the throwing shoulder of healthy professional pitchers. J Sport Rehabil. 2012;21(2):186–93.

101. Spiegl UJ, Warth RJ, Millett PJ. Symptomatic internal impingement of the shoulder in overhead athletes. Sports Med Arthrosc. 2014;22(2):120–9.

102. Dines JS, Frank JB, Akerman M, Yocum LA. Glenohumeral internal rotation deficits in baseball players with ulnar collateral ligament insufficiency. Am J Sports Med. 2009;37(3):566–70.

103. Cools A, Johansson FR, Cambier DC, Velde AV, Palmans T, Witvrouw EE. Descriptive profile of scapulothoracic position, strength, and flexibility variables in adolescent elite tennis players. Br J Sports Med. 2010;44(9):678–84.

104. Cools AM, Witvrouw EE, DeClercq GA, Vanderstraeten GG, Cambier DC. Evaluation of isokinetic force production and associated muscle activity in the scapular rotators during a protraction-retraction movement in overhead athletes with impingement symptoms. Br J Sports Med. 2004;38(1):64–8.

105. Madsen PH, Bak K, Jensen S, Welter U. Training induces scapular dyskinesis in pain-free competitive swimmers: a reliability and observational study. Clin J Sport Med. 2011;21(2):109–13.

106. Ebaugh DD, McClure PW, Karduna AR. Effects of shoulder muscle fatigue caused by repetitive overhead activities on scapulothoracic and glenohumeral kinematics. J Electromyogr Kinesiol. 2006;16(3): 224–35.

107. Reinold MM, Gill TJ. Current concepts in the evaluation and treatment of the shoulder in overhead-throwing athletes. Part 1: physical characteristics and clinical examination. Sports Health. 2010;2(1): 39–50.

108. Reinold MM, Gill TJ, Wilk KE, Andrews JR. Current concepts in the evaluation and treatment of the shoulder in overhead throwing athletes. Part 2: injury prevention and treatment. Sports Health. 2010;2(2):101–5.

109. Manske R, Ellenbecker T. Current concepts in shoulder examination of the overhead athlete. Int J Sports Phys Ther. 2013;8(5):554–78.

110. Seroyer ST, Nho SJ, Bach BR Jr, Bush-Joseph CA, Nicholson GP, Romeo AA. Sports Health. 2009; 1(2):108–20.

10.1 Introduction

The diagnosis of neurovascular-related shoulder dysfunction is a challenging, but necessary component of clinical practice. Although basic screening tests such as Tinel's sign and Hoffman's sign are useful, it is important to identify the precise cause of the patient's symptoms in order to provide an effective treatment protocol. The following sections will describe the pathogenesis and physical examination findings that will aid in the establishment of an effective operative or nonoperative treatment plan.

10.2 Cervical Radiculitis

Cervical radiculitis is one of the most important pathologies to be ruled out in patients presenting with acute or chronic shoulder pain. Degenerative disc disease, disc herniation, spondylolisthesis, and zygoapophyseal joint disease, among others, can all lead to neurogenic neck pain that may or may not radiate to the shoulder. This pain can be indistinguishable from that of many shoulder pathologies and should always be considered in any patient with shoulder pain or dysfunction. It is important to note, however, that cervical spine pathology can coexist with shoulder pathology, making the clinical diagnosis difficult in some cases [1, 2].

10.2.1 Pathogenesis

Many conditions related to the cervical spine can cause impingement of exiting nerve roots, leading to radiating pain towards the ipsilateral shoulder (Fig. 10.1). Oftentimes, patients perceive this pain as coming from the shoulder and radiating towards the neck as if to suggest that a shoulder disorder is causative. However, the difference is that radiating pain from the cervical region will be distributed in a dermatomal pattern whereas that of a shoulder condition would not necessarily be related to any specific dermatome (Fig. 10.2). Cervical spine pathology should always be considered in patients who complain of constant pain regardless of shoulder motion, especially when the pain seems to be isolated to a specific dermatome. On the other hand, patients with a shoulder condition are also more likely to have positional night pain and pain that occurs only with shoulder motion.

10.2.2 Physical Examination

Initial physical findings in patients with cervical spine pathology may include postural imbalances, such as changes in lordosis or forward head positioning, as a result of contracture of paravertebral and/or periscapular musculature. Shoulder muscle atrophy can also be an important clue since the innervation for many of the shoulder muscles are derived from the C5 and C6

R.J. Warth and P.J. Millett, *Physical Examination of the Shoulder: An Evidence-Based Approach*,
DOI 10.1007/978-1-4939-2593-3_10, © Springer Science+Business Media New York 2015

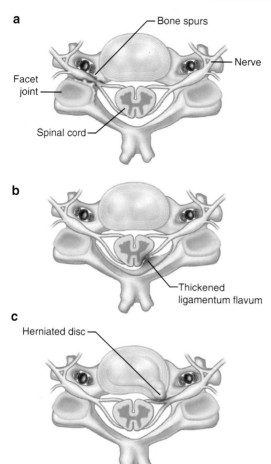

a
Bone spurs
Nerve
Facet joint
Spinal cord

b
Thickened ligamentum flavum

c
Herniated disc

Fig. 10.1 Illustration highlighting the most common causes of cervical radiculopathy. (**a**) Bone spurs can occur along the articular facets which can impinge upon exiting nerve roots. (**b**) Thickening of the ligamentum flavum may also produce a mass effect that can encroach upon the dorsal root ganglion. (**c**) Disc herniation often occurs along the posterolateral aspect of the vertebral disc and may also irritate exiting nerve roots.

nerve roots (especially the suprascapular nerve and the dorsal scapular nerve). Prominence of the scapular spine may indicate atrophy of the supraspinatus or infraspinatus muscles (innervated by the suprascapular nerve) and prominence of the medial scapular border with excessive lateral position of the scapula may indicate the presence of a lesion affecting the dorsal scapular nerve. Tenderness to palpation over the posterior aspect of the cervical spine may also indicate cervical pathology, especially when the pain radiates

towards the shoulder; however, this is not always reliable [3]. Tenderness of the trapezius muscle is not reliable since this can indicate pathology of either the shoulder or the cervical spine; however, trapezius muscle wasting with lateral scapular winging suggests involvement of the spinal accessory nerve (Fig. 10.3).

There are several methods by which physical examination can be used to differentiate between disorders of the shoulder or cervical spine. One method is to simply test the range of motion capacity of the neck and shoulder. Patients who demonstrate full, active, and painless neck range of motion and who demonstrate difficulty with isolated shoulder motion are more likely to have a shoulder condition as opposed to cervical spine pathology. The opposite would also be true for a patient with a disorder related to the cervical spine—that is, painful neck motion with normal shoulder motion. Provocative maneuvers are also designed to differentiate between disorders of the cervical spine and that of the shoulder girdle (see below).

10.2.2.1 Spurling's Test
Spurling's test [5] is performed by bending the neck laterally towards the affected shoulder. The examiner then applies a downward axial force (classically, ~7 kg) to the top of the head, thus narrowing the space for cervical nerve roots to exit the spinal cord (Fig. 10.4). Reproduction of neck and shoulder pain with this maneuver is suggestive of a cervical nerve root lesion. Other authors have suggested various modifications to Spurling's original test, such as the addition of rotation and/or extension prior to applying a downward pressure to the top of the head [3]. L'hermitte's sign, which also indicates cervical spine pathology, occurs when a "shooting" or "electric-like" pain propagates down the neck and down the ipsilateral arm with rotation or flexion of the neck without application of an axial load. Although a few studies have evaluated the validity of L'hermitte's sign, these studies appear to have significant methodological flaws that hinder interpretation of their results [6, 7]. Thus, the value of L'hermitte's sign to detect cervical spine pathology remains anecdotal at best.

Fig. 10.2 Dermatome map of the upper extremity. Because the boundaries of dermatome maps often overlap, clinical correlation is needed before an interpretation can be made.

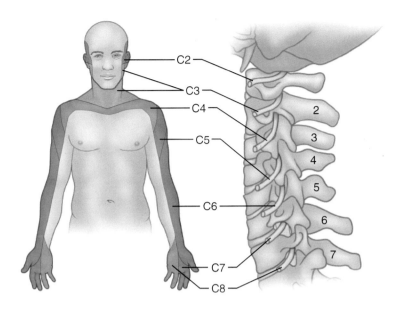

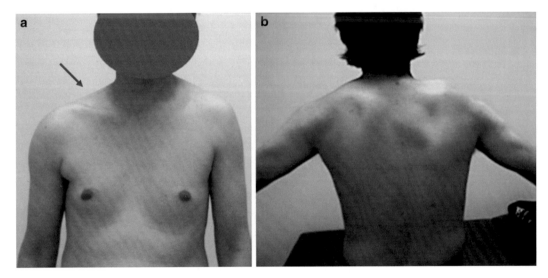

Fig. 10.3 Clinical photographs of a patient with spinal accessory nerve palsy [4]. (**a**) The right trapezius muscle is visibly atrophied (*arrow*) when compared to the contralateral side. (**b**) When viewing from posteriorly, scapular winging can be seen during humeral elevation.

Shah and Rajshekhar [8] studied the reliability of Spurling's test in the diagnosis of cervical disc disease with the reference standard of magnetic resonance imaging (MRI) in 25 patients who were treated nonoperatively and direct visualization at surgery in 25 patients who were treated operatively. The test was performed by extending and laterally bending the neck and then applying an axial load to the top of the head. The investigators did not rotate the head prior to application of an axial load. The sensitivity and specificity of Spurling's test was found to range between 0.90 and 1.00, depending on whether MRI or surgery was used as the reference standard. In contrast, Wainner et al. [9] performed the same test; however, they also rotated the head towards the

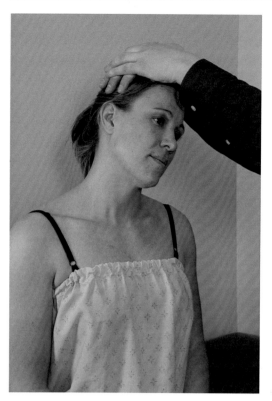

Fig. 10.4 Spurling's test. While sitting, the patient laterally bends the neck towards the affected shoulder. The examiner then applies a downward axial force to the top of the head (approximately 7 kg of force). This maneuver is thought to decrease the space available for cervical nerve roots to exit the spinal cord, thus reproducing the patient's symptoms.

ipsilateral side before applying an axial load. In that study, they used electromyography (EMG) as the reference standard. The investigators calculated a sensitivity of 0.50 and a specificity of 0.93 for this version of Spurling's test. In addition, Tong et al. [10] calculated an even lower sensitivity (0.30) when rotating the neck towards the contralateral shoulder. Combining the results of these three studies, it appears that lateral rotation of the neck decreases the sensitivity of the test for the detection of cervical radiculopathy. This rationale is supported by Anekstein et al. [11] who found the greatest sensitivity with the combination of lateral bending and extension without rotation. Thus, we prefer to perform the Spurling's test in neutral rotation to improve diagnostic efficacy.

10.2.2.2 Shoulder Abduction Test

The shoulder abduction test is performed by simply having the patient abduct the humerus such that the hand is placed on the top of the head (Fig. 10.5). This maneuver is thought to increase the space available for the cervical nerve roots to exit the spinal cord, thus diminishing symptoms. A cadaveric study by Farmer and Wisneski [12] confirmed the theoretical rationale for the test. In their study, pressure transducers were placed within cervical foramina and pressure readings were recorded with the humerus and the neck in various positions. They found that extension of the neck produced the greatest intra-foraminal pressure while abduction of the humerus decreased this pressure, thus further solidifying this maneuver as a viable technique for the detection of cervical nerve root compression. Wainner et al. [9] later found that this maneuver was 17 % sensitive and 92 % specific for the detection of cervical spine-related pathology.

Farshad and Min [13] recently described an abduction extension test that was reported to have a sensitivity of 0.79 and a specificity of 0.98 in the detection of cervical nerve root compression. This test was performed by laterally abducting the humerus to 80° with the neck rotated towards the contralateral shoulder. With the patient in this position, an anteriorly directed pressure was applied to the posterior aspect of the humeral head (Fig. 10.6). Reproduction of symptoms was considered a positive test. In their preliminary cadaveric study using this maneuver, nerve roots were displaced by approximately 4–5 mm in all cases, potentially explaining the resulting high sensitivity and specificity values.

10.2.2.3 Valsalva Maneuver

The Valsalva maneuver is performed with the patient in the seated position. The patient is then asked to take a deep breath and to "bear down" against a closed glottis for 2–3 s. This technique increases intra-abdominal pressure which, in turn, increases pressure within the thecal sac. The test is positive for cervical radiculopathy when neck and shoulder symptoms are reproduced. Wainner et al. found the sensitivity of this test to

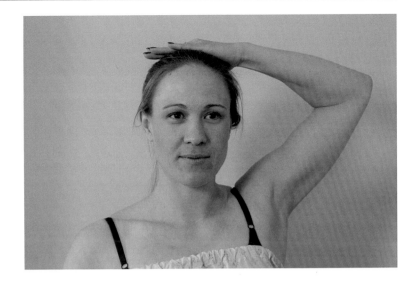

Fig. 10.5 Shoulder abduction Test. In a patient with suspected radiculopathy, asking the patient to place the palm of their hand on top of their head with the elbow pointed laterally may relieve their symptoms by increasing the space available for the cervical nerve roots to exit the spinal cord.

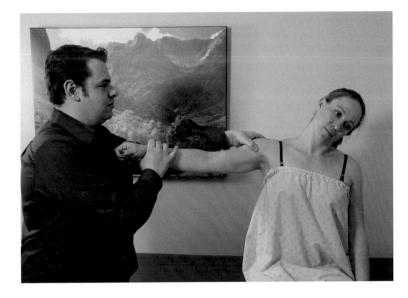

Fig. 10.6 Modified shoulder abduction test proposed by Frashad and Min [13]. In this test, the arm is laterally abducted to approximately 80° and the neck is bent and/or rotated towards the contralateral shoulder. While applying a gentle pressure to the posterior aspect of the humeral head, the examiner applies a gentle traction force along the axis of abduction.

be only 0.22; however, the specificity was 0.94. Therefore, it is suggested to combine this test with a more sensitive test, such as Spurling's test or the upper limb tension test (described below), to improve diagnostic accuracy.

10.2.2.4 Cervical Distraction Test

The cervical distraction test is performed with the patient in the supine position. The examiner cradles the jaw and occiput with their hands and slightly flexes the neck to improve patient comfort. A distraction force is applied gently and gradually until significant resistance is felt (clas-

sically, ~14 kg of force) (Fig. 10.7). This maneuver is thought to increase the space available for exiting nerve roots. Relief of symptoms indicates a positive test and is indicative of cervical pathology. Wainner et al. [9] determined that the cervical distraction test was 44 % sensitive and 90 % specific for the detection of cervical spine pathology. Similarly, Viikari-Juntura [3] calculated a sensitivity of 0.44 and a specificity of 0.97. Thus, similar to the Valsalva maneuver mentioned above, it is important to combine this test with other, more sensitive provocative maneuvers to improve diagnostic efficacy.

Fig. 10.7 Cervical distraction test. With the patient lying supine on the examination table, the examiner cradles the jaw and occiput with their hands. The neck is placed in a slightly flexed position and a gentle superiorly directed distraction force is applied (approximately 14 kg of force). This maneuver is also thought to increase the space available for exiting nerves.

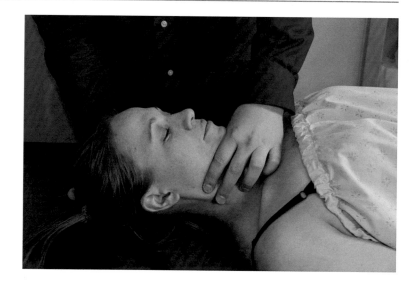

Fig. 10.8 Brachial plexus distraction test. With the patient supine, the examiner uses one hand to stabilize the scapula while the other hand is used to place the humerus in abduction and external rotation, the elbow extended, the forearm supinated, the wrist and fingers extended and the neck bent towards the contralateral shoulder. The neck is then slowly bent laterally towards the affected shoulder which may reproduce the patient's symptoms.

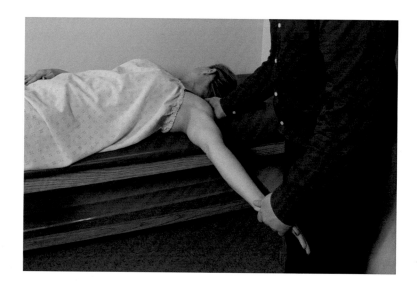

10.2.2.5 Brachial Plexus Tension Test

The brachial plexus tension test was first described by Elvey [14] in 1986 and has been modified on a few occasions [9, 15]. Although less descriptive, some researchers refer to this maneuver as the "upper limb tension test." The test is performed as a series of steps with the patient in the supine position. The first step is to place the hand over the posterior aspect of the scapula and to depress the scapula against the thoracic wall. Sequentially, the shoulder is then abducted, the forearm is supinated, the wrist and fingers are extended, the humerus is externally rotated, the elbow is extended, and the neck is bent towards the contralateral side and then towards the ipsilateral side (Fig. 10.8). Reproduction of the patient's symptoms was considered a positive test. Wainner et al. [9] found that the sensitivity and specificity values for this test were 0.97 and 0.22, respectively. Quintner [15] found slightly lower sensitivity and specificity values; however, they used

Fig. 10.9 Modified brachial plexus distraction test. With the patient supine, the examiner uses one hand to depress the scapula while the other hand is used to place the humerus in 30° of abduction with internal rotation, extend the elbow, and flex the wrist and fingers. The neck is then laterally bent towards the contralateral shoulder. The neck is then slowly bent laterally towards the affected shoulder, potentially reproducing the patient's symptoms.

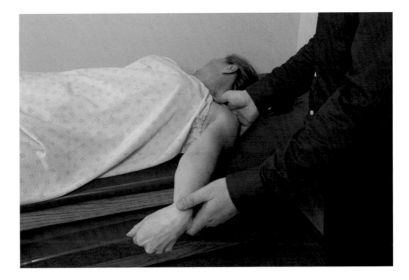

cervical radiography to confirm the diagnosis as opposed to EMG which was performed by Wainner et al. [9].

As an adjunct to this test, Wainner et al. [9] proposed a second method to evaluate for cervical spine pathology. In this maneuver, the patient was positioned supine with the shoulder abducted to 30°. The examiner then sequentially depressed the scapula, internally rotated the humerus, extended the elbow, flexed the wrist and fingers and, finally, contralateral followed by ipsilateral side-bending of the neck (Fig. 10.9). Reproduction of the patient's symptoms was considered a positive test. The sensitivity and specificity values for this maneuver were 0.72 and 0.33, respectively, representing an inferior result compared to Elvey's original test described above.

10.3 Thoracic Outlet Syndrome

In 1956, Peet et al. [16] were the first to coin the term "thoracic outlet syndrome" (TOS) as a result of neurovascular compression between the anterior and middle scalene muscles (i.e., the interscalene triangle). It is one of the most controversial conditions in the orthopedic literature with regard to anatomy, diagnosis, and management. In 2004, Huang and Zager [17] reported that the incidence of TOS was approximately 3–80 cases per 1,000 people. This wide variability is likely due to

Table 10.1 List of possible conditions that may mimic thoracic outlet syndrome

Conditions that can mimic thoracic outlet syndrome	
Cervical radiculitis	Malignancy (e.g. spinal cord tumors)
Brachial plexopathy	Shoulder pathology
Fibromyalgia	Spastic disorders
Angina/acute coronary syndrome	Raynaud's phenomenon/disease
Complex regional pain syndrome	Peripheral nerve entrapment
Neurologic disorders	Vasculitides

misdiagnoses and confusing clinical presentations, especially since there are numerous conditions that can mimic TOS, such as brachial neuritis, peripheral nerve entrapments, and cervical spine disease among many other possibilities (Table 10.1).

10.3.1 Pathogenesis

As the brachial plexus and subclavian vessels course towards the axilla and the upper arm, there are at least four areas of potential narrowing that can result in TOS. The first potential site of compression occurs in patients with a congenital bony or fibrous extension of the transverse process of the seventh cervical vertebra (cervical rib; Fig. 10.10) [18, 19]. The interscalene triangle is

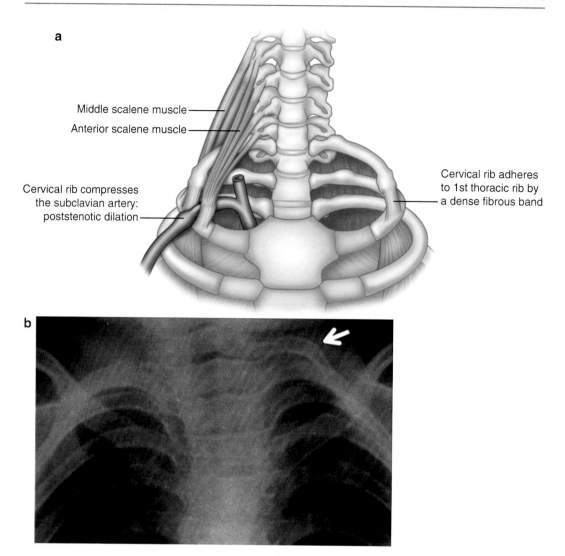

Fig. 10.10 Cervical rib. (**a**) Illustration depicting the anatomy of a cervical rib and its relationship with the nearby subclavian vessels and brachial plexus. (**b**) Radiograph demonstrating a cervical rib arising from the seventh cervical vertebra.

the second of these stenotic areas and is the most common site of compression (scalenus anticus syndrome; Fig. 10.11). The interscalene triangle is bordered by the anterior scalene muscle anteriorly, the middle scalene posteriorly, and the superiomedial aspect of the first rib inferiorly. The subclavian artery, subclavian vein, and the trunks of the brachial plexus are located within this triangle and is thus a potential site of neurovascular impingement. The costoclavicular space is the third site of narrowing and is located between the middle 1/3 of the clavicle and the first rib (costoclavicular syndrome; Fig. 10.12). Impingement in this area primarily involves the subclavian artery and/or vein. The fourth potential site of neurovascular compression is within the subcoracoid space in an area beneath the pectoralis minor muscle-tendon unit (pectoralis minor syndrome; Fig. 10.13).

The numerous potential etiologies for TOS can be divided into static and dynamic causes. Static causes might include cervical ribs, fracture callus, fibrous bands, anomalous or fibrotic musculature (such as pectoralis minor

Fig. 10.11 Illustration depicting the interscalene triangle with the brachial plexus and subclavian vessels situated between the middle and anterior scalene muscles.

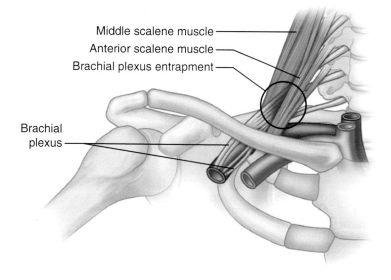

Middle scalene muscle
Anterior scalene muscle
Brachial plexus entrapment

Brachial plexus

Fig. 10.12 Illustration of the contents of the costoclavicular space. Regardless of cause, compression of the neurovascular structures as they pass through the costoclavicular space can result in thoracic outlet syndrome. Vascular symptoms are most common when impingement occurs within the costoclavicular space.

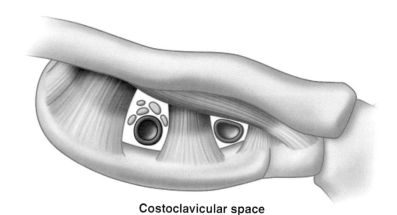

Costoclavicular space

syndrome [20, 21]), poor posture, and pathologic lesions with significant mass effect such as a Pancoast tumor, tuberculosis, or osteomyelitis. Reproduction of symptoms with scapulothoracic or glenohumeral motion typically indicates a dynamic cause which can occur within any of the three typically stenotic areas mentioned above. Repetitive microtrauma, as which occurs commonly in athletes and manual laborers, can also play an important role in the pathogenesis of TOS; however, the exact pathomechanism behind repetitive microtrauma and the development of TOS has not been clearly defined [21, 22].

The potential causes of TOS can also be divided by the structure involved. Neurogenic TOS, which has been reported to account for more than 95 % of all cases of TOS [23], involves compression of the nerves within the brachial plexus and is often the result of neck trauma. Vascular TOS, as the name suggests, involves compression of the subclavian artery and/or vein. Compression of the subclavian artery is typically associated with a cervical rib or rudimentary first rib [24, 25] (see Fig. 10.10). In contrast, compression of the subclavian vein usually occurs within the costoclavicular space [26] (see Fig. 10.12). Mixed TOS is more nonspecific and

Fig. 10.13 Illustration of the mechanism of neurovascular compression beneath the coracoid process and pectoralis minor tendon (within the subcoracoid space) as the humerus is maximally abducted (also known as pectoralis minor syndrome).

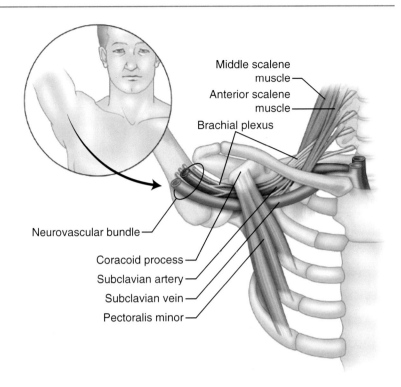

Middle scalene muscle

Anterior scalene muscle

Brachial plexus

Neurovascular bundle

Coracoid process

Subclavian artery

Subclavian vein

Pectoralis minor

may involve compression of nerves, arteries, and/or veins simultaneously with varying magnitudes of compressive force.

Many patients with TOS report an aching sensation over the shoulder or neck accompanied by upper limb paresthesias such as numbness or tingling. Sensory dysfunction of the arm and/or hand often occurs simultaneously with occipital headaches. Compression of the subclavian vein may result in ipsilateral swelling and/or discoloration of the arm whereas compression of the subclavian artery can produce a subclavian bruit. Cold, pale skin distal to the elbow may indicate proximal compression of a sympathetic nerve. In reality, however, most patients with TOS present with vague symptoms that are often difficult to differentiate from other causes of shoulder pain.

10.3.2 Physical Examination

It is important to inspect the entire upper extremity, including the intrinsic muscles of the hand, for muscle atrophy, wasting, or fasciculations since these may suggest the presence of a neuropathy or myelopathy. Hoffman's sign is a useful test for the detection of cervical myelopathy (Fig. 10.14). Combined supraspinatus and infraspinatus atrophy can occur since innervation for both of these muscles is derived from the C5 nerve root of the brachial plexus (suprascapular nerve). Weakness or atrophy of the rhomboid musculature may indicate compression of the dorsal scapular nerve (also from the C5 nerve root). The radial, median, and ulnar nerves are also derived from the brachial plexus, and care must be taken to evaluate the appropriate musculature to potentially locate the site of impingement. Tinel's sign should also be performed to rule out cubital tunnel syndrome at the elbow and carpal tunnel syndrome at the wrist.

There are several provocative maneuvers that can be used to help determine the site of impingement and the structure involved in TOS. However, interpretation of clinical tests for TOS is controversial and there is no individual test that is universally diagnostic. This is due to the wide variation in potential pathomechanisms involved with its development. In addition, the high false positive

Fig. 10.14 Hoffman's sign. The examiner gentle flicks the dorsum of the patient's middle finger in a downward direction. Reflexive thumb flexion is a common indicator of cervical myelopathy.

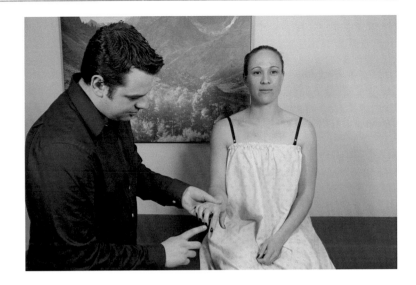

rate for many of these tests calls to question their application in clinical practice [27, 28]. Rayan and Jensen [27] found that 91 % of asymptomatic subjects developed symptoms from at least one of the tests designed to detect TOS.

10.3.2.1 Adson's Test

Adson's test was first described by Adson and Coffey [19] in 1927 as a method to assess for circulatory disruption due to a cervical rib. The test is performed with the patient sitting on the examination table. The radial pulse is then palpated prior to initiating the test. The patient is then asked to rotate the neck towards the affected shoulder, extend the neck, and to take a deep breath while the examiner simultaneously palpates the radial pulse (Fig. 10.15). When there is a decrease in pulse amplitude, the test is positive and indicates that the vascular component of the neurovascular bundle is being compressed within either the interscalene triangle or the costoclavicular triangle. Reproduction of paresthesias with this maneuver can also occur, indicating compression of a neural structure. However, in 1951, Adson [18] suggested that subclavian artery compression can also indicate compression and/or microtrauma of neural elements even in the absence of paresthesias.

Adson's test has been reported to have a sensitivity between 0.79 and 0.94 and a specificity ranging from 0.74 to 1.00 [27, 29–32].

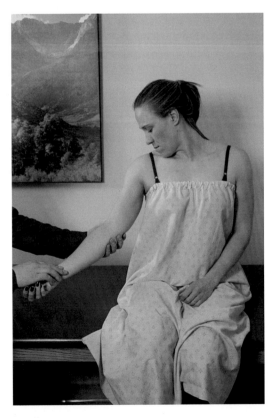

Fig. 10.15 Adson's test. In this test, the examiner first palpates the radial pulse to confirm adequate pulse amplitude. The patient is then asked to rotate the neck towards the affected shoulder and to inhale deeply. The examiner again palpates the radial pulse. A decrease in pulse amplitude suggests that proximal arterial compression, possibly at the interscalene triangle, may be causative of the patient's symptoms.

Fig. 10.16 Halsted maneuver. This test is performed exactly as described for Adson's test; however, rather than rotating the neck, the neck is extended posteriorly. Compression is thought to occur either at the interscalene triangle or the costoclavicular space.

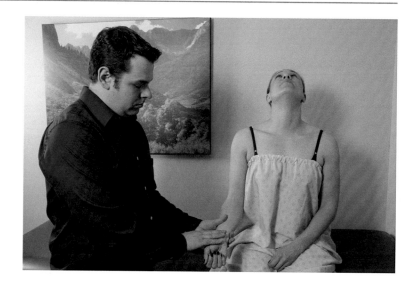

However, the studies by Nord et al. [31] and Plewa and Delinger [32] displayed conflicting results regarding the rate of false positives—Nord et al. [31] calculated a false positive rate of nearly 50 % while Plewa and Delinger [32] calculated a false positive rate of only 7 %. Several other authors have suggested that a positive test result may be associated with worse outcomes after either surgery or rehabilitation, especially in those with mixed neural and vascular symptoms [33, 34]. Clearly, it is important to consider the entire clinical picture before making the diagnosis of TOS using any physical examination maneuver. This includes a combination of the history, other physical findings and, potentially, imaging studies that serve to improve diagnostic accuracy [29, 35].

10.3.2.2 Halsted Maneuver

Dr. William Halsted was the first to identify and treat lesions of the subclavian artery due to the presence of cervical ribs in the late 1910s. The "Halsted maneuver" was developed to induce compression of the subclavian vessels and/or the brachial plexus within the costoclavicular space; however, the test is also purported to identify compression within the interscalene triangle and may be a useful adjunct to Adson's test [36].

The Halsted maneuver is performed with the patient sitting on the examination table with the arms in a neutral position. The patient is then asked to extend the neck while the examiner simultaneously palpates the radial pulse at the wrist. A positive test occurs when the pulse amplitude decreases as the neck is extended and may indicate compression within either the interscalene triangle or the costoclavicular space (Fig. 10.16). The examiner can also apply gentle traction to the arm to help elicit symptoms. An MRI study by Demirbag et al. [35] found that the Halsted maneuver produced a significantly decreased distance between neurovascular structures and the inferior border of the clavicle within the costoclavicular space. Although this test has been widely referenced in the literature, there have been no clinical studies that have evaluated the validity or reliability of the test for diagnosing TOS.

10.3.2.3 Costoclavicular Test

Compression of the subclavian vessels within the costoclavicular space was first described in 1943 by Falconer and Weddel [37]. They described a maneuver in which the sitting patient was asked to retract the scapulae and flex the cervical spine, bringing the chin towards the chest. The examiner simultaneously palpated the radial pulse (Fig. 10.17). A decrease in pulse amplitude during this test indicated that compression of the neurovascular structures between the clavicle and the first rib was likely. Falconer and Weddel [37] found a 60 % false positive rate indicating

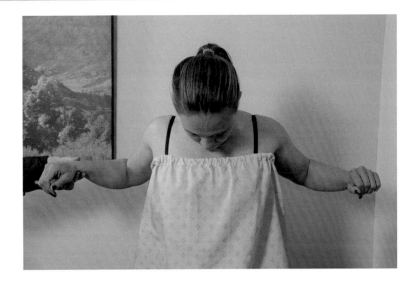

Fig. 10.17 Costoclavicular test. In this test, the patient is asked to maximally retract the shoulders and to simultaneously bend the neck into forward flexion. The radial pulse is palpated both before and after this positioning. Compression is thought to occur within the costoclavicular space.

that this maneuver may cause compression even in the absence of predisposing anatomy. Similarly, Telford and Mottershead [38] found radial pulse diminution in 68 % of normal subjects after shoulder retraction. Although this technique has been used extensively, there have been no studies that have evaluated its actual sensitivity or specificity in the diagnosis of TOS.

10.3.2.4 Wright's Test

In 1945, Wright [39] described the diminution of the radial pulse in 93 % of 150 asymptomatic individuals with the arm hyperabducted to an overhead position and the elbow flexed to 90° (Fig. 10.18). He suggested this finding was the result of axillary artery compression beneath the pectoralis minor tendon within the subcoracoid space (see Fig. 10.13). Along with Raaf [40], Gilroy and Meyer [41] also found positive results in up to 70 % of asymptomatic volunteers. Rayan and Jensen [27] suggested that positive symptoms could be the result of ulnar nerve compression behind the medial epicondyle since the original description of the test involved flexion of the elbow. They proposed that the test be performed with the elbow extended; however, they did not evaluate the reliability or validity of this technique. Tanaka et al. [42] performed a study in which nerve contact pressures were measured with different tests for TOS in a series of eight cadavers without a history of TOS.

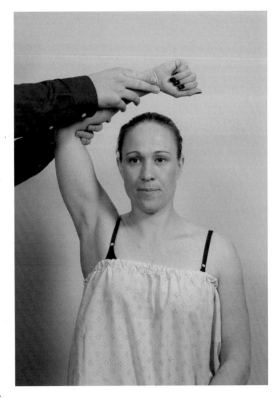

Fig. 10.18 Wright's test. With the elbow flexed to 90°, the humerus is maximally abducted to an overhead position. Reproduction of symptoms may indicate neurovascular compression beneath the coracoid and pectoralis minor tendon.

They found that Wright's test induced the greatest amount of nerve compression compared to any of the other tested positions, further implying

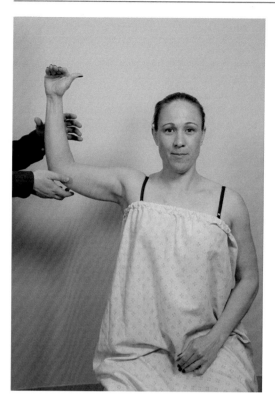

Fig. 10.19 Roos test. With the arm in the 90/90 position (90° of abduction, 90° of external rotation with the elbow flexed 90°), the patient is asked to rapidly open and close their fist for a minimum of 3 min. The clinical utility of this test has not been firmly established.

that nerve compression in the hyperabducted position may be a normal phenomenon—a concept that was originally suggested by Roos [43] in 1976.

10.3.2.5 Roos Test

Roos [43] also developed a test designed to detect vascular compression at the level of the brachial plexus. In this test, the humerus is flexed to 90° and externally rotated with the elbow also flexed to 90°. The patient is then instructed to repeatedly open and close the fist at moderate speed for approximately 3 min (Fig. 10.19). Reproduction of symptoms within the 3-min interval indicates a positive test. However, this test has also been reported to produce a high rate of false positives on at least one occasion [32]. The sensitivity of this test has been reported to range from 0.52 to 0.84 with a specificity between 0.30 and 1.00 [27, 29, 31, 32, 44, 45].

10.4 Quadrilateral Space Syndrome and Axillary Neuropathy

10.4.1 Pathogenesis

There are numerous potential etiologies of axillary nerve palsy, many of which occur as a result of blunt trauma, iatrogenic injury, or nerve compression. The axillary nerve branches from the C5–C6 nerve root and courses towards the quadrilateral space, passing just inferior to the subscapularis and anteroinferolateral to the inferior glenoid rim. The quadrilateral space, as the name suggests, is bordered by four structures—namely, the teres minor superiorly, the teres major inferiorly, the proximal humerus laterally, and the long head of the triceps medially (Fig. 10.20). The posterior circumflex humeral artery, a branch of the axillary artery, travels with the axillary nerve through the quadrilateral space. Compression of the neurovascular bundle within this space, termed the "quadrilateral space syndrome" by Cahill and Palmer [46] in 1983, can occur from anomalous fibrous bands, traumatic scarring, mass lesions, glenolabral cysts, large humeral head osteophytes, and/or muscle hypertrophy [47–51]. Cahill and Palmer [46], along with McKowen and Voorhies [52], observed that axillary nerve compression within the quadrilateral space commonly occurred with the humerus in a hyperabducted and externally rotated position (such as which occurs during the throwing motion). Although uncommon, this position may also cause arterial compression more proximally where the axillary artery travels beneath a hypertrophied pectoralis minor muscle, potentially resulting in thrombosis and distal embolization [53–56].

10.4.2 Physical Examination

Quadrilateral space syndrome typically presents as a vague posterior or lateral pain over the dominant shoulder of young, athletic individuals. Patients may also complain of night pain and mild weakness, especially with forward elevation and/or abduction. The presence of paresthesias

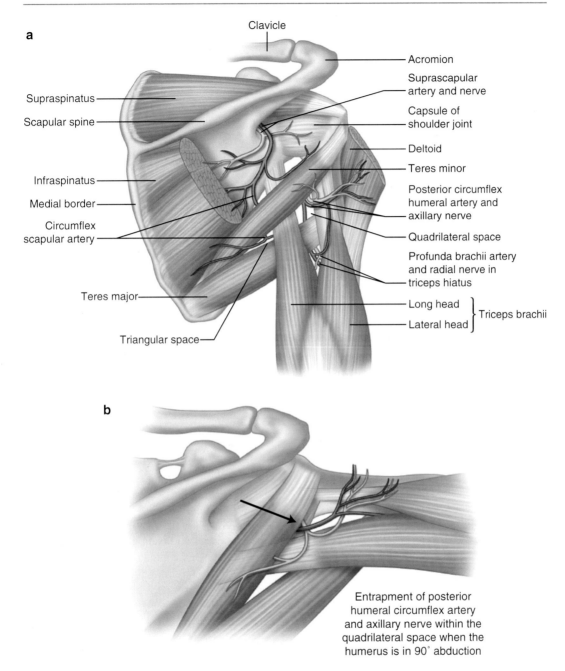

a

Clavicle

Acromion

Suprascapular
artery and nerve

Capsule of
shoulder joint

Deltoid

Teres minor

Posterior circumflex
humeral artery and
axillary nerve

Quadrilateral space

Profunda brachii artery
and radial nerve in
triceps hiatus

Long head ⎤
          ⎬ Triceps brachii
Lateral head ⎦

Supraspinatus

Scapular spine

Infraspinatus

Medial border

Circumflex
scapular artery

Teres major

Triangular space

b

Entrapment of posterior
humeral circumflex artery
and axillary nerve within the
quadrilateral space when the
humerus is in 90° abduction

Fig. 10.20 (**a**) Illustration depicting the anatomy of the quadrilateral space. See text for anatomic description. (**b**) Illustration showing the narrowing of the quadrilateral space as the arm is abducted to approximately 90° in the coronal plane.

over the lateral deltoid is not uncommon and strongly indicates axillary nerve involvement. Aside from these typical complaints, other historical findings are largely nonspecific and generally do not contribute to the diagnosis.

Although physical examination findings are nonspecific in many cases, it is most important to rule out other, more common causes of shoulder pain such as rotator cuff tears and labral lesions, especially in overhead throwing athletes.

Tenderness to palpation directly over the quadrilateral space may occur with concomitant weakness and/or atrophy of the posterior deltoid. This finding should alert the clinician to the potential for neurovascular compromise within the quadrilateral space.

Provocative maneuvers for the diagnosis of quadrilateral space syndrome are rarely reported; however, there are a few techniques that can be used to piece together the diagnosis. Although not always present, the deltoid lag sign may indicate posterior deltoid weakness (see Chap. 3), and the Hornblower's sign (see Chap. 4) may indicate concomitant weakness of the teres minor muscle (both the deltoid and the teres minor muscles are innervated by the axillary nerve). In addition, abnormal sensation may be noted over the lateral deltoid since the sensory branch of the axillary nerve provides innervation to the skin overlying this area. Some authors suggest that forward flexion, abduction, and external rotation of the humerus can reproduce symptoms when the position is held for approximately 2 min; however, this method has not been evaluated in the literature [48]. Because of vague presenting signs and symptoms, a high index of suspicion is needed to correctly diagnose quadrilateral space syndrome by physical examination. Subclavian arteriography demonstrating stenosis or blockage of the posterior circumflex humeral artery with the arm abducted and externally rotated is thought to confirm the suspected diagnosis even though most patients do not have vascular symptoms [46].

10.5   Brachial Neuritis

Brachial plexus injuries, although most commonly idiopathic, have been reported to result from inflammation, trauma, malignancy, and even excessive radiation [49, 57–59]. Parsonage and Turner [60] first described these disorders in 136 patients, labeling the condition as "neuralgic amyotrophy." Others have labeled the condition as a brachial radiculitis, neuropathy, neuritis and, most commonly, Parsonage–Turner syndrome.

10.5.1   Pathogenesis

Several types of brachial neuritis exist and differ in clinical presentation depending on the most likely cause. These include idiopathic, hypertrophic, hereditary, and traumatic types.

Idiopathic brachial neuritis is most commonly asymmetric (bilateral in 1/3 of cases [58]) and affects men more than women at a rate of at least 2:1 [49]. The condition typically has a bimodal age distribution, occurring most commonly in patients in their 20s and 60s [58]. Approximately half of patients report preceding events such as flu-like symptoms [59], recent vaccination [61, 62], and/or recent surgery [63] in the days just prior to the onset of symptoms, leading some to believe the condition may be immune-modulated [58]. Pierre et al. [64] demonstrated oligoclonal banding consisting of elevated IgG titers against herpes simplex and varicella zoster viruses in the cerebrospinal fluid of patients with brachial neuritis. Biopsies of the brachial plexus have also revealed mononuclear infiltrates, further suggesting an immunological basis for the disease [65, 66]. In addition, treatment with immune-modulating drugs such as corticosteroids and IVIg has been helpful on occasion [67–71].

Hypertrophic brachial neuritis has an unknown cause; however, its features differ from that of the above condition in that evidence of demyelination is evident on histologic examination, similar to other demyelinating diseases such as Gullain–Barre syndrome [72, 73]. Signs of generalized polyneuropathy, however, are absent. In addition, brachial plexus edema manifests as an enlarged appearance on MRI that suggests the diagnosis of hypertrophic brachial neuritis (Fig. 10.21) [58, 74].

Hereditary brachial neuritis is a rare autosomal dominant condition that, unlike other forms of brachial neuritis, generally manifests in early childhood with dysmorphic phenotypes such as hypotelorism, facial asymmetry, and/or cleft palate, among others [58]. It is associated with missense mutations and heterogeneous duplications of the SEPT9 gene on chromosome 17q25

Fig. 10.21 Coronal MRI demonstrating brachial plexus hypertrophy in a patient who presented with suspected brachial neuritis [133].

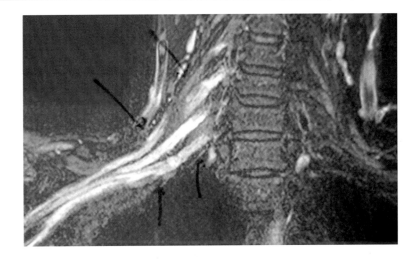

and its prevalence is largely unknown [75, 76]. Klein et al. [76] found intravenous corticosteroids helpful in reducing symptoms thus suggesting a potential immunological mechanism for this condition.

Traumatic injury is probably one of the more common causes of brachial plexopathy (i.e., traumatic brachial neuritis) and usually results from high-energy trauma, such as motorcycle and snowmobiling accidents [50], resulting in traction of the brachial plexus (i.e., the head and neck are stretched away from the affected shoulder) and, potentially, nerve root avulsion from the spinal cord. The brachial plexus can also be injured as a result of a violent hyperabduction motion as it becomes trapped beneath the coracoid process [58, 77]. Midha [50] suggested that injuries occurring more proximally to the clavicle (supraclavicular injury) carry a much poorer prognosis than those that occur distal to the clavicle (infraclavicular injury).

10.5.2 Physical Examination

Although physical examination findings across patients with different brachial plexopathies are often similar, the natural history of the disease can differ widely thus providing a clue to the underlying sub-diagnosis. For example, most patients with idiopathic brachial neuritis experience sudden, intense pain often involving the entire upper extremity which can last from days to weeks. Once the pain subsides (usually within 1 month), significant weakness occurs progressively over several days and finally dissipates with full recovery of function in most patients over time [59]. On the other hand, hypertrophic brachial neuritis is a painless condition that primarily presents as progressive weakness over a period of months to years. Finally, hereditary brachial neuritis begins in childhood and presents as acute "attacks" (similar to the idiopathic form) that can occur throughout the individual's lifetime. The patient will likely have a positive family history, may have cranial nerve involvement, and may have dysmorphic facial features.

Initial inspection of the patient with brachial neuritis may reveal muscle wasting and fasciculations involving the upper arm, forearm, and hand muscles suggesting lower motor neuron involvement, especially during the "weakness" phase of the disease. The axillary, suprascapular, long thoracic, and musculocutaneous nerves are most commonly affected; [78] however, any nerve branching from the brachial plexus, or any nerve passing nearby such as the phrenic nerve, may be involved [79–81]. EMG is most useful in making the diagnosis of brachial neuritis as this typically reveals a pattern consistent with acute demyelination with axonal neuropathy during the acute phase (within 3 weeks) and early regeneration on repeat examination (after approximately 3–4 months) [82].

10.6   Suprascapular Neuropathy

Clinical symptomatology associated with entrapment neuropathy of the suprascapular nerve was first described by Kopell and Thompson [83] in 1959. Suprascapular neuropathy is a relatively uncommon condition in the general population; however, more commonly, it can present as a chronic traction injury in overhead athletes such as volleyball players and baseball players [84–89]. From its origin at the C5 nerve root (Erb's point) to its termination at the infraspinatus muscle, the suprascapular nerve courses a path consisting of several distinct narrow areas including the suprascapular notch and, distal to the supraspinatus, the spinoglenoid notch. The location of nerve entrapment determines clinical signs and symptoms. For example, proximal within the suprascapular notch will result in atrophy and weakness of both the supraspinatus and infraspinatus muscles. On the other hand, entrapment that occurs more distal to the supraspinatus (i.e., within the spinoglenoid notch) will result in isolated atrophy and weakness of the infraspinatus muscle (Fig. 10.22). The spinoglenoid notch may also be a site of "bowstring"

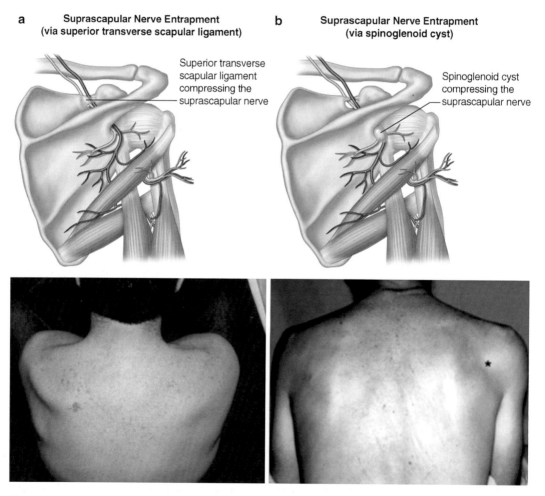

Fig. 10.22 (**a**) Illustration depicting suprascapular nerve entrapment at the level of the transverse scapular ligament. The corresponding clinical photograph demonstrates the observed atrophy of both the supraspinatus and infraspinatus muscles as evidenced by the prominence of the scapular spine. (**b**) Illustration depicting suprascapular nerve compression due to a large glenolabral cyst distal to the spinoglenoid notch. The corresponding clinical photograph demonstrates the observed isolated atrophy of the infraspinatus muscle (*asterisk*) [90].

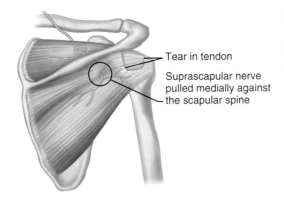

Tear in tendon

Suprascapular nerve
pulled medially against
the scapular spine

Fig. 10.23 Illustration of the bowstring injury to the suprascapular nerve in the presence of a massive, retracted rotator cuff tear. As the muscle retracts, the neurovascular pedicle of the infraspinatus pulls traction on the suprascapular nerve, essentially using the spinoglenoid notch as a fulcrum.

traction of the nerve in massive, retracted rotator cuff tears (Fig. 10.23) [91, 92]. The precise mechanism of injury or entrapment should be determined in all cases as this can affect the viability of treatment options and overall prognosis.

10.6.1 Pathogenesis

Entrapment of the suprascapular nerve can occur anywhere along its course towards the infraspinous fossa; however, the most common sites of entrapment occur in confined areas where there exists limited mobility such as within the suprascapular notch or the spinoglenoid notch. Nerve insult can occur as a result of any pathology that causes increased narrowing of these spaces—some of these might include fractures, ganglion cysts, paralabral cysts with medial extension, spinoglenoid cysts, and even engorged veins [93–97]. The morphologic features of the transverse scapular ligament [98, 99] and the suprascapular notch [100–103] also exhibit significant variability that may increase the propensity to develop a compression neuropathy in this region. In addition, anomalous ligaments and muscles have been described to compress the suprascapular nerve at various sites such as a coracoscapular ligament [104] and subscapularis fascial extensions [105]. Injuries to the suprascapular nerve have been described in overhead athletes, especially as a

result of nerve traction at tethering points, most commonly involving the spinoglenoid notch. Plancher et al. [106] identified increased traction of the suprascapular nerve over the spinoglenoid ligament during the follow-through phase of the overhand throwing motion. Their study suggests that the spinoglenoid notch may provide a fulcrum against which the nerve stretches, thus producing chronic traction injuries in overhead athletes. Ringel et al. [51] suggested that traction forces may produce intimal damage to branches of the suprascapular artery, generating microthrombi and subsequently microemboli that travel distally thus producing ischemia of distal motor nerve branches to the infraspinatus muscle.

Suprascapular neuropathy typically does not occur in isolation: rather, it is often associated with other primary shoulder pathologies. In an EMG study, de Laat et al. [107] reported a 29 % rate of injury to the suprascapular nerve in a series of 101 patients presenting with a shoulder dislocation and/or a proximal humerus fracture—the authors also postulated that the presence of an expanding hematoma after fracture may contribute to neural injury around the shoulder. Patients with massive, retracted rotator cuff tears have also been reported to develop traction injuries to the suprascapular nerve (see Fig. 10.23) [91, 92, 108]. Albritton et al. [91] performed a cadaveric study in which a large supraspinatus tear was made and retraction was simulated. The investigators found that 5 cm of retraction was necessary to significantly increase tension along the first supraspinatus motor branch of the suprascapular nerve. Costouros et al. [92] followed by performing a clinical study in which 10/26 (38 %) patients with massive, retracted supraspinatus tears were found to have isolated suprascapular neuropathy. In this study, the injuries resolved after repair of the rotator cuff and relief of suprascapular nerve tension. The authors also suggested performing routine EMG analysis in patients with massive rotator cuff tears to identify those patients with suprascapular nerve lesions.

Iatrogenic injuries to the suprascapular nerve have also been reported, most commonly involving the development of scar tissue after a surgical procedure or overzealous retraction during a posterior approach to the glenohumeral joint [109].

10.6.2 Physical Examination

Suprascapular neuropathy can present either suddenly or gradually as a constant dull, aching pain over the posterior and lateral aspect of the shoulder that may radiate up the neck or down the lateral arm. Horizontal adduction and internal rotation may exacerbate this pain as a result of the increased tension placed on the suprascapular nerve in this position [106]. Patients may also complain of weakness with motions that involve abduction and external rotation, especially in those patients with suprascapular nerve entrapment proximal to the supraspinatus muscle (i.e., at the suprascapular notch) [110]. In contrast, patients with nerve entrapment distal to the supraspinatus (i.e., at the spinoglenoid notch) may not experience any functional deficits since the teres minor and deltoid muscles can usually compensate for the weakened infraspinatus muscle [86].

Although a distinct traumatic injury is identified in nearly half of patients with suprascapular neuropathy [111], most cases are the result of chronic traction from repeated overhead activity such as those who participate in overhead sports and heavy manual labor. As mentioned above, suprascapular nerve injury should also be suspected in patients with massive, retracted supraspinatus tears [91, 92, 112] in addition to those who have undergone previous shoulder surgery.

Perhaps the most important physical examination findings in patients with suprascapular neuropathy are those obtained via simple inspection of the affected shoulder. The presence of surgical scars over the posterior shoulder should raise concern for nerve entrapment as a result of scar tissue and adhesions. The most common procedures resulting in nerve entrapment include rotator cuff repair, posterior approaches to the glenohumeral joint and, in one case, distal clavicle excision [113]. Prominence of the scapular spine may indicate atrophy of both the supraspinatus and infraspinatus muscle bellies, especially in cases of suprascapular nerve entrapment at the suprascapular notch (see Fig. 10.22). When nerve entrapment occurs more distally at the spinoglenoid notch, isolated atrophy of the infraspinatus muscle belly can be appreciated. If periscapular muscle wasting occurs simultaneously with rota-

tor cuff muscle atrophy, a more proximal lesion should be suspected, such as the C5 nerve root from which the dorsal scapular nerve arises, thus highlighting the importance of a complete neurovascular examination. The supraspinous fossa, infraspinous fossa, and acromioclavicular joint may be tender to palpation in those with nerve entrapment at the suprascapular notch. In contrast, the patient with nerve entrapment at the spinoglenoid notch may be tender to palpation near the posterior joint line. Active and passive range of motion should be tested in all patients to determine the degree of clinical weakness and the potential effects of general shoulder stiffness and scapular dyskinesis on the chief complaint.

There are no specific provocative maneuvers designed specifically for the detection of suprascapular neuropathy; however, it is postulated that humeral adduction and internal rotation may be useful to reproduce symptoms in patients with tension-type suprascapular nerve injuries since a study by Plancher et al. [106] found that this position increased tension across the nerve at the spinoglenoid notch. If the clinician uses this maneuver to detect suprascapular nerve injury, it is important to recognize that this maneuver may induce symptoms related to AC joint pathology (see Chap. 7). When suspected, other provocative maneuvers may be necessary to detect concomitant pathologies such as labral tears, rotator cuff disease, glenohumeral instability, and/or scapular dyskinesis.

10.7 Long Thoracic Nerve Palsy

The long thoracic nerve arises from the C5, C6, and C7 ventral rami of the spinal cord and passes through the muscle belly of the middle scalene muscle to provide motor innervation to all three anatomic divisions of the serratus anterior muscle along its proximal anterior surface. The nerve is tethered to the middle scalene and the neural pedicle of the serratus anterior which explains its high rate of traction-type injuries. As discussed in Chap. 3, contraction of the serratus anterior results in upward rotation and protraction of the scapula and also provides scapular stabilization with various arm motions. Weakness of the serratus anterior produces characteristic scapular winging

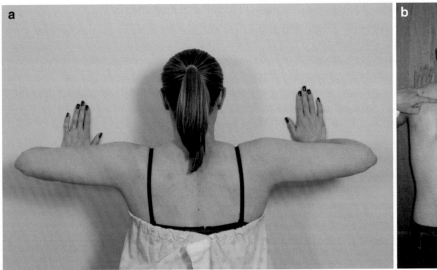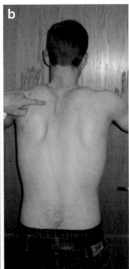

Fig. 10.24 Wall push-up. The patient is asked to perform a push-up against a nearby wall as if the patient were in the prone position. (**a**) Demonstration of the wall push-up in a normal subject. (**b**) Clinical photo of a patient with scapular dyskinesis involving the left shoulder. Note the prominence of the medial scapular border which is a characteristic feature of long thoracic nerve palsy.

which must be differentiated from that which occurs with spinal accessory nerve palsy (see Chaps. 3 and 9).

10.7.1 Pathogenesis

Many cases of long thoracic nerve palsy are the result of non-contact subacute traction in overhead athletes. Typically, the injury occurs when the arm is elevated overhead with the neck rotated towards the contralateral shoulder. This position produces tension across the long thoracic nerve as it passes through the middle scalene muscle. Although direct contact injuries have been reported to cause long thoracic nerve palsy, this mode of injury is relatively uncommon although it is likely underreported. In addition, more generalized neural disorders, such as brachial neuritis, have occasionally been reported to involve the long thoracic nerve [78].

10.7.2 Physical Examination

Patients with serratus anterior weakness often complain of gradually increasing posterior shoulder pain after a distinct traumatic injury. This pain typically occurs along the medial scapular border due to spasm of the unopposed rhomboid musculature. The patient may also complain of mechanical crepitus which can result from scapulothoracic incongruity due to the decreased girth of the atrophied serratus anterior muscle.

On physical examination, the patient may be tender to palpation along the medial scapular border. The patient may also exhibit a decrease in active forward elevation of the humerus [114]. There are a few provocative maneuvers that can be performed to detect serratus anterior weakness (discussed further in Chaps. 3 and 9). The most useful test, however, is the wall push-up since it has been shown to maximally activate the serratus anterior muscle and to provoke medial scapular winging [115]. To perform the wall push-up, the patient places their hands against a nearby wall at approximately shoulder-height and shoulder-width apart. The patient then performs a push-up as if they were in the prone position while the clinician observes scapular motion (Fig. 10.24). The inferior pole of the scapula will rotate medially and away from the chest wall if serratus anterior weakness is present. In addition to physical examination, EMG studies involving the serratus anterior and the trapezius muscle should be performed to confirm the diagnosis and to rule out concomitant spinal accessory nerve palsy which may compromise subsequent surgical outcome if not addressed appropriately [116].

10.8   Spinal Accessory Nerve Palsy

The spinal accessory nerve (cranial nerve XI) provides motor innervation to the entire trapezius muscle and the sternocleidomastoid muscle. The nerve exits the brain stem, travels inferiorly through the jugular foramen of the skull, and receives contributions from the C2, C3, and C4 nerve roots as it enters the posterior triangle of the neck. The posterior triangle is bordered anteriorly by the sternocleidomastoid muscle, posteriorly by the trapezius muscle and inferiorly by the inferior belly of the omohyoid muscle just before its insertion along the distal 1/3 of the clavicle (Fig. 10.25).

10.8.1 Pathogenesis

The spinal accessory nerve travels superficially within the posterior triangle of the neck, leaving it susceptible to traumatic injury especially in contact sports such as hockey and lacrosse [117]. Although less commonly reported, traction injuries to the nerve can also occur as a result of a fall on the shoulder with the neck rotated towards the contralateral shoulder or from excessive traction placed on the arm. Spinal accessory nerve palsy has been reported to occur concomitantly with long thoracic nerve palsy—thus, both nerves should be evaluated during physical examination.

10.8.2 Physical Examination

Patients with spinal accessory nerve palsy often have vague clinical symptoms such as posterior neck pain with or without distal radiation that is made worse by shrugging the shoulders. Patients

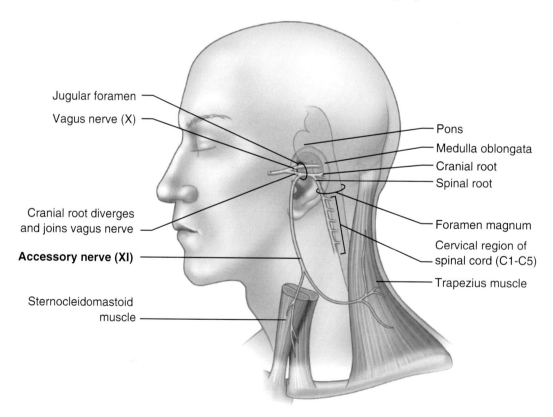

Fig. 10.25 Illustration showing the course of the spinal accessory nerve as it travels from the brainstem, through the jugular notch and through the posterior triangle towards the sternocleidomastoid and trapezius muscles.

may also complain of subjective weakness with forward elevation and abduction; however, this feature is not commonly found on physical examination [118]. The most prominent physical examination findings include scalloping of the lateral neck as a result of upper trapezius atrophy and subtle scapular winging that is reproduced when the patient shrugs the shoulders against resistance (see Fig. 10.3) [119, 120]. More specifically, scapular winging in the setting of accessory nerve palsy manifests as increased lateral scapular tilt and superomedial displacement of the inferomedial border. In any patient with scapular winging, dyskinesis or periscapular weakness, testing for signs of subacromial impingement is necessary since scapular malposition may decrease the space available for the rotator cuff tendons to pass beneath the acromion (see Chap. 4 for more information regarding subacromial impingement) [121–123].

Provocative tests are available for testing each of the three divisions of the trapezius muscle and are discussed in detail in Chap. 3; however, these are generally unnecessary when evaluating a patient for spinal accessory nerve palsy since the entire muscle is likely to be affected. Clinically, it is more useful to simply have the patient shrug their shoulders against resistance to elicit pathologic lateral scapular winging. EMG studies are also useful to confirm the diagnosis and to document functional recovery after operative or nonoperative treatment.

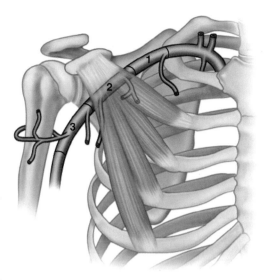

Fig. 10.26 The axillary artery is anatomically divided according to the relative position of the pectoralis minor muscle. The first part of the artery is proximal and medial to the pectoralis minor tendon, the second part of the artery is deep to the pectoralis minor tendon, and the third part of the artery is distal and lateral to the pectoralis minor tendon.

10.9 Axillary Artery Occlusion

The axillary artery is a continuation of the subclavian artery as it exits the thoracic cage inferior to the middle 1/3 of the clavicle and superior to the lateral aspect of the first rib. The axillary artery is anatomically divided into three parts according to its orientation relative to the pectoralis minor muscle (Fig. 10.26). The first portion lies proximal and medial to the muscle, the second portion lies deep to the muscle, and the third portion lies distal and lateral to the muscle. Thrombosis in this area can result in distal embolization and resulting ischemia (most commonly in the digits) which must be identified by history and physical examination.

10.9.1 Pathogenesis

Thrombosis of the second portion of the axillary artery was first reported in 1945 by Wright [39] who also described the pathogenesis of TOS. Wright [39] suggested that hyperabduction of the arms, as which occurs during the late-cocking phase of the throwing motion [55, 124], produces compression of the second part of the axillary nerve from the overlying pectoralis minor muscle (see Figs. 10.13 and 10.18). Turbulent blood flow from intimal hyperplasia, aneurysmal dilatation, and intimal dissection results in eventual arterial thrombosis and, potentially, distal embolization [55]. Since then, many other causes of axillary artery thrombosis have been reported such as shoulder dislocations [125], radiation therapy [126], nearby surgical procedures [127], and arteritides [128], among many others.

10.9.2 Physical Examination

The patient with axillary artery thrombosis may complain of tenderness over the anterior shoulder, specifically over the pectoralis minor muscle. When distal embolization has occurred, the patient may also complain of claudication, night pain, and a cold sensation distal to the embolus. Physical examination should always include a thorough neurovascular examination including capillary refill and the palpation of distal pulses. Provocative maneuvers can be used to elevate suspicion of axillary artery thrombosis and are performed exactly as described for TOS above. However, regardless of the test result, arteriography is necessary to definitively establish the diagnosis of arterial thrombosis.

10.10 Spontaneous Subclavian Vein Occlusion (Effort Thrombosis)

Also known as Paget–Schroetter syndrome, spontaneous subclavian vein thrombosis typically occurs without obvious predisposing factors. The condition is commonly associated with repetitive overhead activities and, therefore, is often referred to as "Effort Thrombosis." Although the condition is rarely seen, the consequences of not recognizing the disorder can be potentially devastating, ranging from pitting edema to life-threatening pulmonary emboli. Most patients who present with the condition are young athletes who may participate in overhead sports such as baseball, tennis, or swimming [129].

10.10.1 Pathogenesis

Similar to TOS which results from compression of the arterial components within the thoracic outlet, effort thrombosis can result from the same mechanism of compression as the subclavian vein exits the thoracic cage beneath the middle 1/3 of the clavicle (see Fig. 10.12). The predisposing anatomic variations are also similar to TOS including cervical ribs, fibrous bands, fracture callus, and stenosis of the interscalene triangle (described above for TOS), among many others. Venous occlusion is thought to be primarily positional in nature. Kunkel and Machleder [130] showed evidence that hyperabduction of the arms produced subclavian vein occlusion in 21/25 patients (84 %) with confirmed effort thrombosis.

10.10.2 Physical Examination

Although there are no provocative maneuvers to detect subclavian vein thrombosis, there are several clinical signs that point to the diagnosis. For example, many patients present with a gradual increase in swelling with dull shoulder and arm pain over a period of several days. Engorgement of surface veins may be evident, especially within the cubital fossa. Swelling may also induce paresthesias as a result of increased hydrostatic pressure and resulting ischemia of peri-neural arterial branches. Some patients also develop mottling and discoloration of the extremity in more severe cases. Treatments that involve preservation of venous patency, such as anticoagulation therapy and venous stents, are most likely to produce the best outcome in these patients [131, 132].

10.11 Summary

The neurovascular conditions related to the shoulder are numerous and complex; however, a systematic, evidence-based approach to physical diagnosis will allow the clinician to develop an effective treatment plan that should lead to a successful treatment outcome.

References

1. Hawkins RJ, Bilco T, Bonutti P. Cervical spine and shoulder pain. Clin Orthop Relat Res. 1990;258: 142–6.
2. Manifold SG, McCann PD. Cervical radiculitis and shoulder disorders. Clin Orthop Relat Res. 1999;368: 105–13.
3. Viikari-Juntura E. Interexaminer reliability of observations in physical examinations of the neck. Phys Ther. 1987;67(10):1526–32.

4. Charopoulos IN, Hadjinicolaou N, Aktselis I, Lyritis GP, Papaioannou N, Kokoroghiannis C. Unusual insidious spinal accessory nerve palsy: a case report. J Med Case Rep. 2010;4:158.

5. Spurling RG, Scoville WB. Lateral rupture of the cervical intervertebral discs: a common cause of shoulder and arm pain. Surg Gynecol Obstet. 1944; 78:350–8.

6. Sandmark H, Nisell R. Validity of five common manual neck pain provoking tests. Scand J Rehabil Med. 1995;27(3):131–6.

7. Uchihara T, Furukawa T, Tsukagoshi H. Compression of brachial plexus as a diagnostic test of cervical cord lesion. Spine (Phila Pa 1976). 1994;19(19):2170–3.

8. Shah KC, Rajshekhar V. Reliability of diagnosis of soft cervical disc prolapse using Spurling's test. Br J Neurosurg. 2004;18(5):480–3.

9. Wainner RS, Fritz JM, Irrgang JJ, Boninger ML, Delitto A, Allison S. Reliability and diagnostic accuracy of the clinical examination and patient self-report measures for cervical radiculopathy. Spine (Phila Pa 1976). 2003;28(1):52–62.

10. Tong HC, Haig AJ, Yamakawa K. The Spurling test and cervical radiculopathy. Spine (Phila Pa 1976). 2002;27(2):156–9.

11. Anekstein Y, Blecher R, Smorgick Y, Mirovsky Y. What is the best way to apply the Spurling test for cervical radiculopathy? Clin Orthop Relat Res. 2012;470(9):2566–72.

12. Farmer JC, Wisneski RJ. Cervical spine nerve root compression. An analysis of neuroforaminal pressure with varying head and arm positions. Spine (Phila Pa 1976). 1994;19(16):1850–5.

13. Farshad M, Min K. Abduction extension cervical nerve root stress test: anatomical basis and clinical relevance. Eur Spine J. 2013;22(7):1522–5.

14. Elvey RL. Treatment of arm pain associated with abnormal brachial plexus tension. Aust J Physiother. 1986;32(4):225–30.

15. Quintner JL. A study of upper limb pain and paraesthesiae following neck injury in motor vehicle accidents: assessment of the brachial plexus tension test of Elvey. Br J Rheumatol. 1989;28(6):528–33.

16. Peet RM, Henriksen JD, Anderson TP, Martin GM. Thoracic-outlet syndrome: evaluation of a therapeutic exercise program. Proc Staff Meet Mayo Clin. 1956;31(9):281–7.

17. Huang JH, Zager EL. Thoracic outlet syndrome. Neurosurgery. 2004;55(4):897–902.

18. Adson AW. Cervical ribs: symptoms, differential diagnosis, and indications for section of the insertion of the scalenus anticus muscle. J Int Coll Surg. 1951;16(5):546–59.

19. Adson AW, Coffey JR. Cervical rib: a method of anterior approach for relief of symptoms by division of the scalenus anticus. Ann Surg. 1927;85(6): 839–57.

20. Fitzgerald G. Thoracic outlet syndrome of pectoralis minor etiology mimicking cardiac symptoms on activity: a case report. J Can Chiropr Assoc. 2012; 56(4):311–5.

21. Sanders RJ. Recurrent neurogenic thoracic outlet syndrome stressing the importance of pectoralis minor syndrome. Vasc Endovascular Surg. 2011;45(1):33–8.

22. Machleder HI, Moll F, Verity A. The anterior scalene muscle in thoracic outlet syndrome: histochemical and morphometric studies. Arch Surg. 1986;121(10): 1141–4.

23. Ombregt L, Bisschop P, ter Veer HJ, Van de Velde T. A system of orthopaedic medicine. London: WB Saunders Co, Ltd; 1995.

24. Dubuisson A, Lamotte C, Foidart-Dessalle M, Nguyen Khac M, Racaru T, Scholtes F, Kaschten B, Lénelle J, Martin D. Post-traumatic thoracic outlet syndrome. Acta Neurochir (Wien). 2012;154(3):517–26.

25. Kemp CD, Rushing GD, Rodic N, McCarthy E, Yang SC. Thoracic outlet syndrome caused by fibrous dysplasia of the first rib. Ann Thorac Surg. 2012;93(3):994–6.

26. Davidović LB, Koncar IB, Pejkić SD, Kuzmanović IB. Arterial complications of thoracic outlet syndrome. Am Surg. 2009;75(3):235–9.

27. Rayan GM, Jensen C. Thoracic outlet syndrome: provocative examination maneuvers in a typical population. J Shoulder Elbow Surg. 1995;4(2):113–7.

28. Warrens AN, Heaton JM. Thoracic outlet compression syndrome: the lack of reliability of its clinical assessment. Ann R Coll Surg Engl. 1987;69(5):203–4.

29. Gillard J, Pérez-Cousin M, Hachulla E, Remy J, Hurtevent JF, Vinckier L, Thévenon A, Duquesnoy B. Diagnosis thoracic outlet syndrome: contribution of provocative tests, ultrasonography, electrophysiology, and helical computed tomography in 48 patients. Joint Bone Spine. 2001;68(5):416–24.

30. Marx RG, Bombardier C, Wright JG. What we know about the reliability and validity of physical examination tests used to examine the upper extremity. J Hand Surg. 1999;24A(1):185–92.

31. Nord KM, Kapoor P, Fisher J, Thomas AG, Sundaram A, Scott K, Kothari MJ. False positive rate of thoracic outlet syndrome diagnostic maneuvers. Electromyogr Clin Neurophysiol. 2008;48(2):67–74.

32. Plewa MC, Delinger M. The false-positive rate of thoracic outlet syndrome shoulder maneuvers in healthy subjects. Acad Emerg Med. 1998;5(4): 337–42.

33. Degeorges R, Reynaud C, Becquemin JP. Thoracic outlet syndrome surgery: long-term functional results. Ann Vasc Surg. 2004;18(5):558–65.

34. Ghoussoub K, Tabet G, Zoghby Z, Jebara V. Rehabilitation of thoracic outlet syndrome: about 60 patients. J Med Liban. 2002;50(5–6):192–6.

35. Demirbag D, Unlu E, Ozdemir F, Genchellac H, Temizoz O, Ozdemir H, Demir MK. The relationship between magnetic resonance imaging findings and postural maneuver and physical examination tests in patients with thoracic outlet syndrome: results of a double-blind, controlled study. Arch Phys Med Rehabil. 2007;88(7):844–51.

36. Talu GK. Thoracic outlet syndrome. Ağri. 2005; 17(2):5–9.

37. Falconer MA, Weddel G. Costoclavicular compression of the subclavian artery and vein. Lancet. 1943;2:539.

38. Telford ED, Mottershead S. Pressure of the cervicobrachial junction; an operative and anatomical study. J Bone Joint Surg (Br). 1948;30B(2):249–65.

39. Wright IS. The neurovascular syndrome produced by hyperabduction of the arms. The immediate changes produced in 150 normal controls, and the effects on some persons of prolonged hyperabduction of the arms; as in sleeping, and in certain occupations. Am Heart J. 1945;29:1–19.

40. Raaf J. Surgery for cervical rib and scalenus anticus syndrome. J Am Med Assoc. 1965;157(3):219–23.

41. Gilroy J, Meyer JS. Compression of the subclavian artery: a cause of ischaemic brachial neuropathy. Brain. 1963;86:733–46.

42. Tanaka Y, Aoki M, Izumi T, Fujimiya M, Yamashita T, Imai T. Measurement of subclavicular pressure on the subclavian artery and brachial plexus in the costoclavicular space during provocative positioning for thoracic outlet syndrome. J Orthop Sci. 2010;15(1):118–24.

43. Roos DB. Congenital anomalies associated with thoracic outlet syndrome: anatomy, symptoms, diagnosis, and treatment. Am J Surg. 1976;132(6):771–8.

44. Howard M, Lee C, Dellon AL. Documentation of brachial plexus compression (in the thoracic inlet) utilizing provocative neurosensory and muscular testing. J Reconstr Microsurg. 2003;19(5):303–12.

45. Smith TM, Sawyer SF, Sizer PS, Brismée JM. The double crush syndrome: a common occurrence in cyclists with ulnar nerve neuropathy – a case-control study. Clin J Sport Med. 2008;18(1):55–61.

46. Cahill BR, Palmer RE. Quadrilateral space syndrome. J Hand Surg [Am]. 1983;8(1):65–9.

47. Apaydin N, Tubbs RS, Loukas M, Duparc F. Review of the surgical anatomy of the axillary nerve and the anatomic basis of its iatrogenic and traumatic injury. Surg Radiol Anat. 2010;32(3):193–201.

48. Aval SM, Durand Jr P, Shankwiler JA. Neurovascular injuries to the athlete's shoulder: part II. J Am Acad Orthop Surg. 2007;15(5):281–9.

49. McCarty EC, Tsairis P, Warren RF. Brachial neuritis. Clin Orthop Relat Res. 1999;368:37–43.

50. Midha R. Epidemiology of brachial plexus injuries in a multitrauma population. Neurosurgery. 1997;40(6):1182–9.

51. Ringel SP, Treihaft M, Carry M, Fisher R, Jacobs P. Suprascapular neuropathy in pitchers. Am J Sports Med. 1990;18(1):80–6.

52. McKowen HC, Voorhies RM. Axillary nerve entrapment in the quadrilateral space. Case report. J Neurosurg. 1987;66(6):932–4.

53. Atema JJ, Unlü C, Reekers JA, Idu MM. Posterior circumflex humeral artery injury with distal embolization in professional volleyball players: a discussion of three cases. Eur J Vasc Endovasc Surg. 2012;44(2):195–8.

54. Durham JR, Yao JS, Pearce WH, Nuber GM, McCarthy 3rd WJ. Arterial injuries in the thoracic outlet syndrome. J Vasc Surg. 1995;21(1):57–69.

55. Duwayri YM, Emery VB, Driskill MR, Earley JA, Wright RW, Paletta Jr GA, Thompson RW. Positional compression of the axillary artery causing upper extremity thrombosis and embolism in the elite overhead throwing athlete. J Vasc Surg. 2011;53(5):1329–40.

56. Ligh CA, Schulman BL, Safran MR. Case reports: unusual cause of shoulder pain in a collegiate baseball player. Clin Orthop Relat Res. 2009;467(10):2744–8.

57. Ha Y, Sung DH, Park Y, du Kim H. Brachial plexopathy due to myeloid sarcoma in a patient with acute myeloid leukemia after allogenic peripheral blood stem cell transplantation. Ann Rehabil Med. 2013;37(2):280–5.

58. Khadilkar SV, Khade SS. Brachial plexopathy. Ann Indian Acad Neurol. 2013;16(1):12–8.

59. Tsairis P, Dyck PJ, Mulder DW. Natural history of brachial plexus neuropathy: report on 99 patients. Arch Neurol. 1972;27(2):109–17.

60. Parsonage MJ, Turner JWA. Neuralgic amyotrophy: the shoulder-girdle syndrome. Lancet. 1948;1(6513):973–8.

61. Shaikh MF, Baqai TJ, Tahir H. Acute brachial neuritis following influenza vaccination. BMJ Case Rep. 2012; 2012.

62. Taras JS, King JJ, Jacoby SM, McCabe LA. Brachial neuritis following quadrivalent human papilloma virus (HPV) vaccination. Hand (N Y). 2011;6(4):454–6.

63. Verhasselt S, Schelfaut S, Battaillie F, Moke L. Postsurgical Parsonage-Turner syndrome: a challenging diagnosis. Acta Orthop Belg. 2013;79(1):20–4.

64. Pierre PA, Laterre CE, Van den Bergh PY. Neuralgic amyotrophy with involvement of cranial nerves IX, X, XI and XII. Muscle Nerve. 1990;13(8):704–7.

65. Suarez GA, Giannini C, Bosche EP, Barohn RJ, Wodak J, Ebeling P, Anderson R, McKeever PE, Bromberg MB, Dyck PJ. Immune brachial plexus neuropathy: suggestive evidence for an inflammatory-immune pathogenesis. Neurology. 1996;46(2):559–61.

66. van Eijk JJ, van Alfen N, Tio-Gillen AP, Maas M, Herbrink P, Portier RP, van Doorn PA, van Engelen BG, Jacobs BC. Screening for antecedent Campylobacter jejuni infections and anti-ganglioside antibodies in idiopathic neuralgic amyotrophy. J Peripher Nerv Syst. 2011;16(2):153–6.

67. Johnson NE, Petraglia AL, Huang JH, Logigian EL. Rapid resolution of severe neuralgic amyotrophy after treatment with corticosteroids and intravenous immunoglobulin. Muscle Nerve. 2011;44(2):304–5.

68. Moriguchi K, Miyamoto K, Takada K, Kusunoki S. Four cases of anti-ganglioside antibody-positive neuralgic amyotrophy with good response to intravenous immunoglobulin infusion therapy. J Neuroimmunol. 2011;238(1–2):107–9.

69. Nakajima M, Fujioka S, Ohno H, Iwamoto K. Partial but rapid recovery from paralysis after immunomodulation during early stage of neuralgic amyotrophy. Eur Neurol. 2006;55(4):227–9.
70. Naito KS, Fukushima K, Suzuki S, Kuwahara M, Morita H, Kusunoki S, Ikeda S. Intravenous immunoglobulin (IVIg) with methylprednisolone pulse therapy for impairment of neuralgic amyotrophy: clinical observations in 10 cases. Intern Med. 2012;51(12):1493–500.
71. Tsao BE, Avery R, Shields RW. Neuralgic amyotrophy precipitated by Epstein-Barr virus. Neurology. 2004;62(7):1234–5.
72. Cusimano MD, Bilbao JM, Cohen SM. Hypertrophic brachial plexus neuritis: a pathological study of two cases. Ann Neurol. 1988;24(5):615–22.
73. Stumpo M, Foschini MP, Poppi M, Cenacchi G, Martinelli P. Hypertrophic inflammatory neuropathy involving bilateral brachial plexus. Surg Neurol. 1999;52(5):458–64.
74. Garosi L, de Lahunta A, Summers B, Dennis R, Scase T. Bilateral, hypertrophic neuritis of the brachial plexus in a cat: magnetic resonance imaging and pathological findings. J Feline Med Surg. 2006;8(1):63–8.
75. Collie AM, Landsverk ML, Ruzzo E, Mefford HC, Buysse K, Adkins JR, Knutzen DM, Barnett K, Brown Jr RH, Parry GJ, Yum SW, Simpson DA, Olney RK, Chinnery PF, Eichler EE, Chance PF, Hannibal MC. Non-recurrent SEPT9 duplications cause hereditary neuralgic amyotrophy. J Med Genet. 2010;47(9):601–7.
76. Klein CJ, Dyck PJ, Friedenberg SM, Burns TM, Windebank AJ, Dyck PJ. Inflammation and neuropathic attacks in hereditary brachial plexus neuropathy. J Neurol Neurosurg Psychiatry. 2002;73(1):45–50.
77. Thatte MR, Babhulkar S, Hiremath A. Brachial plexus injury in adults: diagnosis and surgical treatment strategies. Ann Indian Acad Neurol. 2013;16(1):26–33.
78. Dillin L, Hoaglund FT, Scheck M. Brachial neuritis. J Bone Joint Surg Am. 1985;67(6):878–80.
79. Barraclough A, Triplett J, Tuch P. Brachial neuritis with phrenic nerve involvement. J Clin Neurosci. 2012;19(9):1301–2.
80. Odell JA, Kennelly K, Stauffer J. Phrenic nerve palsy and Parsonage-Turner syndrome. Ann Thorac Surg. 2011;92(1):349–51.
81. Tsao BE, Ostrovskiy DA, Wilbourn AJ, Shields Jr RW. Phrenic neuropathy due to neuralgic amyotrophy. Neurology. 2006;66(10):1582–4.
82. Hershman EB, Wilbourn AJ, Bergeld JA. Acute brachial neuropathy in athletes. Am J Sports Med. 1989;17(5):655–9.
83. Kopell HP, Thompson WA. Pain and the frozen shoulder. Surg Gynecol Obstet. 1959;109(1):92–6.
84. Cummins CA, Messer TM, Schafer MF. Infraspinatus muscle atrophy in professional baseball players. Am J Sports Med. 2004;32(1):116–20.
85. Dramis A, Pimpalnerkar A. Suprascapular neuropathy in volleyball players. Acta Orthop Belg. 2005;71(3):269–72.
86. Ferretti A, Cerullo G, Russo G. Suprascapular neuropathy in volleyball players. J Bone Joint Surg Am. 1987;69(2):260–3.
87. Lajtai G, Wieser K, Ofner M, Raimann G, Aitzetmüller G, Pirkl C, Gerber C, Jost B. The shoulders of professional beach volleyball players: high prevalence of infraspinatus muscle atrophy. Am J Sports Med. 2009;37(7):1375–83.
88. Salles JI, Cossich VR, Amaral MV, Monteiro MT, Cagy M, Motta G, Velazques B, Piedade R, Ribeiro P. Electrophysiological correlates of the threshold to detection of passive motion: an investigation in professional volleyball athletes with and without atrophy of the infraspinatus muscle. Biomed Res Int. 2013;2013:634891.
89. Witvrouw E, Cools A, Lysens R, Cambier D, Vanderstraeten G, Victor J, Sneyers C, Walravens M. Suprascapular neuropathy in volleyball players. Br J Sports Med. 2000;34(3):174–80.
90. Seroyer ST, Nho SJ, Bach Jr BR, Bush-Joseph CA, Nicholson GP, Romeo AA. Shoulder pain in the overhead throwing athlete. Sports Health. 2009;1(2):108–20.
91. Albritton MJ, Graham RD, Richards II RS, Basamania CJ. An anatomic study of the effects on the suprascapular nerve due to retraction of the supraspinatus muscle after a rotator cuff tear. J Shoulder Elbow Surg. 2003;12(5):497–500.
92. Costouros JG, Porramatikul M, Lie DT, Warner JJ. Reversal of suprascapular neuropathy following arthroscopic repair of massive supraspinatus and infraspinatus rotator cuff tears. Arthroscopy. 2007;23(11):1152–61.
93. Carroll KW, Helms CA, Otte MT, Moellken SM, Fritz R. Enlarged spinoglenoid notch veins causing suprascapular nerve compression. Skeletal Radiol. 2003;32(2):72–7.
94. Lee BC, Yegappan M, Thiagarajan P. Suprascapular nerve neuropathy secondary to spinoglenoid notch ganglion cyst: case reports and review of literature. Ann Acad Med Singapore. 2007;36(12):1032–5.
95. Moore TP, Fritts HM, Quick DC, Buss DD. Suprascapular nerve entrapment caused by supraglenoid cyst compression. J Shoulder Elbow Surg. 1997;6(5):455–62.
96. Werner CM, Nagy L, Gerber C. Combined intra- and extra-articulat arthroscopic treatment of entrapment neuropathy of the infraspinatus branches of the suprascapular nerve caused by a periglenoidal ganglion cysts. Arthroscopy. 2007;23(3):328e1–3.
97. Westerheide KJ, Dopirak RM, Karzel RP, Snyder SJ. Suprascapular nerve palsy secondary to spinoglenoid cysts: results of arthroscopic treatment. Arthroscopy. 2006;22(7):721–7.
98. Polguj M, Jędrzejewski K, Podgórski M, Majos A, Topol M. A proposal for classification of the superior transverse scapular ligament: variable morphology

and its potential influence on suprascapular nerve entrapment. J Shoulder Elbow Surg. 2013;22(9): 1265–73.

99. Polguj M, Jędrzejewski K, Majos A, Topol M. Variations in bifid superior transverse scapular ligament as a possible factor of suprascapular entrapment: an anatomical study. Int Orthop. 2012;36(10):2095–100.

100. Polguj M, Jędrzejewski K, Podgórski M, Topol M. Correlation between morphometry of the suprascapular notch and anthropometric measurements of the scapula. Folia Morphol (Warsz). 2011;70(2): 109–15.

101. Polguj M, Jędrzejewski K, Podgórski M, Topol M. Morphometry study of the suprascapular notch: proposal of classification. Surg Radiol Anat. 2011;33(9):781–7.

102. Rengachary SS, Burr D, Lucas S, Hassanein KM, Mohn MP, Matzke H. Suprascapular entrapment neuropathy: a clinical, anatomical and comparative study. Part 2: anatomical study. Neurosurgery. 1979;5(4):447–51.

103. Wang JH, Chen C, Wu LP, Pan CQ, Zhang WJ, Li YK. Variable morphology of the suprascapular notch: an investigation and quantitative measurements in Chinese population. Clin Anat. 2011;24(1):47–55.

104. Avery BW, Fm P, Barclay JK. Anterior coracoscapular ligament and suprascapular nerve entrapment. Clin Anat. 2002;15(6):383–6.

105. Bayramoğlu A, Demiryürek D, Tuccar E, Erbil M, Aldur MM, Tetik O, Doral MN. Variations in anatomy at the suprascapular notch possibly causing suprascapular nerve entrapment: an anatomical study. Knee Surg Sports Traumatol Arthrosc. 2003;11(6):393–8.

106. Plancher KD, Luke TA, Peterson RK, Yacoubian SV. Posterior shoulder pain: a dynamic study of the spinoglenoid ligament and treatment with arthroscopic release of the scapular tunnel. Arthroscopy. 2007;23(9):991–8.

107. de Laat EA, Visser CP, Coene LN, Pahlplatz PV, Tavy DL. Nerve lesions in primary shoulder dislocations and humeral neck fractures. A prospective clinical and EMG study. J Bone Joint Surg Br. 1994;76(3):381–3.

108. Massimini DF, Singh A, Wells JH, Li G, Warner JJ. Suprascapular nerve anatomy during shoulder motion: a cadaveric proof of concept study with implications for neurogenic shoulder pain. J Shoulder Elbow Surg. 2013;22(4):463–70.

109. Shaffer BS, Conway J, Jobe FW, Kvitne RS, Tibone JE. Infraspinatus muscle-splitting incision in posterior shoulder surgery: an anatomic and electromyographic study. Am J Sports Med. 1994;22(1):113–20.

110. Gerber C, Blumenthal S, Curt A, Werner CM. Effect of selective experimental suprascapular nerve block on abduction and external rotation strength of the shoulder. J Shoulder Elbow Surg. 2007;16(6): 815–20.

111. Martin SD, Warren RF, Martin TL, Kennedy K, O'Brien SJ, Wickiewicz TL. Suprascapular neuropathy. Results of non-operative treatment. J Bone Joint Surg Am. 1997;79(8):1159–65.

112. Mallon WJ, Wilson RJ, Basamania CJ. The association of suprascapular neuropathy with massive rotator cuff tears: a preliminary report. J Shoulder Elbow Surg. 2006;15(4):395–8.

113. Mallon WJ, Bronec PR, Spinner RJ, Levin LS. Suprascapular neuropathy after distal clavicle excision. Clin Orthop Relat Res. 1996;329: 207–11.

114. Gregg JR, Labosky D, Harty M, Lotke P, Ecker M, DiStefano V, Das M. Serratus anterior paralysis in the young athlete. J Bone Joint Surg Am. 1979;61(6A):825–32.

115. Ludewig PM, Hoff MS, Osowski EE, Meschke SA, Rundquist PJ. Relative balance of serratus anterior and upper trapezius muscle activity during push-up exercises. Am J Sports Med. 2004;32(2):484–93.

116. Galano GJ, Bigliani LU, Ahmad CS, Levine WN. Surgical treatment of winged scapula. Clin Orthop Relat Res. 2008;466(3):652–60.

117. Aldridge JW, Bruno RJ, Strauch RJ, Rosenwasser MP. Nerve entrapment in athletes. Clin Sports Med. 2001;20(1):95–122.

118. McFarland EG. Examination of the shoulder: the complete guide. New York: Thieme Medical Publishers, Inc; 2006.

119. Ekstrom RA, Soderberg GL, Donatelli RA. Normalization procedures using maximum voluntary isometric contractions for the serratus anterior and trapezius muscles during surface EMG analysis. J Electromyogr Kinesiol. 2005;15(4):418–28.

120. Ekstrom RA, Donatelli RA, Soderberg GL. Surface electromyographic analysis of exercises for the trapezius and serratus anterior muscles. J Orthop Sports Phys Ther. 2003;33(5):247–58.

121. Hébert LJ, Moffet H, McFadyen BJ, Dionne CE. Scapular behavior in shoulder impingement syndrome. Arch Phys Med Rehabil. 2002;83(1): 60–9.

122. Ludewig PM, Cook TM. Alterations in shoulder kinematics and associated muscle activity in people with symptoms of shoulder impingement. Phys Ther. 2000;80(3):276–91.

123. Lukasiewicz AC, McClure P, Michener L, Pratt N, Sennett B. Comparison of 3-dimensional scapular position and orientation between subjects with and without shoulder impingement. J Orthop Sports Phys Ther. 1999;29(10):574–83.

124. Tullos HS, Erwin WD, Woods GW, Wukasch DC, Cooley DA, King JW. Unusual lesions of the pitching arm. Clin Orthop Relat Res. 1972;88:169–82.

125. Rangdal SS, Kantharajanna SB, Daljit S, Bachhal V, Raj N, Krishnan V, Goni V, Singh Dhillon M. Axillary artery thrombosis with anteroinferior shoulder dislocation: a rare case report and review of literature. Chin J Traumatol. 2012;15(4):244–8.

126. Bucci F, Robert F, Fiengo L, Plagnol P. Radiotherapy-related axillary arteriopathy. Interact Cardiovasc Thorac Surg. 2012;15(1):176–7.

127. Bents RT. Axillary artery thrombosis after humeral resurfacing arthroplasty. Am J Orthop (Belle Mead NJ). 2011;40(7):E135–7.

128. Dhaon P, Das SK, Saran RK, Parihar A. Is aorto-arteritis a manifestation of primary antiphospholipid antibody syndrome? Lupus. 2011;20(14):1554–6.

129. DiFelice GS, Paletta GA, Phillips BB, Wright RW. Effort thrombosis in the elite throwing athlete. Am J Sports Med. 2002;30(5):708–12.

130. Kunkel JM, Machleder HI. Treatment of Paget-Schroetter syndrome: a staged, multidisciplinary approach. Arch Surg. 1989;124(10):1153–7.

131. Landry GJ, Liem TK. Endovascular management of Paget-Schroetter syndrome. Vascular. 2007;15(5):290–6.

132. Machleder HI. Evaluation of a new treatment strategy for Paget-Schroetter syndrome: spontaneous thrombosis of the axillary-subclavian vein. J Vasc Surg. 1993;17(2):305–17.

133. Khadilkar SV, Khade SS. Brachial Plexopathy. Ann Indian Acad Neurol. 2013;16(1):12–8.

Index

R.J. Warth and P.J. Millett, *Physical Examination of the Shoulder: An Evidence-Based Approach*,
DOI 10.1007/978-1-4939-2593-3, © Springer Science+Business Media New York 2015